A CASE MANAGER'S STUDY GUIDE

PREPARING FOR CERTIFICATION

DENISE FATTORUSSO, BS, RN, CCM
Crystal Run Healthcare
Rock Hill, New York

CAMPION E. QUINN, MD, FACP, MHA
President, Quinn and Associates Medical Consultants
Rockville Centre, New York

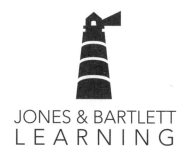

JONES & BARTLETT
LEARNING

World Headquarters
Jones & Bartlett Learning
5 Wall Street
Burlington, MA 01803
978-443-5000
info@jblearning.com
www.jblearning.com

Jones & Bartlett Learning books and products are available through most bookstores and online booksellers. To contact Jones & Bartlett Learning directly, call 800-832-0034, fax 978-443-8000, or visit our website, www.jblearning.com.

> Substantial discounts on bulk quantities of Jones & Bartlett Learning publications are available to corporations, professional associations, and other qualified organizations. For details and specific discount information, contact the special sales department at Jones & Bartlett Learning via the above contact information or send an email to specialsales@jblearning.com.

Copyright © 2013 by Jones & Bartlett Learning, LLC, an Ascend Learning Company

All rights reserved. No part of the material protected by this copyright may be reproduced or utilized in any form, electronic or mechanical, including photocopying, recording, or by any information storage and retrieval system, without written permission from the copyright owner.

A Case Manager's Study Guide: Preparing for Certification, Fourth Edition is an independent publication and has not been authorized, sponsored, or otherwise approved by the owners of the trademarks or service marks referenced in this product.

Some images in this book feature models. These models do not necessarily endorse, represent, or participate in the activities represented in the images.

The authors, editors, and publisher have made every effort to provide accurate information. However, they are not responsible for errors, omissions, or for any outcomes related to the use of the contents of this book and take no responsibility for the use of the products and procedures described. Treatments and side effects described in this book may not be applicable to all people; likewise, some people may require a dose or experience a side effect that is not described herein. Drugs and medical devices are discussed that may have limited availability controlled by the Food and Drug Administration (FDA) for use only in a research study or clinical trial. Research, clinical practice, and government regulations often change the accepted standard in this field. When consideration is being given to use of any drug in the clinical setting, the health care provider or reader is responsible for determining FDA status of the drug, reading the package insert, and reviewing prescribing information for the most up-to-date recommendations on dose, precautions, and contraindications, and determining the appropriate usage for the product. This is especially important in the case of drugs that are new or seldom used.

Production Credits

Publisher: Kevin Sullivan
Acquisitions Editor: Amanda Harvey
Editorial Assistant: Sara Bempkins
Associate Production Editor: Sara Fowles
Marketing Communications Manager: Katie Hennessy
V.P., Manufacturing and Inventory Control:
  Therese Connell
Composition: Arlene Apone
Cover Design: Timothy Dziewit
Cover Images: (Clockwise from left)
  © Stephen Coburn/ShutterStock, Inc.;
  © Monkey Business Images/ShutterStock, Inc.;
  © Jami Garrison/ShutterStock, Inc.;
  © Yuri Arcurs/ShutterStock, Inc.
Printing and Binding: Edwards Brothers Malloy
Cover Printing: Edwards Brothers Malloy

To order this product, use ISBN: 978-1-4496-8335-1

Library of Congress Cataloging-in-Publication Data
Fattorusso, Denise.
  A case manager's study guide : preparing for certification / Denise Fattorusso, Campion Quinn.
  -- 4th ed.
    p. ; cm.
  Includes bibliographical references and index.
  ISBN 978-1-4496-6744-3 (pbk.)
  I. Quinn, Campion. II. Title.
  [DNLM: 1. Case Management--organization & administration--Examination Questions. 2. Health Services Administration--Examination Questions. 3. Managed Care Programs--organization & administration--Examination Questions. W 18.2]
  362.1076--dc23
                              2012011523

6048

Printed in the United States of America
16 15 14   10 9 8 7 6 5 4 3

Contents

Preface   vii

1   Pretest   1
Appendix 1-A: Answers to Pretest   13

2   Case Management Concepts   19
Definition of Case Management   19
Philosophy of Case Management   19
Role of the Case Manager   20
Identifying Patients for Case Management   24
Accountability   26
Negotiation and Conflict Resolutions Strategies   27
Case Manager as a Patient Advocate   32
Communication Skills   33
Interview Techniques   36
Management Strategies for Patients with Comorbidities   40
Motivational Interviewing   41
Case Management Reports   42
Case Management Program Evaluation   44
References   45
Appendix 2-A: Case Management Concept Questions   46
Appendix 2-B: Case Management Concept Answers   62

3 Principles of Practice 67

Medical Records and Confidentiality 67
Medical Records Security 69
Ethical Issues in Case Management 71
Informed Consent 75
Legal Aspects of Case Management 75
Interstate Compact for Nursing 87
References 89
Appendix 3-A: Principles of Practice Questions 90
Appendix 3-B: Principles of Practice Answers 119

4 Psychosocial Aspects 129

Psychosocial and Neurological Assessment 129
Behavioral Health and Psychiatric Disability Concepts 129
Family Dynamics 131
Multicultural Issues and Health Behavior 133
Psychological Aspects of Chronic Illness and Disability 135
Health Coaching 140
Spirituality as It Relates to Health Behavior 141
References 146
Appendix 4-A: Psychosocial Aspects Questions 147
Appendix 4-B: Psychosocial Aspects Answers 157

5 Healthcare Management and Delivery 163

Services and Available Resources 163
Credentials 172
Medical Home Model 174
Accountable Care Organization 175
Transitions of Care 176
References 179
Appendix 5-A: Healthcare Management and Delivery Questions 180
Appendix 5-B: Healthcare Management and Delivery Answers 190

6 Healthcare Reimbursement 193

Private Benefit Programs 193
Healthcare Insurance Principles 201
Case Management Interventions 205

Federal Legislation Important to the Case Manager 210
Public Benefit Programs 220
References 239
Appendix 6-A: Healthcare Reimbursement Questions 240
Appendix 6-B: Healthcare Reimbursement Answers 309

7 Rehabilitation 351

Workers' Compensation Insurance 351
Americans with Disabilities Act of 1990 353
What Is a Work Hardening Program? 355
Assessing the Patient's Level of Physical and Mental Impairment 357
Orthoses, Prostheses, and Assistive Devices 361
Ergonomics 364
Assistive Technology Glossary 368
References 370
Appendix 7-A: Rehabilitation Questions 371
Appendix 7-B: Rehabilitation Answers 381

8 Posttest 387

Appendix 8-A: Answers to Posttest 399

Appendices

A   Consent Agreement Form 405

B   Patient Case Report 407

C   Vendor Progress Report 409

D   Alternate Benefit Plan Form 413

E   CMSA 1996 Statement Regarding Ethical Case Management Practice 415

F   Global Assessment of Functioning (GAF) Scale 417

G   DSM-IV Multiaxial Classification 419

Preface

Managed care is an attempt by private employers and the federal government to gain control of both the cost and the quality of medical care. As healthcare costs have increased, managed care in all its varieties has grown. The field of case management has expanded in parallel with this growth.

Case Managers are on the front lines of both managed care and clinical care, providing information, support, recommendations, and counseling. Case management has been shown to improve clinical outcomes, increase efficiency, and decrease costs associated with complex medical care. Insurers, employers, providers, and patients all use Case Managers' skills; correspondingly, the demand for qualified Case Managers continues to grow.

The current practitioners of case management are not a homogeneous group. They are professionals that come from many disciplines, including nursing, social work, and psychological counseling. Although these varying backgrounds add depth and complexity to a Case Manager's skills, the knowledge base of any individual Case Manager may be incomplete.

Case management certification is aimed at ensuring a uniform knowledge base for all Case Managers. This book was developed to support that goal as follows:

- By providing a source of clear, concise information on case management
- By providing a quick reference resource to Case Managers working in the field
- By providing a study tool for those involved in preparing for case management certification

This book does not represent a compendium of all information needed to pass the Certified Case Manager (CCM) exam. It is hoped that the use of this book will provide a basis from which the readers may expand their studies in case management and identify gaps in their scholarship. The authors refer the readers to the many excellent texts available in case management and related fields to "flesh out" their understanding of the various topics.

HOW TO USE THIS BOOK

Although the book may be read from beginning to end, it has been written so that each chapter comprises information on each of the six knowledge domains in the Certified Case Manager exam. The questions have been written as a tool to help focus your study sessions.

The authors recommend the following approach to using this book:

- Take a practice test before reading the text
- Assess your strengths and weaknesses in each area
- Note those areas in which you need the most work
- Study those areas
- Retest
- Continue this process until you are proficient in all subject areas

INSTRUCTIONS FOR USING THE ONLINE ACCESS CODE CARD

Enclosed within this review guide you will find a printed access code card containing a code providing you access to the new online interactive testing program, Navigate TestPrep.

This program will help you prepare for the CCM exam. The online program includes the same multiple choice questions that are printed in this study guide. You can choose a "practice exam," which allows you to see feedback on your response immediately, or a "final exam," which hides your results until you have completed all the questions in the exam.

Your overall score on the questions you have answered is also compiled. Here are the instructions on how to access Navigate TestPrep, the online interactive testing program:

1. Find the printed access code card bound in this book.
2. Go to http://www.jblearning.com/usecode
3. Review and accept the Terms and Conditions to continue.
4. Enter in your 10-digit access code, which you can find by pulling off the protective tab on the access code card.
5. Follow the instructions on each screen to set up your account profile and password. Please note: Only select a course coordinator if you have been instructed to do so by an institution or an instructor.
6. Contact Jones & Bartlett Learning technical support if you have any questions.
   Call: 1-800-832-0034
   Visit: http://www.jblearning.com and select "Technical Support"
   Email: info@jblearning.com

Good luck with your studies.

Denise Fattorusso, BS, RN, CCM
Campion Quinn, MD, FACP, MHA

CHAPTER 1

Pretest

Read and answer the following questions before you begin your studies. After completing the test, review the answers at the end of this chapter. Take note of those areas that require more attention in your subsequent studies.

1) Of the following, which are common causes of malpractice litigation?
   1. Discourteous behavior by the professional
   2. Provider/patient miscommunication
   3. Lack of patient understanding
   4. Failure to inform a patient's family of pertinent issues
      A. 1, 3
      B. 2, 4
      C. 1, 2, 3
      D. All of the above
      E. None of the above

2) Case Managers may decrease the legal liability associated with patient discharges through which of the following activities?
   1. Reviewing the case with the treating physician
   2. Confirming the integrity of the patient's support network
   3. Reviewing the complete medical record
   4. Confirming the adequacy of follow-up outpatient care
      A. 1, 3
      B. 2, 4
      C. 1, 2, 3
      D. All of the above
      E. None of the above

3) Disclosure of confidential information is mandatory when
   A. It is pursuant to judicial proceedings.
   B. It is government mandated.
   C. A professional has a duty to warn a third party about the illness of a patient.
   D. All of the above
   E. None of the above

CHAPTER ONE

4) Which of the following statements are consistent with the findings of the court case of *Wickline v. State of California?*
   1. Medical doctors have a duty to protest adverse determinations by payers.
   2. Medical doctors can shift their liability to payers if they do protest adverse determinations.
   3. Payers of health care can be held accountable if their adverse decisions are arbitrary, made only for cost containment reasons and are not based on acceptable medical standards of practice in the community.
   4. Case Managers are not liable for their roles in adverse determinations.
      A. 1, 2, 4
      B. 2, 3, 4
      C. 1, 2, 3
      D. None of the above

5) Which of the following statements best defines ethics, as it relates to case management?
   1. The rules of conduct that govern a person or members of a profession
   2. The thoughts that govern a person's conduct
   3. A society's ideal for a person's conduct
   4. The minimal acceptable standards for a person's conduct
      A. 1, 3
      B. 2, 4
      C. 1, 2, 3
      D. All of the above
      E. None of the above

6) Of the following, which activities are associated with a decreased risk of allegations of breach of patient confidentiality?
   1. Understanding applicable federal and state regulations on the disclosure of medical information
   2. Quickly transferring information to any and all parties that request it, without bothering to notify the patient, attorneys, and so on
   3. Informing the patient of his or her right to refuse the disclosure of medical information to any or all parties
   4. Transferring patient information concerning abortions or venereal and psychiatric diseases to third parties without first discussing with the patient or attorneys
      A. 1, 3
      B. 2, 4
      C. 1, 2, 3
      D. All of the above
      E. None of the above

7) A request made by an insured or a provider to re-review a denial of a utilization review organization's decision is also known as
   1. An appeal
   2. A reconsideration
   3. An expedited appeal
   4. An IME
      A. 1, 2
      B. 1, 3
      C. 1, 4
      D. All of the above
      E. None of the above

8) During a case management interview in a workers' compensation case, the patient confides to the Case Manager that he is a recovering alcoholic and has been alcohol free for 5 years. The Case Manager should
   A. Include the information in the psychosocial section of her insurance company report
   B. Immediately notify the patient's attending physician
   C. Make no comment verbally or in writing, as it has no current bearing on a work-related injury
   D. Close the case

9) A Case Manager is frustrated by her inability to get her patient to agree to occupational therapy. The patient was involved in a high-speed motor vehicle accident and suffered severe head injuries. When encouraged to attend therapy sessions the patient refuses, becomes verbally abusive, and hangs up the phone. Likely reason(s) for this patient's reaction is (are)
   A. Head injuries can result in emotional instability.
   B. Head injuries can result in cognitive impairments.
   C. Head injuries can result in prolonged head pain and mood depression.
   D. All of the above
   E. None of the above

10) Which of the following diagnoses should trigger an inquiry for potential case management services?
   1. Blepharitis
   2. Spinal cord injury
   3. Coryza
   4. Non-Hodgkin's lymphoma
      A. 1, 3
      B. 2, 4
      C. 1, 2, 3
      D. All of the above
      E. None of the above

11) Which of the following are "sentinel procedures" that should prompt inquiries for case management services?
   1. Brain biopsy
   2. Bone marrow biopsy
   3. Endocardiac biopsy
   4. Skin biopsy
      A. 1, 3
      B. 2, 4
      C. 1, 2, 3
      D. All of the above
      E. None of the above

12) Of the following, which utilization figure for an individual's medical claims would make an appropriate financial threshold for case management evaluations?
   A. Claims exceeding $500 per year
   B. Claims exceeding $1,000 per year
   C. Claims exceeding $10,000 per year
   D. Claims exceeding $100,000 per year
   E. Claims exceeding $1,000,000 per year

4 CHAPTER ONE

13) Which of the following is needed for the Case Manager to ensure an accurate assessment of the impact an injury will have on a patient and his or her ability to return to work?
    A. The physical requirements of the patient's position
    B. The coworkers'/employer's opinion of the patient's ability
    C. History of childhood diseases
    D. All of the above
    E. None of the above

14) Which of the following statements is (are) true regarding the clinical consequences of head injuries?
    1. A patient may become depressed.
    2. A patient's cognitive ability may be impaired.
    3. Emotional lability is common.
    4. Chronic headaches may result.
        A. 1, 3
        B. 1, 2, 4
        C. 1, 2, 3
        D. All the above
        E. None of the above

15) Of the following methodologies, which are common means that insurers and Case Managers use to identify potential patients for case management services?
    1. Selecting cases with catastrophic diagnoses, such as head or spinal injuries
    2. Selecting cases with "sentinel procedures," such as bone marrow biopsy or brain biopsy
    3. Selecting cases with claims costs of more than $10,000 a year
    4. Selecting cases at random and investigating for potential problems
        A. 1, 3
        B. 2, 4
        C. 1, 2, 3
        D. All of the above
        E. None of the above

16) A variety of cognitive techniques may be used for pain control. Which of the following are examples of these techniques?
    1. Distraction
    2. Pain medication
    3. Relaxation training
    4. Biofeedback
        A. 3, 4
        B. 1, 2, 3
        C. 1, 3, 4
        D. All of the above
        E. None of the above

17) The Case Manager can expect which of the following after ACL reconstruction surgery?
    A. Jogging by the 12th postoperative week
    B. Full weight bearing and range of motion by the 4th postoperative week
    C. Bent knee raises and isometric exercises on the affected leg for the first postoperative week while immobilized in a hinged-type brace
    D. All of the above

18) Which word defines the paralysis of all four limbs?
   A. Hemiplegia
   B. Paraplegia
   C. Quadriplegia
   D. Quadripara

19) Which word defines the inability to swallow or difficulty in swallowing?
   A. Dysphasia
   B. Aphasia
   C. Apraxia
   D. Dysphagia

20) Problems encountered by patients in the early course of a spinal cord injury include which of the following?
   A. Blood pressure control
   B. Depression
   C. Bladder control
   D. Decubitus ulcers
   E. All of the above

21) Which of the following organizations are exempt from the mandates of the Americans with Disabilities Act?
   1. Small businesses with fewer than 15 employees
   2. The federal government
   3. Native American tribes
   4. Software manufacturers
      A. 1, 3
      B. 2, 4
      C. 1, 2, 3
      D. All of the above
      E. None of the above

22) Under the proscriptions of the Americans with Disabilities Act, which of the following are not considered "reasonable accommodations" by the employer?
   1. Making the disabled "typist" a receptionist who answers phones only
   2. Modifying equipment to accommodate disabled employees
   3. Making the paralyzed "ballet dancer" a "theatrical director" of the ballet company
   4. Providing qualified interpreters for the hearing impaired
      A. 1, 3
      B. 2, 4
      C. 1, 2, 3
      D. All of the above
      E. None of the above

CHAPTER ONE

23) Which of the following statements are true regarding the Women's Health and Cancer Rights Act?
   1. It is a law enacted as part of the Omnibus Appropriation Bill.
   2. It ensures coverage for surgery of the contralateral breast to provide a symmetrical appearance after mastectomy.
   3. It amended the Employee Retirement Income Security Act (ERISA) to require both health plans and self-insured plans to provide coverage for mastectomies and certain reconstructive surgeries.
   4. It ensures coverage for breast prostheses after mastectomy.
      A. 1, 3
      B. 2, 4
      C. 1, 2, 3
      D. All of the above
      E. None of the above

24) Which of the following statements are true regarding unemployment insurance?
   1. Financing of unemployment benefits is uniform from state to state.
   2. Unemployment compensation benefits guarantee a replacement of 50% of salary.
   3. Benefits are never extended past the usual maximum length of benefit.
   4. All states pay a minimum of 46 weeks of unemployment benefits.
      A. 1, 3
      B. 2, 4
      C. 1, 2, 3
      D. All of the above
      E. None of the above

25) Which of the following is (are) true regarding workers' compensation insurance?
   1. The scope of coverage varies from state to state.
   2. Benefits generally include the cost of legal bills only.
   3. Employees are entitled to the level of benefit mandated by the state.
   4. Self-funded health insurance programs are exempt from the mandates of workers' compensation regulations.
      A. 1, 3
      B. 2, 4
      C. 1, 2, 3
      D. All of the above
      E. None of the above

26) Which of the following statements about indemnity health insurance plans is (are) not true?
   1. It is a legal entity.
   2. It is licensed by the U.S. Department of the Interior.
   3. It exists to provide health insurance to enrollees.
   4. It reimburses enrollees for the cost of any health care they desire.
      A. 1, 3
      B. 2, 4
      C. 1, 2, 3
      D. All of the above
      E. None of the above

27) Which of the following does not determine minimum policy limits of Personal Injury Protection (PIP) automobile insurance?
1. State insurance department
2. Accident rate in local community
3. State insurance commissioner
4. Driver's record of accidents
    A. 1, 3
    B. 2, 4
    C. 1, 2, 3
    D. All of the above
    E. None of the above

28) A 35-year-old engineer, who is wheelchair bound secondary to a spinal injury, applies for a job in a large engineering firm. The job advertisement calls for candidates with a PhD in engineering, yet he only has a master's degree. The applicant reasons that under the proscriptions of the Americans with Disabilities Act (ADA), the employer must make "reasonable accommodations" to the disabled, and therefore his master's degree should be good enough to get the job. Why is the employer justified (under the ADA) in denying this applicant?
    A. The candidate cannot perform the "essential functions" of the job because he is wheelchair bound and therefore cannot use the existing computer equipment.
    B. The candidate is not "qualified" for the job because he does not have the requirements requested in the written job advertisement.
    C. The candidate cannot enter the building because it lacks a ramp.
    D. The candidate cannot perform the job adequately because it requires adherence to a strict time schedule, and his disability requires advance notice for his transportation.
    E. The candidate cannot work in the building because it lacks appropriate bathroom facilities.

29) Which of the following benefits are usually included under the terms of the Pregnancy Discrimination Act?
1. Home health care
2. Abortions
3. Home physical therapy care
4. Mandatory maternity leave
    A. 1, 3
    B. 2, 4
    C. 1, 2, 3
    D. All of the above
    E. None of the above

30) Which of the following mental health benefit limitations are not allowable under the tenets of the Mental Health Parity Act?
1. Annual dollar limit for mental health care
2. Limited number of annual outpatient visits
3. Lifetime dollar limit on mental health care
4. Limited number of inpatient days annually
    A. 1, 3
    B. 2, 4
    C. 1, 2, 3
    D. All of the above
    E. None of the above

31) Commission for Case Management Certification defines case management as a process involving which of the following?
   1. Managed care
   2. Assessing, planning, and monitoring
   3. Collaboration, coordination, and communication
   4. Implementation and evaluation
      A. All of the above
      B. None of the above
      C. 1, 2, 3
      D. 2, 3, 4

32) Which of the following answers is not included in the six core areas of case management?
   A. The return-to-work process
   B. Case management concepts
   C. Healthcare management and delivery
   D. Rehabilitation

33) Case finding, gathering and assessing information, and problem identification are all part of
   A. Patient advocacy
   B. The return-to-work assessment
   C. The case management process
   D. The precertification process

34) Diagnosis, high costs, and multiple admissions or treatments are red flags for
   A. Preexisting HMO exclusions
   B. Utilization management review
   C. Case management evaluation
   D. Disability hearings

35) The Case Manager should never contact
   A. The patient
   B. The caregivers
   C. The employer
   D. The patient's coworkers

36) A case management consent agreement provides for which of the following?
   1. Release of clinical information to the Case Manager
   2. Claims payment
   3. Permission to review the case information with the parties involved in the care of the patient or the payment of services
   4. Provision of durable medical equipment
      A. 1, 2
      B. 2, 3
      C. 1, 3
      D. 3, 4

37) In the case management process, the stage of "obtaining approval" refers to
   A. Permission from the patient to implement case management
   B. Permission from the payer to implement a care plan
   C. Permission from claims to negotiate fees
   D. None of the above

38) Case Managers perform their function in the following four areas: medical, financial, rehabilitation, and
   A. Workers' compensation
   B. Social
   C. Legal
   D. Behavioral/motivational

39) Continual assessment of the care plan is part of which of the following process(es)?
   A. Initial evaluation
   B. Goal setting
   C. Implementation
   D. Monitoring and evaluation

40) Which of the following is (are) true regarding the purposes of an orthosis?
   1. It can be used to support body parts.
   2. It can be used to position body parts.
   3. It can be used to immobilize body parts.
   4. It can be used to modify muscle tone.
      A. 1, 3
      B. 2, 4
      C. 1, 2, 3
      D. All of the above
      E. None of the above

41) Which of the following is (are) true regarding a prosthesis?
   1. It may restore or replace all or part of a missing body part.
   2. It may improve a person's sense of wholeness or body image.
   3. It has as its goals increased function and cosmesis.
   4. It may result in injury or illness if improperly fitted.
      A. 1, 3
      B. 2, 4
      C. 1, 2, 3
      D. All of the above
      E. None of the above

42) Which of the following is (are) true regarding assistive devices?
   1. They are products that substitute for an impaired function.
   2. They are a substitute for rehabilitation services.
   3. They allow an individual to perform an activity more independently.
   4. When prescribing one, little input is needed from the patient or the patient's family.
      A. 1, 3
      B. 2, 4
      C. 1, 2, 3
      D. All of the above
      E. None of the above

43) Which of the following factors may influence the rate of prosthesis replacement?
1. Activity level
2. Age of user
3. Type of prosthesis
4. Impact resistance of materials used
    A. 1, 3
    B. 2, 4
    C. 1, 2, 3
    D. All of the above
    E. None of the above

44) Which of the following is (are) considered an assistive device?
1. Text-to-speech synthesizer
2. Phone receiver volume control
3. Quad cane
4. Grab bars in the tub
    A. 1, 3
    B. 2, 4
    C. 1, 2, 3
    D. All of the above
    E. None of the above

45) The three basic goals of a patient interview are to
1. Provide information
2. Establish rapport
3. Provide a care plan
4. Collect information
5. Formulate a care plan
    A. 1, 2, 3
    B. 2, 3, 4
    C. 1, 4, 5
    D. 2, 4, 5

46) When the Case Manager is arranging for discharge to a traumatic brain injury rehabilitation facility, he or she should
1. Confirm that the facility can provide the therapies, by credentialed providers, that the patient requires
2. Verify there is a board-certified medical director at the facility
3. Ensure the facility is accredited by the Joint Commission on Accreditation of Healthcare Organizations (Joint Commission or JCAHO) and the Commission on Accreditation of Rehabilitation Facilities (CARF)
4. Certify an unlimited length of stay to ensure the patient gets the care he or she needs
    A. 1, 2, 3
    B. 2, 3, 4
    C. All of the above
    D. None of the above

47) The Case Manager will find which of the following services difficult to arrange at home?
   A. Homemaker services
   B. Durable medical equipment
   C. Personal care
   D. All of the above
   E. None of the above

48) When conducting an interview, it is important that the Case Manager ask about the medical history of the patient. To get the most from the interview, questions should be of what type?
   A. Open ended
   B. Who, what, where, when, why, and how
   C. Direct
   D. Leading

49) Case Managers should follow up on arrangements they have made for durable medical equipment to
   A. Determine if it is being used
   B. Determine if it was delivered
   C. Determine if the patient and caregiver are satisfied with the equipment
   D. Determine if it meets the current need of the patient
   E. All of the above

NOTES

Appendix 1-A

Answers to Pretest

1) **ANSWER: D**
Discourteous behaviors, communication failures, lack of patient understanding, and lack of family understanding are the most common causes of malpractice litigation. Malpractice litigation stems more commonly from poor relationships with patients than from negligent medical care.

2) **ANSWER: D**
The Case Manager has an obligation of "reasonable care" to the patient. Failing to ensure the discharge is "safe" is negligent on the part of the Case Manager.

3) **ANSWER: D**
Case Managers are required by both legal statues and tenets of ethical behavior to release medical information to courts, healthcare authorities, and other people who are put at risk of physical harm by failure to disclose that information.

4) **ANSWER: C**
Case Managers are liable for damages if their referral of patients to providers is negligently performed and harm comes to the patient as a direct result of that referral.

5) **ANSWER: A**
Ethics refers to the rules or standards that govern the conduct of a person or members of a profession. Ethical rules describe a society's ideal of how a person or professional should conduct himself or herself.

6) **ANSWER: A**
A Case Manager can decrease the risk of allegations of breach of confidentiality by fully understanding the following: the implications of federal and state regulations on the disclosure of medical information; that venereal diseases, abortion, mental illness, and substance abuse are very sensitive topics and transferring such information should be done only after discussing it with patients and attorneys; and that a patient has the right to refuse all information release.

7) **ANSWER: A**
An appeal and reconsideration. An expedited appeal may be requested if an urgent need exists for a particular service or treatment. An IME is an independent medical exam and is most often used in workers' compensation or disability cases.

8) **ANSWER: C**
According to the Code of Professional Ethics, it is the responsibility of the Case Manager to safeguard the patient's confidentiality unless there is a legal requirement to disclose the information.

9) **ANSWER: D**

10) **ANSWER: B**
Both spinal cord injuries and lymphomas are complex, high-cost, and life-threatening illnesses that may potentially benefit from case management. Coryza is a common cold, and blepharitis is a minor infection of the eyelid.

11) **ANSWER: C**
Although biopsies of the endocardium, the brain, and bone marrow involve high risk and are done infrequently, biopsies of the skin are low risk, are commonly performed, and require case management services in a small minority of cases.

12) **ANSWER: C**
Screening all patients with claims over $500 and $1,000 per year would yield too many claims and too few catastrophic illnesses. Those patients with claims of $100,000 and over would no doubt be well known to the insurers and Case Managers long before the patients hit those thresholds. Thresholds of $5,000 to $10,000 are most commonly seen in the industry.

13) **ANSWER: A**
To make an accurate determination in regard to a patient's ability to return to work, the Case Manager and the team involved in the care of the patient must know the physical requirements of the patient's job.

14) **ANSWER: D**

15) **ANSWER: C**
Common methodologies include screening claims of catastrophic diagnoses, sentinel procedures, high-claims cost, and direct case referral from community physicians.

16) **ANSWER: C**
Pain medication is not a cognitive technique.

17) **ANSWER: C**
Postoperatively, the knee is immobilized in a hinged brace in a flexed position.

18) **ANSWER: C**

19) **ANSWER: D**

20) **ANSWER: E**
The micturition reflex center is located in the sacral region of the spinal cord. As a result, bladder function may be impaired with a lower spinal cord injury. Depression, problems controlling blood pressure, and decubitus ulcers are common problems that need to be dealt with early in spinal cord injuries.

21) **ANSWER: C**
The exceptions to the American with Disabilities Act are

- Religious organizations or private membership clubs, except when these organizations sponsor a public event
- The federal government or corporations owned by the federal government
- Native American tribes
- Compliance with this Act can prove a hardship for small employers; therefore, if an employer has fewer than 15 employees, he or she is exempt. (Note: An accommodation's expense for an employer does not automatically make it a "hardship.")

22) **ANSWER: A**
The employer is obligated to make "reasonable accommodations" to an individual's disability that allows the employee to perform his job. Reasonable accommodations in employment may include

- Making existing facilities readily accessible to and usable by an individual with disabilities
- Job restructuring, part-time or modified work schedules, reassignment to a vacant position
- Acquiring or modifying equipment or devices
- Appropriately adjusting or modifying examinations, training materials, or policies
- Providing qualified readers or interpreters and other similar accommodations for individuals with disabilities

In the previous examples the individual hired as a typist must be able to type; similarly, a ballet dancer must be able to dance. Changing the essential job function, although laudatory, is not mandated by the ADA.

23) **ANSWER: D**
The Women's Health and Cancer Rights Act is a law that was enacted as part of an Omnibus Appropriation Bill and became effective for plan years beginning on or after October 21, 1998. This Act amended the Employee Retirement Income Security Act (ERISA) to require group health plans, including self-insured plans, which provide coverage for mastectomies, to provide certain reconstructive and related services following mastectomies. The services mandated by the Act include

- Reconstruction of the breast upon which the mastectomy has been performed
- Surgery and reconstruction of the other breast to produce a symmetrical appearance
- Prosthesis and treatment for physical complications attendant to the mastectomy, for example, lymphedema

24) **ANSWER: E**
State financing and benefit laws vary widely. In general, unemployment compensation benefits under state laws are intended to replace about 50% of an average worker's previous wages. Maximum weekly benefits provisions, however, result in benefits of less than 50% for most higher-earning workers. All states pay benefits to some unemployed persons for 26 weeks. In some states the duration of benefits depends on the amount earned and the number of weeks worked in a previous year. In others, all recipients are entitled to benefits for the same length of time. During periods of heavy unemployment, federal law authorizes extended benefits, in some cases up to 39 weeks; in 1975 extended benefits were payable for up to 65 weeks. Extended benefits are financed in part by federal employer taxes.

25) **ANSWER: A**
The scope of coverage for workers' compensation benefits varies by state, with respect to benefits payable in case of death, of total disability, and of partial disability due to specific injuries or continuing during specified periods. Although they vary among states, these benefits generally include the cost of medical bills attendant to treating the illness or injury as well as some percentage of lost wages. The compensation benefits, set forth by the state, take precedence over the funding source. Employees are entitled to the level of benefits mandated by the state without regard to the financial status or desires of the employer. Therefore, even if the employer is self-funded or self-administered, he or she is required to offer the full level of benefits required by the state's workers' compensation commission. Self-funded

group health insurance plans may be exempt from mandated benefits under the Employee Retirement Income Security Act (ERISA) guidelines but are not exempt under workers' compensation regulations.

26) **ANSWER: B**
An indemnity health insurance plan is a legal entity licensed by the state insurance department. It exists to provide health insurance to its enrollees. An indemnity health insurer "indemnifies" or reimburses the enrollee for the costs of healthcare claims that are medically necessary and appropriate for his or her care. Indemnity insurers historically had not spent money or time on utilization or quality management. Now, because of savings demonstrated by the managed care companies, some indemnity companies have adopted these cost-saving approaches.

27) **ANSWER: B**
Each state determines what the minimum level of liability insurance will be for drivers in that state. Although the costs of car insurance premiums may vary by the cost of the automobile, the community accident experience, or the driving record of the owner, the minimum policy limits for personal injury protection do not vary.

28) **ANSWER: B**
The American with Disabilities Act (ADA) offers protection for "qualified disabled" individuals. In this case the candidate for the job is not qualified for the job. The ADA does not consider a change in the essential functions of the job to be a "reasonable accommodation."

29) **ANSWER: A**
Although its scope is large, the Pregnancy Discrimination Act does exclude some benefits. Those benefits are abortions and mandatory maternity leave. When home health and home physical therapy are allowed under medical benefits, they are included under maternity benefits also.

30) **ANSWER: A**
Although annual or lifetime dollar limits cannot be set under the provisions of the Mental Health Parity Act, other limits are allowed. Examples of other allowable limits are

- Limited number of annual outpatient visits
- Limited number of inpatient days annually
- A per-visit fee limit
- Higher deductibles and copayments are allowed in mental health benefits under the Mental Health Parity Act, without parity in medical and surgical benefits. If an employer does not offer medical benefits, he or she does not have to offer mental health benefits; said differently, if an employer chooses not to offer mental health benefits, he or she must also choose not to offer medical benefits.

31) **ANSWER: D**

32) **ANSWER: A**
The return-to-work process is part of workers' compensation case management, not a core component of case management. The six core areas consist of B, C, D, case management principles and strategies, psychosocial and support systems, and healthcare reimbursement.

33) **ANSWER: C**
These are all part of the case management process, which also includes planning, reporting, obtaining approval, coordination, follow-up, monitoring, and evaluation.

34) **ANSWER: C**
These are the three criteria for case management referrals.

35) **ANSWER: D**
The first three choices are involved in the patient's care or benefit payment. The caregivers are contacted for the assessment of the patient and his progress. The employer is contacted for approval of benefit plans or return-to-work information. The patient is contacted to collaborate with the Case Manager on his care plan.

36) **ANSWER: C**

37) **ANSWER: B**

38) **ANSWER: D**

39) **ANSWER: D**

40) **ANSWER: D**
An orthosis is a device that is added to a person's body to achieve one or more of the following ends: support, position, immobilize, correct deformities, assist weak muscles, restore muscle function, and modify muscle tone.

The term "orthosis" generally encompasses such devices as slings, braces, and splints. Orthoses are used to support or aid in the functioning of the upper and lower extremities, hands and feet, and the trunk and spine.

41) **ANSWER: D**
A prosthesis is a device that restores or replaces all or part of a missing body part. The science of prosthetics addresses the mechanical, physiological, and cosmetic functions of restorations. Orthoses, on the other hand, are aimed at assisting the body to restore function; prostheses restore or replace those parts of the human body that are absent or no longer function. The need for replacement and cosmesis, rather than a simple increase in functionality, stems from a person's need for "wholeness" and a "positive body image." With this in mind, the professional prosthetist has as his or her goals to increase both functionality and cosmesis. Poorly fitted prostheses can cause injury or illness.

42) **ANSWER: A**
Assistive or adaptive devices are products that substitute for an impaired function and allow the individual to perform an activity more independently. Adaptive devices should be used only if other methods of performing the task are not available or cannot be learned. A reasonable effort should be made to teach the patient a method of performing the task in question, before an adaptive device is suggested. Mastery of a task, for example, walking, allows the patient greater independence and flexibility in that he or she does not need a wheelchair to move around and is not limited by lack of ramps, and so on. The device may serve as a useful supplement, however, or permit a function to be performed if the adapted method cannot be learned or requires too much effort. The type of assistive device is determined by the needs of the individual patient, his or her abilities and functional limitations, and his or her environment.

43) **ANSWER: D**
Many factors influence replacement frequency. For example, lower extremity prostheses bear weight, sustain high impact, and are exposed to the elements. Damage to the prostheses acquired by these activities demands maintenance, repair, and replacement. Replacement

frequency depends on the activity level of the patient and the demands he or she puts on the prosthesis, as well as the complexity of the prosthesis and the properties of the materials used. Further, an individual's prosthetic needs may change. For example, a sedentary individual may become more active, requiring a new prosthesis with more features and flexibility. Conversely, an active individual may become more sedentary with advancing age or disease, requiring a replacement prosthesis that is lighter and more stable. Finally, the younger patient will require successively larger prostheses to compensate for growth.

44) **ANSWER: D**

45) **ANSWER: D**
Providing information is not one of the basic goals of the interview. Providing a care plan does not allow the patient to be an active participant in the care-planning process.

46) **ANSWER: A**
Certifications should be time-limited, and progress reports should be evaluated before extending lengths of stay. Verifying the credentials of the facility and the providers is important in choosing an appropriate facility for the patient.

47) **ANSWER: E**

48) **ANSWER: A**
Open ended. All other answers neither leave room for the patient to introduce new information nor leave the door open for free communication.

49) **ANSWER: E**

CHAPTER 2

Case Management Concepts

DEFINITION OF CASE MANAGEMENT

Case management can generally be viewed as a process where licensed professionals identify covered patients with explicit healthcare needs and then formulate an efficient treatment plan that is implemented to produce the most cost-effective outcomes.

The Commission for Case Management Certification (CCMC) has their own specific definition, defining case management as a collaborative process that assesses, plans, implements, coordinates, monitors, and evaluates the options and services required to meet the client's health and human service needs.[1] This process is characterized by advocacy, communication, and resource management. It creates quality, cost-effective interventions and promotes improved clinical outcomes.

In addition to assessment, planning, implementation, coordination, monitoring, evaluation, and outcomes, the CCMC states that case management has general activities such as adherence to regulatory standards. These activities comprise the eight essential activities of case management. Case management is practiced by licensed health professionals in each of six fundamental areas: case management concepts, principles of practice, psychosocial aspects, healthcare management and delivery, healthcare reimbursement, and rehabilitation.

PHILOSOPHY OF CASE MANAGEMENT

Case management is an area of specialty practice within one's health and human services profession. The practice of case management involves the clients being served, their support systems, the healthcare delivery systems, and the various payers.[2] Its underlying premise is that everyone benefits when clients reach their optimum level of wellness, self-management, and functional capability. Case management certification[3] determines that the Case Manager possesses the education, skills, knowledge, and experience required to render appropriate services delivered according to sound principles of practice.

19

ROLE OF THE CASE MANAGER

CM Role

The Case Manager's role is the same across a variety of settings. Whether working in an acute care hospital, subacute care setting, rehabilitation facility, psychiatric milieu, home care agency, hospice, patient-centered medical home, insurance industry, or as an independent Case Manager, the goals and duties are the same. The role of the Case Manager is that of an assessor, planner, facilitator, and patient advocate.

The method of managing a patient's care progresses through the following eight stages[4]:

1. Case finding/case identification
2. Gathering and assessing information to identify problems
3. Planning
4. Reporting
5. Obtaining approval
6. Coordination
7. Follow-up/monitoring
8. Evaluation

Although all Case Managers may perform these processes, not all Case Managers function in all settings. Case management is as specialized as the various professions that comprise it. Although some Case Managers deal with discharge planning and never follow a patient after discharge, others may follow a patient from preadmission through various admissions and treatments until case management services are no longer required. The common denominators for Case Managers are their commitment to patient advocacy, educating patients and others involved in their care, facilitating a patient's optimal outcome, and empowering patients to be active decision makers in their health care.

Case Managers work in four major areas:

- Medical
- Financial
- Behavioral/motivational
- Rehabilitation

Medical activity refers to all those activities generally performed by a nurse Case Manager: following a patient throughout his or her hospital stay or treatment course, contacting and coordinating his or her care with a team of medical professionals, arranging for discharge needs, and so on. Financial activity deals with assisting the patient to cope with the insurance company and claim payers, negotiating with vendors, and assisting with applications for Medicare, Medicaid, skilled nursing facilities, medication assistance programs, and other entities. Behavioral/motivational activity includes assisting the patient and family to manage the stress brought about by the disease process/injury, offering counseling (if qualified), or arranging for social work or other intervention as needed.

Vocational activity is more often done in the setting of rehabilitation or workers' compensation case management. However, it may be required in the group health setting, when Case Managers deal with catastrophic illness or injury. Rehabilitation activities can involve testing for function, abilities, limitations, aptitude, and interests. Return-to-work strategies can be developed based on this rehabilitation testing. Finally, vocational activities of the Case Manager involve working with an employer to get an employee back to work.

Case Finding

The case management process begins with case identification. This can occur in the following ways: self-referral, referral by an employer, referral by a provider, referral by an insurer/third-party administrator via a claims person/computer system, referral by a discharge planner, or referral by a utilization reviewer. The three basic criteria for referring patients for case management evaluation are diagnosis-driven referrals, high-dollar referrals, or high utilization referrals, as is seen in patients with multiple or repeated service requests.

Assessment

After a potential case has been identified, the assessment phase begins. The CCMC[5] defines assessment as the process of collecting in-depth information about a person's situation and functioning to identify individual needs to develop a comprehensive case management plan to address those needs. In addition to direct client contact, information should be gathered from other relevant sources (patient/client, professional caregivers, nonprofessional caregivers, employers, health records, educational/military records, etc.).[5] The goal of assessment is to gather enough information regarding the current and prior status of the patient to enable the creation of a care plan to assist the patient in obtaining the optimal level of wellness and autonomy.

The Case Manager should evaluate the information that triggered the referral. It may be a diagnostic test, a clinical treatment or hospitalization history, a catastrophic or chronic diagnosis, or a high-dollar claim. If the information warrants further action, the Case Manager should then contact the patient. This call identifies the case management function to the patient, gathers more information, and assesses the patient's needs. All case management information gathered from the point of referral until discharge needs to be systematically documented. The patient should be sent a consent agreement (see Appendix A) so the Case Manager may contact the physician and other providers on behalf of the patient. The consent form should be clear on the issue of confidentiality, stating that the information gathered will be shared only with those professionals involved in the care of the patient or in payment of services. The consent form also serves to involve the patient in the case management process. It empowers the patient to participate in decision making and the planning of his or her health care. All contacts with the patient and family can be used to develop a rapport and a sense of cooperation and trust.

The Case Manager should be respectful of the patient's time and disabilities. For example, the patient should be asked at the beginning of all contacts if it is a good time to talk. If not, a better time can be scheduled so the patient may speak freely with the Case Manager. The success of the case management plan and the ultimate outcome depends on the cooperation and involvement of the patient and his or her support network. Therefore, taking the time to understand the patient's grasp of his or her disease process, value system and beliefs, and ultimate goals for treatment engender cooperation and positive outcomes.

After the patient has been contacted and agrees to accept the Case Manager's services, it is appropriate for the Case Manager to contact the patient's physicians and other healthcare providers. The signed consent agreement makes this process easier. To create a plan with the patient, it is necessary to review the evaluation, treatment plans, and goals from each provider. The Case Manager should become acquainted with the patient's previous health status, the patient's physical and mental abilities, and the patient's goals for therapy.

Planning

CCMC defines the care management plan as a timeline of patient care activities and expected outcomes of care of each discipline involved in the care of a particular patient.[6] It is usually developed prospectively by an interdisciplinary healthcare team in relation to a patient's diagnosis, health problem, or surgical procedure.[6] Good case management plans are objective and have goals that are both attainable and tailored to the individual patient's needs. Plans of care should always have a definable beginning and end. Some cases may end with the patient's death, such as in terminal cancer patients. Other cases have a happier endpoint, such as return to work after a patient undergoes a hip replacement. In these instances case management intervention should conclude with the end of the rehabilitation period. All treatment goals require written time frames for achievement or reevaluation of the goal, if it is unmet.

Goal setting is a priority in effective case management. The characteristics of an effective goal can be recalled using the mnemonic SMART.[7] All case management goals should be

- **S** *Specific:* Goals should be specific; for example, a physical therapy goal may be to ambulate 100 feet without assistance.
- **M** *Measurable:* Goals should be measured; for example, after having physical therapy three times a week for 1 week, the patient can ambulate 50 feet with a walker and supervision.
- **A** *Achievable:* Goals should be achievable; for example, if the patient was unable to ambulate before hospitalization and was only able to transfer with assistance, the goal of ambulating 100 feet is not achievable.
- **R** *Realistic:* Goals should be realistic; for example, in the above case the goal of ambulating 100 feet is not realistic.
- **T** *Timely:* Goals should be set at the appropriate time; for example, the physical therapy goal of ambulating 100 feet is not timely if set within 24 hours of a cardiovascular accident before the patient is stabilized or 10 years after a cardiovascular accident.

The Case Manager must have communication and interviewing skills that encourage the patient to participate in his or her own health management and goal setting. By focusing on the patient and his or her health goals, the Case Manager builds rapport and sets the stage for attainment of future goals. The patient's active participation in his or her case management plan optimizes clinical and psychological outcomes.

Implementation

CCMC defines implementation as the process of executing specific case management activities and/or interventions that will lead to accomplishing the goals set forth in the case management plan.[8] The Case Manager implements a care plan after the assessment and goals have been set. The plan should be agreeable to all concerned parties, especially the patient.

Coordination

Case Managers do not act in a void. They are the care coordinators for a team of professionals involved in a patient's health care. The Case Manager works as the liaison between all groups interested in the patient's care. These groups include the patient, the patient's family and friends, the physicians and allied health professionals, the employer, and the insurer. The Case Manager coordinates the care being rendered between the patient and the healthcare system across the various healthcare settings, such as hospital care, rehabilitation, subacute facilities, hospice, home care, pharmacy, infusion therapy, primary care, subspecialty care, and ambulatory care.

As a result of acting as the coordinator, the Case Manager also has the role of liaison and communicator to all parties involved in the care of the patient from the healthcare team to the patient/family. This is true whether he or she works for an insurance company (payer sector), in the private sector, in the provider sector, or as an independent Case Manager.

Monitoring and Evaluation

Monitoring is the ongoing process of gathering information about the patient's progress toward his or her goals as defined in the care management plan. The processes of monitoring and evaluating a patient's care plan are dynamic and continuous. With every patient contact and every progress report received from the patient and caregivers, the plan needs to be reevaluated. Are the strategies working? Is the patient progressing as expected? If not, the Case Manager needs to reassess the goals and set new ones in collaboration with the patient, provider, and care team.

Outcomes Assessment

Outcomes are the result of the cumulative interventions by the Case Manager. The Case Manager is responsible for measuring the effects of her or his interventions on outcomes in every case managed. For example, how did the case management intervention influence the clinical progress, financial impact, quality of care provided, patient's quality of life, and client satisfaction? Outcomes are reviewed and evaluated on an ongoing basis, and changes are made to the process as needed.

There is a difference between this type of case-specific outcome monitoring and the monitoring defined as outcome monitoring for a specific population. In "case-specific" monitoring the Case Manager may measure, for example, the effects of a particular type of orthopedic surgery on a patient with a hip fracture. In a "population-specific" outcome measure the Case Manager may measure, for example, the effects of an intensive course of diabetic education on all newly diagnosed diabetics.

General Assessment

General assessment refers to the evaluation of case management activities/interventions that are not contained in the previous activities, such as maintaining patient privacy and confidentiality; advocacy; and compliance with ethical, legal, accreditation, and regulatory standards.

IDENTIFYING PATIENTS FOR CASE MANAGEMENT

Patients who will benefit the most from case management are identified through a series of proactive and often overlapping processes, including catastrophic diagnosis selection, high-cost diagnosis selection, sentinel procedures, high-cost case selection, chronic disease/multiple comorbidities selection, passive case acquisition, and direct case referral.

Catastrophic Diagnosis Selection

A payer's software system can be programmed to "flag" those diagnoses and procedures that historically result in high utilization of medical resources. These cases are often complex, require multiple care providers, and are very costly for the payer and the patient alike. Individual insurers, managed care corporations, and Case Managers have unique lists of diagnoses and procedures. These lists often are based on community or corporate experience; however, all lists will have diagnoses in common. The following is a short list of diagnoses and procedures that fit this category:

- HIV infection/AIDS
- Adult respiratory distress syndrome
- Renal failure
- Hepatic failure
- Head injuries
- Spinal cord injuries
- Cancer/leukemia
- Multiple-trauma cases
- Neurological surgery
- Back surgery
- Solid organ transplants
- Bone marrow transplants
- Premature delivery
- Respiratory distress syndrome of infancy

High-Risk Diagnosis Selection

Although some diagnoses do not necessarily result in high medical utilization rates, they are placed on these lists because they are often the harbinger of high-cost cases. For example, although diagnoses such as pregnancy-induced diabetes or uncontrolled hypertension do not, in themselves, result in high utilization rates, that small minority of patients who have complications are exorbitantly expensive. Some examples of high-risk diagnosis and procedures are as follows:

- Seizure disorder, new onset
- Transient ischemic attack
- Syncope
- Malignant cardiac arrhythmia
- Gestational diabetes (the diabetes of pregnancy)
- Pregnancy-induced hypertension
- Premature labor

Sentinel Procedures

The term "sentinel procedure" refers to those procedures associated with catastrophic diseases. The procedures themselves do not imply grave diagnoses, per se, but are associated with them often enough to merit investigation by the Case Manager for potential case management services. The following are some examples of these procedures:

- Exploratory laparotomy
- Mediastinoscopy
- Lung biopsy
- Kidney biopsy
- Bone marrow biopsy
- Brain biopsy
- Liver biopsy
- Electrophysiological testing
- Thalidotomy
- Arteriovenous shunt placement
- Lymph node biopsy

High-Cost Case Selection

Experienced Case Managers realize that admitting diagnoses alone can be misleading. An admitting diagnosis of diabetic ketoacidosis may be masking other, more complex diagnoses such as acute myocardial infarction, sepsis, and occult wound infection. Therefore, Case Managers benefit from reviewing those cases whose cost rises above a predetermined dollar limit. The cost limit acts as a proxy for case complexity that would otherwise not be searchable by computer software. For example, a weekly report can be generated that lists all patients whose claims have exceeded $10,000 in the previous 6 to 12 months. Reviewing this list will reveal cases that had escaped the Case Manager's notice because of irregularities in diagnosis reporting or bill submission.

Chronic Disease and Multiple Comorbidities Selections

Ninety-nine percent of Medicare spending is for patients with one or more chronic conditions, and 66% of Medicare spending is for patients with five or more chronic conditions.[9] The Patient Protection and Affordable Care Act incentivizes healthcare providers and provider groups to improve healthcare outcomes while reducing healthcare costs. Case Managers have an exceptional opportunity, in every setting, to coordinate care across the continuum of care, particularly those patients with multiple comorbidities. Providers of health care with electronic health records are able to run reports identifying patients individually and to monitor outcomes for the individual as well as the disease and age-specific population. Case Managers can then focus their efforts on patients who fall out of acceptable parameters to assist patients in meeting their healthcare goals, toward self-management and optimal wellness.

Passive Case Acquisition and Direct Case Referral

Passive case acquisition refers to the way a Case Manager receives cases by persons in the community, not in the employ of the Case Manager or her or his company, requesting the Case Manager's services for themselves or for their patients. These persons in the community can be physicians, therapists, nurses, and lay persons. These cases are referred to as "passive" because the Case Manager does not actively solicit the cases and is not involved in case selection.

Direct case referral is a method of case acquisition in which the Case Manager or his or her employers have established criteria and rules for case referrals. Direct case referrals occur in the managed care setting, where cases can be selected based on claims data and referred directly to the Case Manager.

Established Case Managers have cases sent to them from the community. Knowledgeable physicians and other healthcare providers refer patients who they believe will benefit from case management. These patients can have a newly identified catastrophic diagnosis or a more common diagnosis with unusual clinical or social complexity. This method of passive case acquisition has historically been responsible for only a minority of the Case Manager's caseload. The increased emphasis on accountable care and patient-centered care has highlighted the Case Manager as an invaluable member of the care team, resulting in an increasing number of passive referrals.

ACCOUNTABILITY

Accountability is the acknowledgment and assumption of responsibility for actions and decisions that are made in your role as a Case Manager. It encompasses the obligation to report, explain, and be answerable for the resulting consequences. The responsibility for achieving the case management goals rests with the Case Manager alone. The Case Manager is frequently called on to explain how the patient is progressing toward these goals or why certain goals have not been achieved. The requests may come from the patient, treating physicians, family members, or payers. Clear documentation of all Case Manager decisions and changes in the patient's status is therefore imperative. It is important to document these data from the initial contact with the patient until discharge from case management. There is critical information to document:

- Discharge planning goals
- The medical stability of the patient within 24 hours of discharge
- The plan of care agreed on with the patient and his or her family
- Falls, injuries, restraints, medication reactions/problems
- Justification of the need for referrals to specific providers
- Ongoing evaluation of the patient's condition and progress in light of the treatment
- Evidence of properly credentialed and competent healthcare providers
- Evidence of continuity of care when transitioning from one level of care to another
- Summary of nursing and medical history
- Patient and family education
- Informed consent
- All patient communications, including acceptance or refusal of case management services
- Consultation with the treating physician
- Precertification and the time it took to obtain a precertification
- Advanced directives, living wills, healthcare proxies, do not resuscitate orders, and medical durable power of attorney

Case Managers can be held liable when inappropriate decisions are made regarding medical services. Case Managers are held to a "reasonable standard" of care and are expected to be the patient's advocate, especially if they work for the payer. Case Managers must be aware of national standards and of new treatments and their appropriateness. If an incident should occur with a vendor they put in place, the Case Manager must document the results of her or his investigation and subsequent actions.

NEGOTIATION AND CONFLICT RESOLUTION STRATEGIES

Negotiation skills are necessary for anyone working within the healthcare setting. Learning how to effectively negotiate with physicians, colleagues, managers, patients, payers, vendors, and regulators can make case management easier and more enjoyable. The negotiations between patients and Case Managers regarding their best course of treatment, or the best provider of treatment, are as frequent as they are challenging. Effective negotiating with payers regarding the best care for a patient can be rewarding, because it assists patients in reducing their healthcare costs while obtaining the care they require.

Negotiation is not a skill used exclusively by lawyers, businesspeople, and diplomats. It is an ever-present process used daily in professional and business settings as well as in the home and at school. When a teenager asks to stay out later on a Saturday night and offers to call home at 9:00 p.m. to tell who he is with and how and when he will get home, he is negotiating. When a husband and wife discuss what movie and restaurant to attend, they often negotiate. For example, the husband may give up his choice of movie in order to eat at his favorite restaurant. The wife would rather not eat at the restaurant but is happy to go if she can see the movie she wants. They are negotiating. When a physician suggests a patient exercise more and lose weight rather than starting the patient on antihypertensive medication, negotiation is taking place.

What Is Negotiation?

Negotiation may be defined as the action or process of communication, whereby two or more parties advance mutual interests and reconcile differences to achieve a common goal or solve a common problem. Note in this definition neither demands nor threats are mentioned. The definition implies that negotiation is a reciprocal process aimed at a mutually satisfactory conclusion. It is not a contest with winners and losers. No one gets "beaten" or "out-foxed" in a successful negotiation.

What Is a Successful Negotiation?

A successful negotiation is a mutually satisfactory resolution to a conflict in desires or needs between two or more parties. A successful negotiation results in the following:

- *An agreement that satisfactorily accomplishes the goals of both parties:* If all parties involved in the negotiation do not have their interests served, the negotiation has not been successful.
- *A completion without an excess of time or expense:* Most parties with legitimate common interests want a quick resolution to negotiations. For example, although both the Case Manager and the physician want to arrive at a satisfactory price for a procedure, neither has the time to waste on haggling. Although complicated, multifaceted arrangements may take a long time to work out and may require

"teams" of negotiators (think of SALT II treaties!). The average negotiation for a Case Manager, if handled appropriately, should be completed with a minimum of time and personnel.

- *An agreement that is "workable and enduring":* The agreements that are the result of successful negotiations take into account both the abilities of the parties to comply with the agreement and the predictable changes in the situation surrounding the agreement over time.

- *An agreement that fosters an environment for future, successful negotiations:* A successful negotiation, if handled professionally, does not ensure that all parties will be happy with the outcome or get everything they wanted. However, if there is clear communication of the true interests of both parties, if an agreement is made that serves those true interests, and if the agreement is made with a minimum of time and expense, future negotiations will be easier for both parties. The parties will have developed an informal "partnership" for advancing their common goals. Keep in mind that many, if not most, of the agreements that Case Managers make with physicians, hospitals, and vendors are only one of many agreements they will make with those parties in the future. Treating those other parties with professionalism and respect will make future negotiations easier and more pleasant.

- *An agreement that is workable:* A workable agreement is an agreement whose obligations can be fully satisfied by both parties in the time allotted. Surprisingly, it is not uncommon for parties to enter into unworkable agreements. Many times this happens not because of malice but because of naive miscalculation or presumption born of desperation. For example, a financially desperate vendor, in an effort to gain new business customers to save his failing business, may ensure a level of service or a price structure that he cannot sustain. Common examples of unworkable agreements for a Case Manager may involve overly ambitious turnaround times for claims processing, or providing clinical reports, or even promising durable medical equipment at prices below their acquisition costs. This can be avoided if the purchaser practices due diligence. That is, the purchaser must spend time finding out what the "industry standard" is for reasonable prices or levels of service. If a price or service seems too good to be true, it often is. If the Case Manager discovers what the other party's capabilities, resources, and client history are, he or she may save time and embarrassment in his or her business dealings.

- *An agreement that is enduring:* An enduring agreement can be defined as an agreement that functions successfully over the term of the agreement. Enduring agreements have to be flexible enough to accommodate the variability of the patient's health, finances, and family situation. For example, a private duty nursing agency negotiates an agreement to accept a patient whose service needs are expected to last 6 months or less for a certain hourly rate. Although this is workable upon the start of care, what happens if the patient is still on service 2 or 3 years later? What are the costs if the patient becomes more ill and needs more hours of care per day or specialty nursing care? Will the original payment cover the legitimate expenses for caring for the patient? A successful negotiation in this case would take this predictable outcome into account or be flexible to future negotiations as the healthcare needs continue or change.

What Is an Unsuccessful Negotiation?

An unsuccessful negotiation has the following characteristics:

- *An unsuccessful agreement is based on a win/lose mentality:* People who state they "really got the best of the other party" or who took the other party to the "cleaners" or "beat them to a pulp at the negotiation table" are unlikely to have addressed all the interests and desires of the other party. One-sided "wins" are not the hallmark of a successful negotiation and plant the seeds for future conflict.
- *An unsuccessful agreement results in one or more aggrieved parties:* Persons or groups who believe they have been taken advantage of during a negotiation are likely to remember this when the next negotiation arises. This future negotiation is liable to be characterized by anger and intransigence, even if the point of contention is minor and easily solved.
- *An unsuccessful agreement fails to seek opportunities for "increasing the whole pie" rather than just one's share of the pie:* When two parties discuss openly and intelligently their goals for the negotiation, opportunities arise for not only apportioning the pie fairly but also for increasing the size of the pie. For example, a Case Manager and a vendor of electronic wheelchairs are discussing the price of a wheelchair for one of the Case Manager's patients. There is the usual discussion of what constitutes an appropriate price for the desired wheelchair. The Case Manager states that finding a good-quality wheelchair at a fair price is a problem for her. Every time a patient has a need for a wheelchair, she is forced into spending a lot of time shopping around for the various options she needs and then negotiating a price. She complains this is time-consuming and aggravating. The vendor, seeing an opportunity, asks, "How many patients do you see like this a month?" The Case Manager responds "Oh, 20 or so per month." The discussion then moves from haggling over the price of a single chair to arranging volume discounts and faster delivery for 20 chairs per month. The Case Manager now has a "partner" upon whom she can rely for an agreed-upon price and advice on options and enhancements for her many patients. The vendor has increased the volume and profitability of his business; he can concentrate on improving his customer service rather than on increasing his sales and marketing budget. Both parties are relieved of the cost and burden of further price negotiations.

What You Need (and Don't Need) to Negotiate Successfully

The published "techniques of successful negotiations" fill many volumes in the average library. Some techniques are more appropriate for unique negotiation settings, such as international diplomacy or collective bargaining with labor unions. Not all techniques are sound or appropriate in the setting of the average Case Manager. However, the following examples of techniques or actions are considered necessary to carry on most successful negotiations.

Information

The coin of the realm in negotiations is information, not power, influence, or advantage. A successful negotiator knows what his or her interest is in the discussion with the other party. A successful negotiator knows what she or he hopes to get out of the discussion with the other party. Here are some questions a successful negotiator might ask when preparing for the negotiation:

- Is it merely a lower price the other party wants, or does the speed of delivery or quality of service matter?
- Does the party want a visiting nurse to check a patient's vital signs at home on a daily basis, or does he or she want the visiting nurse to improve the patient's health and keep the patient from being readmitted to the hospital? Is the party willing to pay for that difference?
- Does the party want a facility that has the lowest bed rate for a hospitalization, or the facility that has vast experience with the patient's disease and will treat the patient efficiently and, thereby, decrease the overall length of stay and costs?
- Does the Case Manager want the absolute lowest price on a piece of durable medical equipment, or does he or she want a fair price and a responsive partner in serving the many needs of his or her patients?

Other examples of important information to know before a negotiation starts are as follows:

- Who else in the area provides this service or sells these items?
- Is the vendor accredited or bonded?
- What is their service like?
- Do they deliver on time?
- Do their nurses show up late at a client's home, or not at all?
- What are the "usual and customary" charges for these services?
- Are there other benchmarks for these charges? (Medicare fee schedule? Major insurer's fee schedule?)
- Have these vendors been used before?
- What price was paid in the past?
- Were there quality issues then?

Obviously, there is a large amount of information. Is it worth tracking this information for future negotiations? Most negotiation experts would say so.

Best Alternative to a Negotiated Agreement

A very important piece of information for the Case Manager to have during a negotiation is the best alternative to a negotiated agreement, or BATNA. This concept was explained in the book *Getting to Yes* by Roger Fisher and William Ury.[10] BATNA is an exercise in imagination and research that should occur before any substantive negotiation. It is an exploration of what happens when there is a negotiation impasse and no agreement can be reached. For example, assume surgical services are necessary for a patient who is 3 years old. In preparation for a negotiation with a provider, it is discovered that there are more than 30 pediatric surgeons in the community who perform this type of surgery regularly. Thus, the best alternative to an impasse in negotiation with the first surgeon is to go to another surgeon for this surgery. This is a powerful piece of information during the negotiation and will affect how aggressively the surgeon's fee can be negotiated. If, on the other hand, the prenegotiation research indicates the patient requires a unique type of surgery and only one provider on the East Coast regularly performs this rare type of surgery, the BATNA is to either pay the surgeon her "full charges" or incur the cost of sending the patient to the West Coast for the procedure. A Case Manager would then negotiate the procedure cost much less aggressively.

The use of BATNA in these situations allows the negotiator to anticipate the outcome to a failure in negotiations and think of alternatives to likely unfavorable outcomes. For example, in the case of the only provider of the surgical service who wants a fee that is much higher than is usual and customary, she may be the only provider of the service, but she is interested in getting paid as soon as possible with as little additional effort as possible. In discussing with the provider the complex process necessary for authorization of her nonstandard fee, the additional reports she will have to provide, and the expected delays in payment, the provider may be encouraged to accept a lesser fee to expedite the payment. Using BATNA on both sides of the negotiating table allows the parties to explore these alternatives for their mutual benefit.

Trust/Trustworthiness

When negotiating with another party, a certain level of trust must exist or the scope of the negotiation becomes very narrow and bogged down with needs for assurances and indemnifications on both sides. Trust can be built over time with a history of successful negotiations. From the Case Manager's perspective, this means scrupulous adherence to the tenets of the agreement. Be timely; look to streamline further approvals or payments if appropriate. Mail, fax, or e-mail a written copy of the verbal agreement as soon as possible to the other party. Act rapidly on all agreed on approvals or the issuance of checks. This should be easy for a Case Manager, and it will win points with the other party. A Case Manager should expect the same treatment from the other party. If a Case Manager finds his or her trust is misplaced, he or she should find another vendor or provider of services.

Respect for the Other Party

A good negotiator respects the other party. For a Case Manager, this means timing the negotiation so it is most convenient for both parties. For example, calling a physician in the middle of the day while she's seeing patients and expecting her to drop everything to enter into a lengthy discussion about prices or services may be unfair. Calling beforehand and setting up an appointment so both parties are prepared to discuss the issue is ideal.

Avoidance of "Irritators" in Communications

"Irritators" are terms that, intentionally or not, are judgmental and cause the other party pain or embarrassment. They are not conducive to a dispassionate discussion of the items of interest and do not advance a mutual goal. For example, during a price negotiation on a surgical procedure the Case Manager states the surgeon should accept the offered price because it is "fair" or "reasonable" (implying that the surgeon's charge for the procedure is unfair or unreasonable). This would irritate the surgeon and make him less willing to work with the Case Manager to arrive at a mutually satisfactory price. As an alternative, the Case Manager might explain that the surgeon's fees deviate from the usual and customary charges and that company policy only authorizes prompt payment for usual and customary charges. This allows both parties to save face and continue negotiations. Another example of the use of irritators in negotiation occurs when a Case Manager wants to negotiate an increase in performance from a provider of care. To characterize a provider's work as "unprofessional" or "shoddy" will only anger the provider and not resolve the quality issue. Stating specifics, such as "the respiratory therapist arrived late and left paper wrappers and puddles of water on the patient's floor" provides the other party with information he or she can use to improve the provider's care and avoids emotional reactions and further conflict.

Active Listening

Inherent in the process of communication is listening to the interests of the other party. Often, these are not stated directly but must be culled from facial expressions, body language, and tone and nuances of speech. It is common for an inexperienced negotiator to be busy formulating another argument while he or she quietly waits for the other party to stop speaking. Active listening requires more than just silence on the part of the listener. It requires the listener to hear and understand what is being said and to think about the content and the implications of the other party's statements. When actively listening, encourage the other party to fully explain his or her ideas and then restate them in your own words. This not only ensures you have heard the other party correctly, but tells the other party you were listening closely. Repeating the major points stated by the other party also allows you to rephrase their statements slightly to explore possible alternatives: for example, "You have mentioned price and service as important to you, is there anything else?" or, "You mentioned promptness of delivery as something that is very important to you. Do you want to expand on that topic?"

CASE MANAGER AS A PATIENT ADVOCATE

The Case Manager's foremost role is that of patient advocate. The case selection process identifies a group of critically or chronically ill patients. Frequently, because of the physical and emotional effects of their disease process or as a result of being overwhelmed by the magnitude and complexity of their treatment plan, these patients and their families have no idea what their needs are. They may not be intellectually or emotionally capable of dealing with the issues or the people involved in their care. This is when a Case Manager is most needed. The Case Manager can assist the patient and his or her family in attaining autonomy and self-determination by empowering them. This can be done through education on the disease process (or injury), offering and explaining the available options to the patient, clarifying the available insurance benefits and community resources, and listening to the patient verbalize his or her views and perceived needs. The Case Manager can intercede on behalf of the patient with the physician and other service providers. He or she can negotiate treatment or procedure rates to minimize the patient's expenses, assist the patient in finding physician specialists or specialty services, and help identify resources for those needs not covered by insurance.

The Case Manager also has a legal and ethical responsibility to protect patients from misinformation and errors in comprehension. The Case Manager can fill in gaps in knowledge, clarify misunderstandings, and communicate with providers when the patient requires more information or further clarification regarding the treatment plan and options. The Case Manager can play a central role in helping patients and their families examine their views and feelings on the difficult subject of end-of-life treatment and plans. The Case Manager is in the unique position of being able to obtain information regarding the patient's end-of-life treatment decisions. For a competent patient the Case Manager can help explain the patient's wishes to his or her family and caregivers. For the incompetent patient the Case Manager can find a family member who will make decisions or gain consensus on an end-of-life treatment plan from loved ones. Generally, it is the Case Manager who assists the patient in documenting his or her wishes regarding withdrawal of care or end-of-life decisions. The Case Manager then has a major advocacy role in ensuring the patient's wishes are documented and observed.

For the Case Manager to effectively advocate for his or her patients, he or she must have adequate contact with the patient. He or she must spend the time required to understand the patient's concerns and to educate the patient and the patient's family regarding options. The Case Manager must also be able to convey the patient's and the family's concerns to the appropriate providers, obtain answers or possible solutions, and report back to the patient or family. The Case Manager must be fully aware of the patient's bill of rights and state laws and mandates pertaining to health care. The Case Manager is charged with the responsibility of explaining all of these things to the patient and family, advocating for the patient, alleviating their worries, providing emotional support, and obtaining information for the patient when he or she does not have the answer.

COMMUNICATION SKILLS

Most of a Case Manager's day is spent communicating. Conversations held face to face or via phone, fax, or mail need to be as clear, complete, and concise as possible. Educating the patient, caregivers, and referral source is a vital case management function. Explaining the full clinical picture, especially when requesting extracontractual benefits, allows the referral source to make the best possible decision. Long and windy explanations waste time and tax the listener's patience. Jumbled stories and fuzzy plans can lead to delays and clinical errors. Clear communication is an essential skill of case management. So, what exactly is communication, and what are good communication skills?

Communication is an act or instance of transmitting information. Effective communication is further defined as the successful exchange of information between individuals. An effective communicator is also successful in establishing an active relationship or "two-way link" with another person, so information can flow in two directions. These statements imply that not all communication or communicators are successful. Case Managers cannot afford to be poor communicators and should work to improve their communication skills.

An effective communication has four components[11]:

1. *Sender:* The person sending the communication.
2. *Message:* All information transferred, including verbal and nonverbal content.
3. *Receiver:* The person to whom the message is sent.
4. *Context:* The surroundings in which the communication takes place. The environment is identified by such factors as the patient's condition (is he or she concentrating on the pain and not the Case Manager?), cultural background, health beliefs, and values. When making a call for a telephone interview the Case

Manager should allocate time exclusively for the patient, rather than continuing to answer the phone, scan paperwork, or handle other cases. A distracted Case Manager sends another message in addition to the intended message.

The method of sending a message is also important to the communication process. Some messages are better communicated in person than by letter or telephone. Some are better communicated in groups or by specific individuals. Certain types of information require written communication. For example, an exercise plan explained to the patient by a physical therapist is reinforced between physical therapy visits when a written description and pictures of the exercises are left with the patient. In the same way a complex medication regimen explained to the patient is enhanced when a written schedule of administration is left with the patient. If there is an attorney involved on a case, the Case Manager should get the attorney's permission before contacting the patient. The Case Manager should assure the patient and family that all communications are confidential and that certain information will not be communicated to the employer. All communications (verbal and written) should be documented.

Barriers to Communication

There are several areas in which communication between a Case Manager and a patient is hindered. These barriers[12] to good communication are

- Physical interference
- Psychological noise
- Information processing barriers
- Perceptual barriers
- Structural barriers

Physical Interference

Ideally, the Case Manager and the patient communicate in a quiet space and during a time when neither is distracted. For example, if the patient is being served lunch, watching a favorite television show, or surrounded by visitors, the ability to effectively communicate is diminished.

Psychological Noise

Is the patient thinking about something else? Is the patient in pain, hungry, depressed, anxious about the outcome of a test, or just angry with his or her situation? If the patient's psychological barrier can be addressed, then the likelihood that effective communication can take place has increased. Sometimes the issue bothering the patient is as simple as who is paying for the Case Manager's services. Many patients refuse case management services because they believe it is an additional cost to them. Explaining that it is already a part of their benefit package, at no additional cost, can free the way to effective communication and a commitment to the case management process. A Case Manager should inquire about the patient's state of mind (or mood) in the beginning of important conversations, that is, conversations in which important information is provided or where significant clinical decisions are made. If the patient manifests signs of psychological problems or distractions, those problems or distractions should be explored to see if they will interfere with clear communication.

Information Processing Barriers

Discussions with patients often involve unfamiliar medical terms or complex information regarding their treatment. Not all patients are able to absorb this information easily and use it to make informed decisions. This inability to absorb and use complex information is called an information processing barrier. Information processing barriers can include

- Information overload
- Cognitive deficits
- Intellectual/educational deficits

Information overload occurs when too much information is being sent and the patient cannot process it all. A large volume of information can be overwhelming to the patient, causing him or her to stop listening. The patient may be too embarrassed to mention this and the Case Manager continues to talk, unaware of the growing communication barrier.

Information processing barriers are also a problem for patients who suffer from cognitive deficits. Information needs to be sent at a rate and in a fashion that the patient can process effectively. By observing physical cues, such as the patient's eye contact or the number and type of questions asked, the Case Manager can determine the patient's level of attention to the message delivered. The Case Manager may assess the patient's understanding of an issue discussed by asking the patient to explain the issue back to the Case Manager in his or her own words.

Most patients are unfamiliar with the causes and treatment of their disease. Even the most intelligent patient may be lost when discussing these unfamiliar topics. Patients with intellectual or cognitive deficits are at a particular disadvantage. These patients may become passive and disinterested in their care or become fearful and uncooperative with the care plan. Therefore, the Case Manager must be aware of possible intellectual or educational deficits that may constitute a barrier to good communication. The Case Manager should avoid medical jargon and overtly technical words and frequently ask the patient for feedback to ensure she or he has been understood. Nothing impairs communication like using a vocabulary the patient does not understand.

Perceptual Barriers

Perceptual barriers are impediments to communication based on the prejudices of the listener. These barriers result in unintended and unwarranted interpretations of information provided by another person. That is, the Case Manager and the patient can sometimes see the same situation from a different point of view, and this can affect understanding and decision making. Perceptual barriers are formed by the patient's unique experiences, cultural background, educational level, and value system. Everything the patient experiences is subject to interpretation based on past experiences (e.g., Will this experience be good or bad, right or wrong, or pleasurable or painful? What experience in my past that was the same or similar?). If the patient has had negative experiences with Case Managers, everything the Case Manager does or says will be filtered through this perception. If the patient comes from a cultural background in which seeking assistance is frowned upon or admitting illness or debility is equated with failure, this will affect communication. The Case Manager needs to have an understanding of the patient's intellectual, religious, and cultural background and adjust his or her communication style accordingly.

Structural Barriers

Structural barriers occur due to bureaucratic, procedural, technologic, or geographical barriers. If a patient must pass through several layers of bureaucracy or speak to several intermediaries before each conversation with the Case Manager, patient frustration and anger is likely. In a similar vein, Case Managers who communicate important information through one or more intermediaries risk a critical miscommunication, like when playing the children's game of telephone. This is true whether the communication is with the patient, family, caregivers, or the Case Manager's own peers.

The best way to avoid this type of miscommunication is to have a communication plan. The plan should identify the time and method for direct communication with interested parties. For some this will be telephone calls in the morning; for others it will be e-mails during the evening; for still others it is a face-to-face conversation at the bedside. If the Case Manager is able to ensure that all interested parties can contact him or her directly, then the level of frustration will be much lower.

Another structural barrier is a geographical and time barrier. When team members are not in the same place at the same time, critical information about a case may be missed by some or all decision makers. A possible solution to this structural problem is to establish team conferences. Team conferences are meetings of all the decision makers whose purpose it is to exchange information, answer questions, and come to a consensus on critical clinical issues. Although a face-to-face meeting is desirable, team conferences can be held over the telephone or Internet. The Internet allows for asynchronous communication, wherein individual team members can leave messages or updates for all the members when new information is available. This allows faster information transfer without the challenges of setting up a team meeting.

If a team meeting is not possible, the Case Manager should personally communicate with members of the treating team and then with the patient and family members. Speaking to each team member does not guarantee the message sent is the message received; the Case Manager still must test for feedback. Important information should be written down and mailed to the patient or clinical team member. Do not leave important information to the vagaries of a poor memory.

The most important aspect in communication is the Case Manager's ability to listen. A rule of thumb for the Case Manager is to do less talking and more listening. This sends the message that the Case Manager places the needs of the patient above his or her own needs.

INTERVIEW TECHNIQUES

The three basic goals of an interview are to establish a rapport, to collect information, and to formulate a care plan.[13] The case management process begins with gathering and assessing information. The information gathered will become the basis for the case management plan. The more information known before planning, the better the plan will be. It is essential, therefore, that the information collected is complete and accurate. Toward that end, the Case Manager needs to use good interview and communication skills. The following steps are applicable regardless of whom the Case Manager is interviewing[14]:

- *Introduction:* The Case Manager should introduce him- or herself and explain the reason he or she will be asking so many questions. He or she should ask if it is a good time to talk. If not, he or she should call back at a more convenient time. The Case Manager should explain his or her role in the patient's case and assure the patient that the information collected will remain confidential. After this, the Case Manager should ask permission to proceed.
- *Empowerment:* Patient empowerment is an important interview technique. One way to empower the patient is for the Case Manager to allow the patient to do most of the talking, use his or her own words and expressions, and speak at his or her own pace and to finish thoughts. This makes the patient feel in control of the interview and a partner in the management process. It also allows the Case Manager to assess the patient's comprehension of the disease process and treatment plan.
- *Trust:* Trust is defined as a firm reliance on the integrity, ability, or character of a person. It is difficult to establish such a relationship over the phone. However, a few techniques can improve a Case Manager's chances of meeting this challenge:
  - Be sensitive to the emotional content of the issues being discussed. Allow time for the patient to absorb painful information and assess his or her ability to continue to actively listen.
  - Always use layman's terms when discussing medical problems. It helps to establish a rapport with the patient. Remember that confusing medical terminology may be a barrier to effective communication and trust.
  - Patients suffering from severe illness or injury are often fearful for the future and can be concerned about the abilities of those caring for them. The Case Manager should offer reassurance to the patient concerning the training and experience of the clinical team handling the case. Further, the Case Manager should reaffirm that he or she is the patient's advocate and will always act in the patient's best interest. The Case Manager should explain that he or she is available to the patient for any questions or concerns the patient may have.
- *Respect:* The Case Manager should maintain a respectful demeanor when speaking with the patient. This is especially important when the patient's value system is different from that of the Case Manager. When acting as the patient's advocate, the Case Manager may find differences between the patient's idea of what is appropriate and the Case Manager's idea of what is appropriate. A perceived lack of respect for the patient's beliefs or decisions can be another barrier to effective communication and interviewing. By demonstrating empathy and understanding of their differences but a commitment to their shared goals, a Case Manager can further his or her rapport. This well-developed rapport may encourage the patient or family to call the Case Manager early enough to make timely interventions, perhaps avoiding costly hospitalizations or complex treatments.
- *Body language:* If the Case Manager is interviewing the patient in person (rather than by telephone), he or she should be careful of his or her own body language. Nonverbal body language can reveal a judgmental attitude to the patient. During the in-person interview the Case Manager should also observe the patient's general appearance and body language. Does the patient's body language suggest he or she is tired or in pain? Is the patient unshaven and in stained clothing,

suggesting depression. Alternatively, does the Case Manager's body language confirm his or her attentiveness? If the interview is by telephone, a careful Case Manager will take note of the tone of his or her voice. The voice used with patients should always be calm, professional, and empathetic. A Case Manager should also test discrepancies between a patient's body language and actual statements. Sometimes, a patient's words and body language do not match. In general, words are easier to change than the way they are expressed. A Case Manager should explore these discrepancies with the patient. If the patient is uncommunicative, the issue should be noted and discussed at a later date.

- *Listening:* Listening (as opposed to just hearing) is an active, cognitive process requiring sensitivity and focused attention. Active listening requires real participation and uses attending behaviors, such as facial gestures, head nodding, note taking, and repeating back what is said. This assures the patient that the Case Manager is listening and encourages the patient to continue.
- *Note taking:* By using a pad and pencil to take notes during the interview, a Case Manager can prevent omissions. However, note taking should be kept to a minimum during the interview because it is distracting and can be viewed with suspicion by the patient. As soon as the interview is over, a Case Manager can complete his or her notes while the interview is fresh in his or her mind.
- *Interviewing style:* An interview should start by asking about the patient's major problem. The details may be filled in as the patient talks about other topics, without the necessity of asking indelicate questions. Open-ended questions should be used (i.e., those that require more than a one-word answer). A Case Manager should try to avoid "why" questions, as they often sound accusatory. Rapid-fire questions and cutting off answers that appear irrelevant or nonresponsive on the surface appear to be ways to make the exchange of information go faster. However, for some patients the conversation takes on the characteristics of an interrogation, which can be unpleasant for the patient and can make them shorten answers or avoid mentioning concerns for fear of "wasting the interviewer's time." For some patients getting information is a slow process that can be approached only with patience and understanding. A helpful technique is to ask "combination questions." By asking combination questions the patient isn't always answering rapid-fire questions and can reveal his or her interests and concerns by what he or she chooses to respond to and what questions are avoided (e.g., "Tell me about your family, employment, and what you like to do to relax and enjoy yourself").
- *Closing the interview:* An excellent way for a Case Manager to close the interview is by sharing his or her summary with the patient. This summary should capture the essence of the interview and explain the care plan. After this review the patient should be encouraged to add information or correct any misunderstandings. This act demonstrates to the patient that the Case Manager was actively listening and helps to develop a consensus on the plan goals.

Initial Assessment

The initial assessment interview should evaluate the following clinical categories[15]:

- Cognitive function
- Diagnosis/medical conditions
- Medications

- Care access
- Functional status
- Social situation
- Nutritional status
- Emotional status

Cognitive Function

Cognitive deficits are associated with many diseases of the neurological system, such as dementias, infections, tumors, cerebral vascular accidents, and traumatic brain injuries. If, during the interview, the Case Manager notices the patient is cognitively impaired, the Case Manager should seek a patient proxy, such as a family member or caregiver, to answer questions. This person should have the legal authority to make healthcare decisions for the patient. This authority should be established by having a signed and witnessed statement to the effect (i.e., medical power of attorney, medical proxy, living will naming the person as proxy). A copy of the formal proxy statement should be kept with the patient record. The cognitive deficit should be addressed in the care plan that is developed.

Diagnosis/Medical Conditions

The Case Manager should elicit from the patient his or her understanding of the disease process or injury. Questions should bring to light areas of concern for the patient that may require the Case Manager's intervention.

Medications

Medications are a large area often overlooked when multiple providers care for a patient. Case Managers are in the unique position of being able to detect potential problems with drug administration, such as pharmacy misunderstandings, prescription duplications, drug–disease interactions, and drug–drug interactions. The Case Manager is also able to improve drug compliance by explaining or reinforcing information about drug dosing and side effects. The Case Manager can educate the patient about how the drug works to improve his or her health and can explore any financial barriers the patient has in acquiring the medications.

Care Access

The Case Manager evaluates the health services the patient is using, looking for appropriateness of service type, service location, and provider. Based on these findings the Case Manager can assist in filling gaps, eliminating duplicate services, arranging for credentialed providers, and negotiating appropriate costs on behalf of the patient.

Functional Status

The evaluation of functional status is an important part of the assessment process. This evaluation has several parts, including activities of daily living, instrumental activities of daily living, and fall prevention:

- Activities of daily living include items such as whether the patient can bathe, feed, dress, and toilet him- or herself. Can she or he do these activities within certain parameters? For instance, can the patient dress her- or himself if she or he has assistive devices? Is she or he mobile? If so, how? Does the patient need

assistance or need equipment to be mobile; is she or he independent on flat surfaces but not able to climb stairs safely?
- Instrumental activities of daily living are a group of activities that include the ability to do housework, shop, and prepare meals. Questions such as "Is the patient subsisting on 'tea and toast' because he or she cannot carry heavier groceries home?" "Is the environment a barrier to effective wound healing due to the inability to clean house?" should be asked.
- Fall prevention is another important aspect of the assessment process. Is there a potential for falls? Does the patient have a history of falls? Do new medical circumstances put the patient at risk for falls? For example, the following conditions have been associated with an increased risk for falls: blindness, vestibular problems, syncope, leg or arm weakness, new bandages, and casts. Certain medications have been associated with falls, such as benzodiazepines or barbiturates. Does the patient need an assessment and assistance in creating a barrier-free environment to prevent falls? Common household improvements include pulling up slippery carpets, marking the edges of steps, improving lighting, and installing handrails in the bath. Does the patient require a quad cane, a walker, or another assistive device for safety? These improvements or supplies may not always be covered under insurance, but the Case Manager has the option of presenting alternate benefit plans to the referral source and using community resources.

Social Situation

This area of assessment involves an evaluation of the patient's support system. The Case Manager determines who is available, able, and willing to participate in the patient's care plan. If the family is having difficulty coping with the patient's illness or dependent status, the Case Manager can arrange for social work intervention.

Nutritional Status

Nutritional deficits can be the cause of, or exacerbate, many health problems. In particular, they delay wound healing and adversely affect cognitive function. Poor nutrition affects many disease states, such as diabetes mellitus. It also impairs the effectiveness of medication. A Case Manager should assess the nutritional status of patients in his or her care and incorporate improvement of nutrition into the care plan when appropriate.

Emotional Status

The Case Manager can recognize depression and other emotional disorders during the assessment or in subsequent patient interactions. Emotional disorders negatively affect the well-being of the patient, the care plan, and the desired outcomes. The Case Manager is in a position to observe emotional changes in the patient and to have them assessed by the primary care physician. She or he can also arrange for psychological interventions, if necessary.

MANAGEMENT STRATEGIES FOR PATIENTS WITH COMORBIDITIES

As our population ages patients increasingly have multiple chronic conditions. Some are concordant and go hand in hand, such as diabetes and hypertension; others are not, such as diabetes and lung cancer. For most patients with diabetes this is their top health priority, for others with more severe conditions, like stage 4 lung cancer, the long-term effects of diabetes are not a priority for them.

Patients with multiple chronic conditions have more healthcare needs and as a result more healthcare goals and associated costs than patients with one disease process. Prioritizing these goals must be done with the patient as well as the physician to have optimal outcomes. Initially, it is important to focus on two to three goals the patient identifies as the most important to him or her. It is overwhelming for the patient to work on everything at once. Having success on a few goals that are important to the patient helps build rapport and a foundation for future goal setting and successes.

The Case Manager should be mindful of financial issues that may keep the patient from being amenable with the treatment regime. Whenever possible, generic medications or formulary medications should be prescribed. If this is an issue for the patient, the Case Manager should intercede on his or her behalf with the prescribing provider. Also, an abundance of drug store chains offer generic drugs at inexpensive copays, such as $4 for a 30-day supply and $9.99 for a 90-day supply. When necessary, the Case Manager can assist the patient with applications to drug company assistance programs.

Patients with multiple diagnoses such as diabetes, high blood pressure, and high cholesterol will have several dietary changes as part of their care plan. If their significant other is the main cook, it may be helpful to get the patient's permission to meet with them and their significant other to review dietary goals.

Information and handouts should be kept to a minimum at any one time. Beware of overwhelming your patient with too much information. Ask the patient if there is anything he or she would like to have as a reference and supply that, or give the patient a handout and agree to review it with him or her the next time you speak. Remember, if the patient is seeing several healthcare professionals, he or she might be in information overload already.

Patients with multiple chronic conditions generally need to make multiple lifestyle changes to meet their goals. When working with these patients it is important that you acknowledge their successes—no matter how small. Recognizing and affirming their progress helps build positive outcomes and sets the stage for future goal setting.

MOTIVATIONAL INTERVIEWING

When dealing with patients with chronic conditions the Case Manager's main role is to assist the patient to identify the goals most important to him or her for self-management of the disease state. Motivational interviewing is used to help identify patient preferences and help patients develop and maintain healthy behaviors. It is focused on those patients with chronic conditions that need help optimizing their health status. Motivational interviewing is better applied to ongoing monitoring and coaching than initial assessment. It is based on asking open-ended questions, affirmations, and summarizing what the patient has said. Motivational interviewing is especially useful for ongoing monitoring of your patient in relation to a chronic disease.

The thought process behind motivational interviewing is that empathy promotes change and patient awareness of the discrepancies between his or her behavior and personal values creates change. Using this style of interviewing, the Case Manager tries to draw out the patient's values or preferences and clarifies how the patient's behavior fits

42 CHAPTER TWO

(or doesn't fit) with his or her expressed values/preferences. Self-recognition of these discrepancies assists patients with goal setting and real change.

CASE MANAGEMENT REPORTS

Reports that are commonly made available to the Case Manager should include those on the patient's medical care, cost-to-benefit analysis, summary, and vendor progress. Case Managers should receive regular reports of the patient's progress or status from the vendors and providers in place. Likewise, regular patient case reports should be provided to the payer (see Appendix B). In some cases this will be to the insurer, whereas in others it will be the employer.

Patient case reports should clearly state the following:

- Desired outcomes
- Progress toward the outcomes
- Cost of care without case management intervention
- Cost of care with case management intervention
- Savings due to case management intervention

Specific patient reports should be produced monthly and upon case closure. Additionally, a cost-to-benefit analysis report should be produced upon closure of a case and should contain the following:

- Diagnosis
- Summary of intervention
- Total time in case management
- Total cost without case management intervention
- Total cost with case management intervention
- Total savings

A Case Manager should produce a cost-to-benefit analysis report for his or her client on a regular basis. This report should include all the activity on the client's employees in the past reporting period. Quarterly reporting is usually sufficient, unless there is unusually heavy activity with a client. This cost-to-benefit report gives the client an understanding of what the Case Manager is doing for his or her employees and just how valuable the Case Manager's services are. A review of the literature demonstrates varied reported case management savings: ratios of four to six dollars saved per one dollar spent on case management services to percentages saved after subtracting the cost of case management services. Regardless of how the savings were calculated, they were attributed to Case Managers coordinating the best treatment, at the appropriate time, at the appropriate level of care, at the best cost across the continuum of care.

Summary reports from the Case Manager to the payer should contain the following:

- A summary of the activity of a particular client
- The number of cases in case management
- The number of cases referred
- The number of cases closed

- The fees for case management services
- The savings generated by case management intervention
- The ratio of savings per dollar billed

Progress reports should be submitted regularly to the Case Manager (see Appendix C). These reports should communicate the results of the provider's most recent evaluation, goals, and progress toward the patient's goals. Like the case management plan, they should be specific, measurable, achievable, realistic, and timely. They should include time frames for goal reevaluation if the goals are unmet.

Alternate Benefit Plans

At times, benefit plan limitations and exclusions can hinder efficient and cost-effective medical care. In these cases, offering extracontractual benefits (also known as "alternate benefit plans" or "flexed benefits") is helpful. For instance, a patient's benefit plan may only pay for nursing visits after a hospitalization. A newly diagnosed diabetic with this limited benefit plan may require nursing visits for diabetic education, for initial insulin injections and for glucometer instruction. Although this patient clearly can be managed at home without a costly hospitalization, his or her only recourse under the limitations of his or her health plan is to enter the hospital for this care or pay significant out-of-pocket expenses for home nursing care. The Case Manager needs to present to the payer the rationale for extending the extracontractual benefit of home nursing care in lieu of a hospitalization. The request should indicate the desired outcomes and the cost-effectiveness of managing the patient at home while avoiding a costly hospitalization. Extracontractual benefits should be approved by the payer before their implementation. These extracontractual benefits and confirmation of the payer's approval need to be communicated to the insurance plan's claims adjuster. The claims adjuster will then ensure a smooth payment process and avoid unintended claims denials. See Appendix D for a sample alternate benefit plan.

Extracontractual benefits are a powerful tool in the Case Manager's armamentarium but are insufficient to meet all the challenges presented by a catastrophic injury or chronic debilitating illness. A Case Manager must be able to maximize the resources the patient has at his or her disposal. These resources include family, friends, neighbors, community-based philanthropies, religious and other charitable organizations, and federal entitlements, as well as any private insurance coverage. Maximizing resources requires prudent planning, such as instructing the patient and significant others on certain aspects of care, using lending closets, encouraging the use of generic drugs, and exploring programs for indigent patients that pay for part or all the costs of pharmaceutical medications. It is the Case Manager's responsibility to keep apprised of available family, community, and governmental resources. An excellent reference is the *Case Management Resource Guide*.[16] Additionally; the Case Manager should compile and keep his or her own file of facilities and specialists to whom he or she can refer. This file should include specialized programs and providers with accredited expertise.

Documentation

As was mentioned under Accountability, earlier, documentation is essential. Not only should the Case Manager document all discussions with healthcare providers and vendors, but it is important to document all conversations with the patient from initial contact until discharge from case management. This documentation aids the Case Manager in clinical management, justifies expenditures, and defends from allegations of negligence. Some critical information to document is as follows:

- Discharge planning goals
- The medical stability of the patient within 24 hours of discharge
- The plan of care agreed on with the patient and his or her family
- Any falls, injuries, restraints, or medication reactions/problems
- Justification of the need for referrals to specific providers
- Ongoing evaluation of the patient's condition
- Progress in light of treatment
- Evidence of properly credentialed and competent healthcare providers
- Evidence of continuity of care upon discharge from the inpatient setting
- Summary of nursing and medical history
- Patient and family education
- Informed consent
- All patient communications, including acceptance or refusal of case management services
- Consultation with the treating physician and/or other providers
- Precertification for procedures and the time it took to obtain it
- Advanced directives, living wills, healthcare proxies, do not resuscitate orders, and medical durable power of attorney

Patient Advocates

As the patient's advocate the Case Manager is obligated to act in the patient's best interest. In this role Case Managers are held to a "reasonable standard of care." To be the best advocate possible, the Case Manager needs to know what the standard of care is for many conditions. He or she must be well informed on current trends in medical, surgical, and rehabilitation therapeutics. The Case Manager is not only responsible for his or her own actions, but also for those of the vendors he or she recommends. If an incident should occur with a vendor he or she puts in place, there must be documentation of the investigation of the incident, the findings of the investigation, and subsequent corrective action plans that derive from it.

CASE MANAGEMENT PROGRAM EVALUATION

The Case Management Society of America created the Case Management Model Act in 2009 to put forth the key elements that should be included in a comprehensive case management program for state and federal legislators to use as a guideline when drafting public policy.[17] This document addresses definitions, staff qualifications, case management functions, authorized scope of services, payment of services, other program requirements (such as information management), training, quality management, consumer protections, handling of complaints, and general oversight and implementation. Using the Case Management Model Act to establish a case management program should ensure quality, cost-effective, and improved clinical outcomes from qualified

Case Managers through an evidence-based, data-driven program with clinical oversight and quality management activities.

Case management programs should have written, evidence-based criteria, ongoing evaluation standards, and monitoring of their activities. There should be guidelines for identifying patients for case management services, comprehensive assessments, guidelines for accepting cases, ongoing assessments, and guidelines for closing cases. Patients should know the procedure to submit complaints about medical care and other services. Case Managers should conduct regular case audits and patient surveys. Clinical outcomes should be reviewed on individual case as well as population levels. This can be done for a particular employer group, service level (i.e., Has the incidence of hospital readmissions within 30 days decreased since focusing on transition of care issues?), or disease entity (i.e., Has the number of patients with a measured hemoglobin A_{1c} greater than 9 been reduced since directing case management services toward this population?).

REFERENCES

1. Commission for Case Management Certification (CCMC). Certification guide published 1992, revised 2004. Retrieved August 21, 2011, from http://www.cmsa.org/portals/0/pdf/MemberOnly/CCMCertificationGuide.pdf
2. Ibid.
3. Ibid.
4. Mullahy, C. (2010). *The Case Manager's handbook* (4th ed.). Sudbury, MA: Jones & Bartlett Learning.
5. Commission for Case Management Certification (CCMC). (2005). Glossary of terms. Retrieved February 24, 2012, from http://www.ccmcertification.org/sites/default/files/downloads/2011/CCMC%20Glossary.pdf
6. Ibid.
7. Covey, S. (2004). *The 8th habit: From effectiveness to greatness.* New York: Free Press.
8. Commission for Case Management Certification (CCMC). (2005). Glossary of terms. Retrieved February 24, 2012, from http://www.ccmcertification.org/sites/default/files/downloads/2011/CCMC%20Glossary.pdf
9. Anderson, G., & Horvath, J. (2002). *Chronic conditions: Making the case for ongoing care.* Baltimore, MD: Partnership for Solutions.
10. Fisher, R., & Ury, W. (1981). *Getting to yes: Negotiating agreement without giving in.* Boston: Houghton Mifflin Company.
11. Cesta, T., Tahan, H., & Fink, L. (1998). *The Case Manager's survival guide: Winning strategies for clinical practice.* St. Louis: Mosby.
12. Ibid.
13. Mullahy, C. (2010). *The Case Manager's handbook* (4th ed.). Sudbury, MA: Jones & Bartlett Learning.
14. Powell, S. K. (1996). *Nursing case management: A practical guide to success in managed care.* New York: Lippincott.
15. Aliotta, S. L., Clarke, J., & Paulwan, T. F. (1998). Case management assessment and planning for high-risk Medicare HMO members. *Journal of Care Management, 4*(2), 86–94.
16. 2011 *Case management resource guide* (21st ed.). Rockville, MD: Dorland Health.
17. Case Management Society of America. Retrieved September 25, 2011, from http://www.cmsa.org

Appendix 2-A

Case Management Concepts Questions

1) Case management is defined by the CCMC as an activity that includes which of the following processes?
   1. Advocacy and resource management
   2. Assessing, planning, and monitoring
   3. Collaboration, coordination, and communication
   4. Implementation and evaluation
      A. All of the above
      B. None of the above
      C. 1, 2, 3
      D. 2, 3, 4

2) Arranging for continuity of care upon discharge from the hospital is also known as
   A. Discharge status
   B. Effective utilization review
   C. Discharge planning
   D. Timeliness

3) Of the following answers, which is not included in the six core areas of case management?
   A. The return-to-work process
   B. Case management concepts
   C. Healthcare management and delivery
   D. Rehabilitation

4) Case management documentation should
   1. Be completed upon closure of the case
   2. Be completed as close to the time of all contacts as possible
   3. Be thorough
   4. Reflect the patient's level of involvement in care planning
      A. 1, 2, 3
      B. 1, 3, 4
      C. 2, 3, 4
      D. All of the above

5) Assessment, planning, implementation, coordination, monitoring, evaluation, outcomes, and general are referred to as
   A. The nursing process
   B. The scientific method
   C. The eight essential activities of case management
   D. None of the above

6) **Accurate and thorough case management documentation**
   A. Limits or reduces liability
   B. Is a legal medical record subject to state record retention laws
   C. Is confidential
   D. None of the above
   E. All of the above

7) **The role of the Case Manager is that of**
   A. Educator, facilitator, insurance advocate
   B. Assessor, planner, educator, facilitator, patient advocate
   C. Claims adjuster, planner, educator, facilitator
   D. Assessor, medical planner, facilitator

8) **Case finding, gathering, and assessing information and problem identification are all part of**
   A. Patient advocacy
   B. The return-to-work assessment
   C. The case management process
   D. The precertification process

9) **Diagnosis, high costs, and multiple admissions or treatments are red flags for**
   A. Preexisting HMO exclusions
   B. Utilization management review
   C. Case management evaluation
   D. Disability hearings

10) **The Case Manager never contacts**
    A. The patient
    B. The caregivers
    C. The employer
    D. The patient's coworkers

11) **Which of the following is not true about case management?**
    A. It is a new profession.
    B. It is an area of practice within one's profession.
    C. It is performed by a variety of healthcare providers.
    D. It is performed in a variety of settings.

12) **Case Managers work in a variety of settings. Which of the following are examples of the provider sector?**
    1. Third-party administrators
    2. Infusion company
    3. Rehabilitation center
    4. Hospital
        A. 1, 2, 3
        B. 2, 3, 4
        C. None of the above
        D. All of the above

13) Case Managers perform their function in the following four areas: medical, financial, rehabilitation, and
    A. Workers' compensation
    B. Social
    C. Legal
    D. Behavioral/motivational

14) Although Case Managers work in a variety of settings, they all have a common denominator of patient advocacy, educating patients, and facilitating the patients' optimal outcomes. However, the focal point of their work is
    A. Empowering physicians to be gatekeepers
    B. Empowering patients to be active decision makers in their health care
    C. Mandating care plans to patients and their families
    D. Mandating services to be provided by their physicians

15) Case Managers deal with vocational activity most often in a
    A. Subacute setting
    B. Acute care facility
    C. Rehabilitation center
    D. None of the above

16) Continual assessment of the care plan is part of which process(es)?
    A. Initial evaluation
    B. Goal setting
    C. Implementation
    D. Monitoring and evaluation

17) The following information should be included in which report?
    - Desired outcomes
    - Progress toward outcomes
    - Cost without case management intervention
    - Cost with case management intervention
    - Savings due to case management intervention
        A. Cost-to-benefit analysis reports
        B. Patient case reports
        C. Summary reports
        D. Vendor progress reports

18) The savings derived from case management activity is attributed to Case Managers
    A. Coordinating the best treatment, at the best cost, across the continuum of care
    B. Coordinating at the appropriate time, at the appropriate level of care
    C. Coordinating at the appropriate time, across the continuum of care
    D. All of the above

19) Which of the following is (are) true regarding client cost-to-benefit analysis reporting?
    1. Reports should be generated only when requested.
    2. Regular reports should be generated.
    3. Reports should include specific cases.
    4. Reports should include the ratio of savings per dollar billed.
    5. Reports should never include billed amounts for case management services.

Case Management Concepts

A. 1, 2, 3
B. 3, 4, 5
C. 2, 4
D. None of the above
E. All of the above

20) Which of the following are important areas for Case Managers to document?
1. Medical stability of patient upon discharge
2. Refusal of case management services
3. Social history
4. Living wills
   A. 1, 2, 3
   B. 2, 3, 4
   C. None of the above
   D. All of the above

21) Alternate benefit plans are also known as
A. A secondary insurance plan
B. A plan option when electing coverage
C. Extracontractual benefits
D. None of the above

22) Which of the following is (are) true of alternate benefit plans?
1. They require preapproval by the patient.
2. They require preapproval by the payer.
3. They require cost-effectiveness justification.
4. They require prior hospitalization.
5. They require claims notification.
   A. 1, 2, 3
   B. 2, 3, 5
   C. 2, 3, 4
   D. All of the above

23) Which of the following is (are) not true regarding the planning process?
1. The coordinator is the primary care physician.
2. Care plans should be objective.
3. Care plans should be individualized by disease process.
4. Case Managers act as coordinators and liaisons.
5. Care plans should have time frames for reaching and reevaluating goals.
   A. 2, 4
   B. 1, 2, 3
   C. None of the above
   D. All of the above

24) In goal setting, the mnemonic SMART should be used. This refers to goals being
A. Specific, Measurable, Achievable, Realistic, and Timely
B. Standardized, Medical, Action Oriented, Reasonable, and Timely
C. None of the above
D. A, B

25) Which of the following is (are) true regarding the practice of case management?
1. It is a relatively new profession.
2. Certification ensures appropriate care plans.
3. All Case Managers are nurses.
4. Case management is based on the premise that when an individual reaches his or her optimal level of wellness and functional capability, everyone benefits.
    A. 1
    B. 2
    C. 1, 3
    D. 2, 4
    E. All of the above

26) Assessment, problem definition, selecting/planning the solution, implementation, and evaluation/monitoring are all part of which process?
    A. Coordination and service delivery
    B. Problem solving
    C. Life-care planning
    D. None of the above

27) Accurate, thorough case management documentation
    A. Limits or reduces liability
    B. Is a legal medical record subject to state record retention laws
    C. Is confidential
    D. None of the above
    E. All of the above

28) Reports that demonstrate case management savings to the payer of services in terms of dollars spent as compared with dollars saved are
    A. Outcome reports
    B. Cost-to-benefit analysis reports
    C. Case closure reports
    D. Claims reports

29) Identification of potential high-risk or high-cost patients is known as
    A. Case finding and targeting
    B. Planning
    C. Gathering and assessing information
    D. None of the above

30) During the _____, the Case Manager determines how the family members see their role.
    A. Implementation phase
    B. Initial assessment
    C. Referral process
    D. All of the above

31) In evaluating a medical plan, what are the main considerations?
    1. Quality of life
    2. Number of treating providers
    3. Quantity of money spent on health care
    4. Progress of patient

A. 1, 2, 3
B. 1, 3, 4
C. All of the above
D. None of the above

32) The process of case management includes which of the following categories?
1. Case finding and targeting
2. Planning, reporting, and obtaining approval
3. Gathering and assessing information
4. Coordination, follow-up, and evaluation
    A. 1, 2, 3
    B. 2, 3, 4
    C. All of the above
    D. None of the above

33) Items a Case Manager should review in his or her initial assessment are
    A. Vocational status
    B. Leisure activities
    C. Socioeconomic and psychological factors
    D. All of the above

34) Case management is
    A. A way of reducing costs.
    B. A method of following the referral source instructions.
    C. A profitable business.
    D. A collaborative process that assesses, plans, implements, coordinates, monitors, and evaluates the options and services required to meet the client's health and human service needs. It is characterized by advocacy, communication, and resource management and promotes quality and cost-effective interventions and outcomes.

35) The focus of case management is to
    A. Save money
    B. Report to the referral source
    C. Empower patients
    D. All of the above

36) The Case Manager needs to keep the referral source informed regarding
    A. Total case management charges
    B. Case management interventions and outcomes
    C. Large cases in terms of money and time
    D. All of the above

37) **A Case Manager's records should be scrupulously accurate, unbiased, and completed in a timely fashion because**
    A. Orderliness of records is scored by state inspectors during reviews and therefore can affect state reimbursement rates.
    B. A client may become involved in litigation that may require the testimony or written records of the Case Manager.
    C. A Case Manager's records have an impact on the policy limits of Personal Injury Protection (PIP) coverage.
    D. All of the above
    E. None of the above

52 CHAPTER TWO

38) After a case management plan is implemented, the Case Manager should
    1. Monitor compliance and communicate noncompliance to the treating physician.
    2. Always arrange for a second opinion to determine if the treatment plan is medically necessary.
    3. Monitor the patient's progress and change the patient's goals as necessary.
    4. Cancel the physician's orders if the insurer disagrees with the care plan.
        A. 1, 2
        B. 1, 3
        C. 1, 2, 3
        D. All of the above
        E. None of the above

39) The Case Manager can facilitate the treatment plan ordered by the physician and the patient's recovery by
    1. Facilitating approval for all authorizations required
    2. Arranging for all medically necessary services in a timely fashion
    3. Evaluating the effectiveness of the services or care plan on a regular basis
    4. Communicating with the providers of services and the physician regularly and as needed
    5. Providing hands-on care when needed
        A. 1, 2, 3
        B. 2, 3, 4
        C. 1, 2, 3, 4
        D. All of the above
        E. None of the above

40) The effectiveness of the entire case management process depends on which of the following?
    1. Physician cooperation
    2. Patient cooperation
    3. Obtaining an accurate history
    4. Family cooperation
        A. 1, 2
        B. 1, 2, 3
        C. 1, 3
        D. All of the above
        E. None of the above

41) To assess the appropriateness of the treatment plan, the Case Manager should
    1. Discuss job requirements and whether the possibility for light duty or modified duty exists.
    2. Interview the injured worker to obtain information regarding the injury and response to treatment to date.
    3. Obtain medical information from the attending physician.
    4. Complete an in-person assessment.
        A. 1, 2, 3
        B. 2, 3, 4
        C. All of the above
        D. None of the above

42) Case Managers spend most of their time managing high-cost cases. In this role, the focus of the Case Manager is
1. To arrange services and supplies with vendors that the physician has a relationship with
2. To obtain supplies from the closest and most convenient vendor
3. To contact several vendors and select the lowest cost vendor
4. To obtain specifics regarding credentials, accreditation status, scope of services, dependability, and costs to select the best vendor for cost, availability, and dependability
    A. 1, 2, 3
    B. 2, 3, 4
    C. 4
    D. 3
    E. All of the above

43) Case management care plans should be continually reevaluated to ensure
1. The treatment is cost-effective.
2. The treatment meets the patient's needs.
3. The treatment is effective.
4. The patient is progressing.
    A. 1, 2
    B. 1, 3
    C. 3, 4
    D. All of the above
    E. None of the above

44) Case management care plans should
1. Be included in case reports
2. Include specific goals and time frames for achieving them
3. Include short- and long-term goals and objectives
4. Be followed without deviation once implemented
    A. 1, 2, 3
    B. 2, 3, 4
    C. All of the above
    D. None of the above

45) Case management care plans are constantly reevaluated and revised. Which of the following statements is the most precise?
    A. Care plans remain constant once implemented and do not change because the patient's status has changed.
    B. Care plans are revised whenever the patient's status changes.
    C. Short-term case management problems are always short-lived.
    D. Short-term case management problems always turn into long-term problems.

46) When the Case Manager reports to the referral source regarding alternate treatment options, he or she should include
    A. Availability of options
    B. Expected costs of options
    C. Approval of the attending physician
    D. All of the above
    E. None of the above

47) Case Managers can receive cases from the following referral sources:
1. Insurers
2. Employers
3. Third-party administrators (TPAs)
4. Attorneys
5. Providers
    A. 1, 2, 3, 5
    B. 1, 2, 4, 5
    C. 1, 2, 3, 4
    D. All of the above
    E. None of the above

48) A case management report should contain which of the following?
1. The physician's recommendations for optimal recovery
2. The diagnosis
3. The prognosis
4. The employer's assessment of the patient
5. The expected length of the disability
    A. 1, 2, 3, 4
    B. 1, 2, 3, 5
    C. 1, 2, 4, 5
    D. All of the above
    E. None of the above

49) _____ is a systematic process of data collection and analysis involving multiple components and sources.
    A. Assessment
    B. Evaluation
    C. Implementation
    D. Planning

50) Diagnosis, high costs, and multiple admissions or treatments are red flags for
    A. Preexisting HMO exclusions
    B. Utilization management review
    C. Case management evaluation
    D. Disability hearings

51) Which of the following diagnoses should trigger an inquiry for potential case management services?
1. Blepharitis
2. Spinal cord injury
3. Coryza
4. Non-Hodgkin's lymphoma
    A. 1, 3
    B. 2, 4
    C. 1, 2, 3
    D. All of the above
    E. None of the above

52) Of the following, which are "sentinel procedures" that should prompt inquiries for case management services?
   1. Brain biopsy
   2. Bone marrow biopsy
   3. Endocardiac biopsy
   4. Skin biopsy
      A. 1, 3
      B. 2, 4
      C. 1, 2, 3
      D. All of the above
      E. None of the above

53) Of the following, which utilization figure for an individual's medical claims would make an appropriate financial threshold for case management evaluations?
   A. Claims exceeding $500 per year
   B. Claims exceeding $1,000 per year
   C. Claims exceeding $10,000 per year
   D. Claims exceeding $100,000 per year
   E. Claims exceeding $1,000,000 per year

54) Of the following methodologies, which are common means that insurers and Case Managers use for identifying potential patients for case management services?
   1. Selecting cases with catastrophic diagnoses, such as head or spinal injury
   2. Selecting cases with "sentinel procedures," such as bone marrow biopsy or brain biopsy
   3. Selecting cases with claims costs over $10,000 in a year
   4. Selecting cases at random and investigating for potential problems
      A. 1, 3
      B. 2, 4
      C. 1, 2, 3
      D. All of the above
      E. None of the above

55) The primary goals of medical case management include all of the following *except*
   A. To ensure the effectiveness of medical treatment and that rehabilitative services are arranged for in a timely and progressive manner
   B. To assist in cost containment
   C. To minimize the recovery period without jeopardizing medical stability or quality of care
   D. To provide hands-on nursing care

56) Motivational interviewing is based on
   A. Clarifying how a patient's behavior fits with expressed values/preferences
   B. Self-recognition of discrepancies between values and behaviors
   C. Setting goals based on what is most important to the patient
   D. None of the above
   E. All of the above

57) _____ is used to help identify patient preferences.
   A. Assessment
   B. Coaching
   C. Coordination
   D. Motivational interviewing

58) The Case Management Model Act of 2009 was created by Case Management Society of America
   A. To be a reference for Case Manager behavior
   B. As a mandate for Case Manager program development
   C. As a guideline for our legislators to utilize when drafting public policy
   D. None of the above

59) Using the Case Management Model Act to create a comprehensive case management program would include the following key elements:
   A. Evidence-based criteria
   B. Data driven
   C. Clinical oversight
   D. Credentialed Case Managers
   E. Quality management activities
   F. None of the above
   G. All of the above

60) The Case Management Society of America drafted the Case Management Model Act of 2009 to ensure quality, cost-effective, and improved clinical outcomes from qualified Case Managers.
   A. True
   B. False

61) Which of the following choices best defines negotiation?
   A. The action or process of communication whereby two or more parties advance mutual interests and reconcile differences to achieve a common goal or solve a common problem
   B. The process of reciprocally voicing demands
   C. The process of communication whereby two or more parties attempt to gain advantage in a dispute
   D. The action whereby two or more parties contest a mutually sought after goal

62) Which of the following choices is the most important thing to have in a negotiation?
   A. Physical presence
   B. Financial advantage
   C. Information
   D. Influence in the business community

63) The acronym BATNA is best defined by which of the following?
   A. Business aptitude training for negotiators in America
   B. Business attitude testing for negotiators in the Americas
   C. Best answer in negotiated alliances
   D. Best alternative to a negotiated agreement

64) Which of the following is not true of BATNA?
   A. BATNA is an exercise in imagination and research.
   B. BATNA should occur before any substantive negotiation.
   C. BATNA is an exploration of what happens when there is a negotiation impasse and no agreement can be reached.
   D. BATNA allows you to beat the other party at its own game.

65) **Which of the following is not considered necessary in most negotiations involving Case Managers?**
   A. Respect between the parties
   B. Trust and trustworthiness
   C. Team negotiation
   D. Information

66) **Which of the following does not characterize the end of an unsuccessful negotiation?**
   A. One or more aggrieved parties
   B. A "winner" and a "loser"
   C. A tendency toward conflict in the future
   D. A situation in which both parties have benefited and increased their opportunities for profitable business relations in the future

67) **Which of the following is an example of active listening during a negotiation?**
   A. "Okay, I've heard your side, now listen to what I've got to say!"
   B. "Yeah, yeah, yeah, but what about my issues?"
   C. "You've mentioned quality of service twice now. Do you want to give me some examples of what good quality means to you?"
   D. "Hey, when do I get a chance to air my grievances?"

68) **An "irritator" in the setting of a negotiation is best described by which of the following?**
   A. Any physical action by one party that the other party finds annoying, such as sneezing or scratching.
   B. A statement of fact that the other party finds unpleasant, such as "Your delivery occurred 4 days after the agreed upon delivery date."
   C. Any negotiation position that one party takes that the other party finds distressing, such as "a price higher than usual and customary."
   D. Any characterization by one party of the other party's facts, positions, or issues that implies a negative judgment, such as "That's an insulting offer!" or "We've been more than generous!" or "We've been nothing, if not cooperative."

69) **Negotiated services and verbal agreements with vendors of medical equipment or services should be confirmed in writing and include which of the following?**
   A. Time frame of the negotiation
   B. Service approved, number of units approved, frequency approved
   C. Fees negotiated (itemized)
   D. B, C
   E. All of the above

70) **When conducting an interview to obtain an accurate history after a work-related accident, which of the following is (are) essential?**
   1. Investigating the legal issues of the accident
   2. Current treatment and medications
   3. Employment history and job requirements
   4. Description of the accident
   5. Previous medical history
      A. 1, 2, 3, 4
      B. 2, 3, 4, 5
      C. 3 only
      D. All of the above
      E. None of the above

58 CHAPTER TWO

71) When establishing working relationships with referral sources, it is important to describe
1. Reporting expectations
2. Role expectations of the referral source
3. Business lines involved
4. Workflow processes
   A. 1, 2, 3
   B. 2, 3, 4
   C. All of the above
   D. None of the above

72) Introductions, empowerment, trust, active listening, questioning, and testing discrepancies are all part of
   A. Determining functional status
   B. Interviewing
   C. The communication process
   D. None of the above

73) The three basic goals of a patient interview are to
1. Provide information
2. Establish rapport
3. Provide a care plan
4. Collect information
5. Formulate a care plan
   A 1, 2, 3
   B. 2, 3, 4
   C. 1, 4, 5
   D. 2, 4, 5

74) When conducting an interview, it is important that the Case Manager ask about the medical history of the patient. To get the most from the interview, questions should be of what type?
   A. Open ended
   B. Who, what, where, when, why, and how
   C. Direct
   D. Leading

75) A thorough interview and assessment enables the Case Manager to assist the patient and family to
   A. Make informed healthcare decisions
   B. Make informed financial decisions
   C. Cope with the complex healthcare system
   D. All of the above

76) When conducting an interview with the patient, it is important to encourage the patient to use his or her own _____. This assists the Case Manager in discerning the patient's level of understanding or denial of his or her situation.
   A. Goals
   B. Values
   C. Words
   D. Beliefs

77) The Case Manager has the roles of communicator and liaison. This requires that he or she be familiar with certain aspects of which of the following disciplines?
   A. Insurance
   B. Legislation
   C. Rehabilitation
   D. All of the above
   E. None of the above

78) Which statement(s) describes good negotiating skill?
   1. Be brief and precise as you state your main point.
   2. Be aware of male and female communication styles and match your style to that of the vendor.
   3. Speak in a businesslike fashion, being both assured and assertive.
      A. 1, 2
      B. 2, 3
      C. All of the above
      D. None of the above

79) Which statement(s) does not describe good negotiating skill?
   1. Be brief and precise as you state your main point.
   2. Be aware of male and female communication styles and match your style to that of the vendor.
   3. Speak tentatively and communicate to build friendship and agreement.
      A. 1
      B. 2
      C. 3
      D. All of the above
      E. None of the above

80) During a case management interview in a workers' compensation case, the patient confides to the Case Manager that he is a recovering alcoholic and has been alcohol free for 5 years. The Case Manager should
   A. Include the information in the psychosocial section of his or her insurance company report.
   B. Immediately notify the patient's attending physician.
   C. Make no comment verbally or in writing, as it has no current bearing on a work-related injury.
   D. Close the case.

81) Which of the following is (are) needed for the Case Manager to ensure an accurate assessment of the impact an injury will have on a patient and his or her ability to return to work?
   A. The physical requirements of the patient's position
   B. The coworkers'/employer's opinion of the patient's ability
   C. A history of childhood diseases
   D. All of the above
   E. None of the above

82) When interviewing a patient, the Case Manager is aware that the patient is being overtly and verbally hostile. The most appropriate response by the Case Manager is
   A. Verbal defense
   B. Complete withdrawal from the patient
   C. Acceptance of the patient's behavior in silence
   D. A, B
   E. All of the above

83) The Case Manager has a patient who continues to focus on his functional loss. Which of the following would be the best response by the Case Manager?
   1. "You should be making faster progress than this in PT."
   2. "Your last physical therapy report states you have increased your strength and flexibility."
   3. "Other patients with this injury returned to work 2 weeks ago."
      A. 1, 2
      B. 2, 3
      C. 2
      D. All of the above
      E. None of the above

84) A patient with chronic back pain needs hospital admission
   A. For immediate surgery
   B. For IV pain administration
   C. Only in an emergency situation
   D. Every 6 weeks for evaluation

85) Patients with musculoskeletal disorders frequently require physical therapy as part of the case management care plan. The goal(s) of physical therapy is (are)
   1. To develop strength and endurance above and beyond the patient's condition before getting ill or injured
   2. To learn massage techniques and other passive modalities
   3. To progress to work hardening
   4. To improve range of motion, strength, and pain and to teach a home exercise program to the patient
      A. 1, 2, 3
      B. 4
      C. All of the above
      D. None of the above

86) Which treatment(s) would be the most appropriate for reflex sympathetic dystrophy?
   A. Physical therapy and anti-inflammatory medications
   B. Anti-inflammatory medications only
   C. Physical therapy and anesthetic or nerve blocks of sympathetic nerve function
   D. Physical therapy: heat or cold therapy
   E. All of the above

87) Which of the following is (are) part of the treatment for a rotator cuff tendonitis?
   1. Exercises that bring objects toward the body
   2. Exercises that push objects away from the body
   3. Surgical correction for severe injuries
   4. Rest of the injured tendons
      A. All except 1
      B. All except 2
      C. All of the above
      D. None of the above

88) The Case Manager is following a CVA patient at home. In speaking with the family the Case Manager discovers that the patient can no longer feed himself and is having difficulty swallowing. What should the Case Manager do?
   A. Call the physical therapist on the case.
   B. Call the physician on the case.
   C. Arrange for a swallowing consult by a speech therapist.
   D. Arrange for an assistive device.

89) Case Managers know that motivating a patient with a knowledge deficit can be problematic. As the Case Manager evaluating the duration and progress of occupational services, what questions should be asked if informed the patient was making little progress and was noncompliant with his or her instructions?
   1. Has anyone explored the reasons for his or her resistance?
   2. Has anyone discussed his or her lack of progress and cooperation with the family?
   3. What time of day is he or she receiving teaching?
   4. Is there a time of day when he or she is more cooperative and compliant?
      A. 1, 2, 3
      B. 2, 3, 4
      C. All of the above
      D. None of the above

NOTES

Appendix 2-B

Case Management Concepts Answers

1) **ANSWER: A**

2) **ANSWER: C**

3) **ANSWER: A**
   The return-to-work process is part of workers' compensation case management, not a core component of case management. The six core areas consist of B, C, D, principle of practice, psychosocial aspects, and healthcare reimbursement.

4) **ANSWER: D**
   Proper documentation minimizes a Case Manager's liability risk.

5) **ANSWER: C**

6) **ANSWER: E**

7) **ANSWER: B**
   Case Managers are patient advocates, not insurance advocates. They do not adjust claims, and they are not medical planners—that is the physician's role.

8) **ANSWER: C**
   These are all part of the case management process, which also includes planning, reporting, obtaining approval, coordination, follow-up, monitoring, and evaluation.

9) **ANSWER: C**
   These are the three criteria for case management referrals.

10) **ANSWER: D**
    The first three choices are involved in the patient's care or benefit payment. The caregivers are contacted for the assessment of the patient and his or her progress. The employer is contacted for approval of benefit plans or return-to-work information. The patient is contacted to collaborate with the Case Manager on his or her care plan.

11) **ANSWER: A**
    Case management by itself is not a profession but an area of practice within one's profession.

12) **ANSWER: B**
    HMOs, insurance companies, and third-party administrators are examples of the payer sector.

13) **ANSWER: D**

14) **ANSWER: B**

15) **ANSWER: C**
Vocational activity is most often necessary in rehabilitation centers and workers' compensation cases.

16) **ANSWER: D**

17) **ANSWER: B**

18) **ANSWER: D**

19) **ANSWER: C**

20) **ANSWER: D**
The medical stability of a patient upon discharge is important in ensuring a safe discharge. Refusal of case management services with an explanation and an offer for the patient to call if he or she changes his or her mind protects the Case Manager from claims of negligence. Information regarding social history is important in setting up the care plan. Knowledge of living wills also helps the Case Manager and the patient develop a plan of care that is consistent with the patient's wishes.

21) **ANSWER: C**

22) **ANSWER: B**
Alternate benefit plans include services that are not normally part of the benefit package. Therefore, they need preapproval by the payer, cost justification, and claims notification to prevent denial of benefits.

23) **ANSWER: B**

24) **ANSWER: A**

25) **ANSWER: D**

26) **ANSWER: B**

27) **ANSWER: E**

28) **ANSWER: B**

29) **ANSWER: A**

30) **ANSWER: B**

31) **ANSWER: B**
Case management is concerned with quality and cost. Additionally, all medical plans should evaluate the progress of the patient.

32) **ANSWER: C**

33) **ANSWER: D**

34) **ANSWER: D**

35) **ANSWER: C**
Although A and B can be outcomes of case management, choice C, empowering the patient, is the focus of case management.

36) **ANSWER: D**

37) **ANSWER: B**
During litigation all medical records are subpoenaed for review by the courts. The quality or orderliness of a Case Manager's record has no effect on the policy limits of Personal Injury Protection (PIP) coverage, nor does the state change reimbursement rates based on this.

38) **ANSWER: B**
The role of the Case Manager, after implementing a care plan, includes monitoring for compliance, reevaluating goals, and communicating with the treating physician. Second opinions are not necessary on every case, and the Case Manager has no authority to "cancel" physicians' orders.

39) **ANSWER: C**
Case Managers do not provide hands-on care.

40) **ANSWER: D**

41) **ANSWER: A**
An onsite review of a case should be saved for the very complex cases. The Case Manager can assess the treatment plan, in most cases, by discussing and obtaining information from the employer, the injured worker, and the attending physician.

42) **ANSWER: C**
Arranging services based on prior physician relationships, convenience, and lowest cost is not in the best interests of the patient. Although cost and convenience are factors, it is more important to deal with a reputable, dependable, and credentialed vendor.

43) **ANSWER: D**

44) **ANSWER: A**
Case management plans need to be evaluated frequently and changed as the patient's needs change. It is in the patient's best interest to change the care plan whenever reevaluation demonstrates a need to do so. Care plans should be specific, have target dates for achieving goals, and should be part of the standard reports.

45) **ANSWER: B**

46) **ANSWER: D**

47) **ANSWER: D**

48) **ANSWER: B**
The medical and clinical issues are relevant in evaluating the appropriateness of the treatment plan, anticipated length of disability, and costs involved. The employer is not equipped to assess the patient's medical condition.

49) **ANSWER: A**

50) **ANSWER: C**
These are the three criteria for case management referrals.

51) **ANSWER: B**
Both spinal cord injuries and lymphomas are complex, high-cost, and life-threatening illnesses that may potentially benefit from case management. Coryza is a common cold, and blepharitis is a minor infection of the eyelid.

66 CHAPTER TWO

52) **ANSWER: C**
Although biopsies of the endocardium, the brain, and bone marrow involve high risk and are performed infrequently, biopsies of the skin are low risk, are commonly performed, and require case management services in a small minority of cases.

53) **ANSWER: C**
Screening all patients with claims over $500 and $1,000 per year would yield too many claims and too few catastrophic illnesses. Those patients with claims of $100,000 and over would no doubt be well known to the insurers and Case Managers long before the patients hit those thresholds. Thresholds of $5,000 to $10,000 are most commonly seen in the industry.

54) **ANSWER: C**
Common methodologies include screening claims with catastrophic diagnoses, sentinel procedures, high-claims cost, and through direct case referral from community physicians.

55) **ANSWER: D**
Case Managers do not provide hands-on care.

56) **ANSWER: E**

57) **ANSWER: D**

58) **ANSWER: C**

59) **ANSWER: C**

60) **ANSWER: A**

61) **ANSWER: A**

62) **ANSWER: C**

63) **ANSWER: D**

64) **ANSWER: D**

65) **ANSWER: C**

66) **ANSWER: D**

67) **ANSWER: C**

68) **ANSWER: D**

69) **ANSWER: E**
The date of the negotiation and the signature and title of the agreeing party should also be included.

70) **ANSWER: B**
The Case Manager should not get into any discussions regarding legal issues. They are not pertinent to his or her case management role.

71) **ANSWER: C**

72) **ANSWER: B**

73) **ANSWER: D**
Providing information is not one of the basic goals of the interview. Providing a care plan does not allow the patient to be an active participant in the care-planning process.

74) **ANSWER: A**
The other answer choices do not leave room for the patient to introduce new information, nor do they leave the door open for free communication.

75) **ANSWER: D**
A thorough interview and assessment allow for the collection of data required to assist the patient in formulating his or her case management plan.

76) **ANSWER: C**
The other answers are important in developing a care plan; however, the best answer for the Case Manager to comprehend what the patient understands about his or her situation is C, words.

77) **ANSWER: D**

78) **ANSWER: A**
The Case Manager should be brief and precise and should be aware of male and female communication styles to be an effective negotiator. She should not speak tentatively, but should speak in a businesslike manner with both assurance and assertiveness.

79) **ANSWER: C**
The Case Manager should not speak tentatively but should speak in a businesslike manner, with assurance and assertiveness.

80) **ANSWER: C**
According to the Code of Professional Ethics, it is the responsibility of the Case Manager to safeguard the patient's confidentiality unless there is a legal requirement to disclose the information.

81) **ANSWER: A**
To make an accurate determination in regards to a patient's ability to return to work, the Case Manager and the team involved in the care of the patient must know the physical requirements of the patient's job.

82) **ANSWER: C**
Acceptance of the behavior in silence is an effective interpersonal skill demonstrating a nonjudgmental attitude. As the patient may be exhibiting a defensive behavior, this is the most appropriate way to begin a nonthreatening relationship with the patient.

83) **ANSWER: C**
The Case Manager should be motivating the patient by focusing on his or her progress, not lack of progress.

84) **ANSWER: C**
A patient with chronic back pain generally requires hospitalization only during an emergency situation or when incapacitating, intractable pain occurs. Chronic conditions are best handled on an outpatient basis.

85) **ANSWER: B**
Work hardening is not always appropriate or necessary. It is not medically necessary to set goals beyond the starting point of the patient. The goals of therapy are not to learn passive modalities but to increase range of motion and strength while decreasing pain and learning self-management.

86) **ANSWER: C**

87) **ANSWER: B**
Exercises that push objects away from the body should be avoided.

88) **ANSWER: B**
Call the physician on the case. Although a swallowing consult may be appropriate, it is more appropriate to inform the physician so he or she can evaluate the patient and order whatever services or diagnostic testing he or she believes appropriate.

89) **ANSWER: C**
All the previous questions can help shed light on the reason for the patient's resistance and assist the team in formulating a more effective care plan.

CHAPTER 3

Principles of Practice

MEDICAL RECORDS AND CONFIDENTIALITY

Why Case Managers Need to Record and Manage Medical Records

Case Managers record patient information for many reasons:

- To provide the rationale for the actions taken by Case Managers
- To form the basis of case management costs and savings reports
- To allow supervisors or coworkers to assume management of a case in the absence of the original reviewer
- To provide a longitudinal perspective and continuity on long and complex cases
- To provide the foundation of a legal defense when questions of propriety of the care are raised

A medical record documents the privileged conversations between a patient and a provider. Communications with a patient fall within the patient–provider privilege and (with limitations) are protected from disclosure. This confidentiality is a right held by the patient and may be waived by the (fully informed) patient but not by the provider. Generally speaking, the patient's medical records are private, and it is the responsibility of medical professionals to ensure they remain private, unless otherwise directed by the patient or the courts.

Who Usually Has Access to a Patient's Medical Records?

Although it is assumed that only the patient's primary healthcare provider has access to confidential medical information, a surprising number of others have regular and legal access to it. The following list contains the parties who have access to a patient's medical record and the reasons for that access:

- *Professional medical colleagues:* Partners in a medical group, who may care for the patient in the primary provider's absence
- *Clinical experts and consultants:* May aid the primary provider with determining the diagnosis or treatment of the patient

- *Hospitals:* When the spread of communicable diseases may endanger other patients, for billing purposes, or when discussions of the quality improvement committee require an examination of disease states, treatments, and so on
- *Insurance companies and managed care companies:* Who have to determine the medical necessity of care
- *Third-party administrators and utilization management agents:* Who examine medical records for compliance with allowable benefits, medical necessity, and medical appropriateness
- *Pharmacy benefits administrators:* Responsible for adjudicating pharmaceutical claims and drug benefits, as an agent of the insurer
- *Specialty management or "carve out" organizations:* Adjudicate claims in specialized areas of care for insurers and health maintenance organizations (HMOs); services provided by these organizations range from optometry and podiatry to cancer and HIV care
- *Government agencies:* The Centers for Disease Control and Prevention, the National Institutes of Health, and the National Cancer Institute, when they are engaged in epidemiological research and providing for the public health.
- *The Medical Information Bureau:* A central medical information database sponsored by insurance companies; exists to collect, analyze, and distribute information about life insurance policy applicants
- *Pharmaceutical companies:* Charged by the U.S. Food and Drug Administration to collect patient-specific medical information concerning adverse reactions to drugs, biotech agents, and vaccines

Despite the fact that medical information is shared regularly with all these agents and organizations, comprehensive laws regarding medical record privacy did not exist before the Health Insurance Portability and Accountability Act (HIPAA) regulations were enacted.

Circumstances in Which a Case Manager May Release Confidential Patient Information

There are special circumstances under which a Case Manager may release patient information:

- After receiving a written authorization or waiver from the patient
- When required by law (civil, criminal, or public health law); licensed practitioners in most states have an affirmative duty to report the following and are not required to seek the patient's permission before doing so:
  - Suspected child abuse, neglect, or exploitation
  - Suspected elder abuse, neglect, or exploitation
  - Abuse, neglect, or exploitation of a resident of a long-term care facility
  - Information regarding treatment of patients with physical injury that have been inflicted by nonaccidental means (e.g., gunshot wounds, stab wounds)
  - Births
  - Unusual or suspicious deaths
  - Specific diseases; public health laws in many states require the reporting of certain diagnoses, such as animal bites, sexually transmitted diseases including HIV/AIDS, tuberculosis, head or spinal injuries, meningitis, etc.
  - Upon receipt of court order or subpoena

When releasing information pursuant to the preceding list, the Case Manager is usually held harmless from legal liability. However, when a request for "sensitive" information is received, the prudent Case Manager will review the case with his or her corporate counsel before releasing it. Sensitive information includes, but is not restricted to, the following topics: mental health, substance abuse, sexually transmitted diseases, cancer, and HIV/AIDS.

What Medical Information Should Not Be Regularly Released?

Communications between a psychiatrist and patient are absolutely privileged. A psychiatrist cannot be compelled to reveal those communications, even by a subpoena. Case Managers should not release this information without signed consent forms from the patient and explicit direction from their corporation's legal counsel.

MEDICAL RECORDS SECURITY

The first step to be taken in the management of the confidentiality of medical records is to set the expectations for the staff:

- Develop confidentiality policies
- Distribute the confidentiality policies to all staff
- Review and update the policies as needed

The case management staff should then sign statements affirming they have read and understood the corporation's confidentiality policies, the corporation's expectations regarding handling of confidential material, and what penalties exist for violation of these policies.

Development of Confidentiality Policies

These policies should include, but are not limited to, the security of electronic and paper records and the release and transmittal of patient information.

Security of Electronic Records

Access to electronic records should be limited to those who "need to know." The primary way to limit access is by restricting access to Case Managers' computers. The computers should be placed in separate work areas that have locking doors, and access to Case Managers' electronic files should be restricted by using passwords known only to the Case Managers. Case Managers should be aware of all areas where electronic information is stored and take appropriate precautions to secure it (e.g., voice mail, faxes, recorded conversations, medical and radiological images, e-mail, text messages, patient or physician videos). Electronic storage mediums, such as computer hard drives, flash drives, portable hard drives, CDs, and other electronic storage media containing sensitive information, should be secured in a locked cabinet when not in use.

When possible, medical information should be recorded in encrypted files. A secure audit trail built into the computer's software should record the name, time, and date of all those who access the medical files, and the software should record any alteration of data.

Computer files containing medical records that are no longer useful should be erased—not just deleted. Deleted documents can easily be "undeleted" by computer-savvy users. Use of names and other identifying data should be limited to situations in which they are necessary. Utilization of telecommunication firewalls that prevent unauthorized parties, especially those outside the organization, from gaining electronic access to medical information systems should be part of the electronic system's software package.

Securing medical records does not only mean to protect their confidentiality but also their physical security. Lost, unreadable, or unrecoverable records are a disaster that slows or stops good care management. Case Managers should make sure patient information they collect is protected against computer failure, theft, fire damage, water damage, or natural disaster.

The manager of health information systems should be able to provide the Case Manager with formal data protection and recovery plan. At its most basic data should be backed up at least daily. The backup storage site should be at a distant location, where data are adequately protected from non-natural and natural disasters. The information should be stored in an encrypted form. In the event of data loss, the stored data should be able to be reconstituted on new computer quickly so that care is not interrupted.

It should be noted that remote backup services are HIPAA compliant because they do not involve the use or disclosure of private health information to another party. Access to personal health information by a remote backup service provider should be precluded by well-designed software and the encryption of medical data. Remote backup service providers are not considered to be business associates and are therefore not covered by the HIPAA Privacy Rule. As a precautionary measure, some covered entities may wish to have a business associate contract in place regardless.

Security of Paper Records

Limit the use of paper records when possible. Know where all paper records are generated and stored (e.g., mail, faxes, memos, and clinical notes), and take proper precautions to secure them. Limit the use of patient and provider names on paper records when possible (the use of file numbers and/or provider and patient code numbers is helpful).

Case Managers should personally destroy (not simply discard) paper records when they are no longer needed. Paper shredders should be readily available in the case management area, preferably at each Case Manager's workstation. Alternatively, a certified document destruction service can be employed to handle these sensitive files. Access to the area in which paper records are stored should be limited. Only those who "need to know" should have this access. The area in which paper records are stored should be locked when not in use. Paper records in the possession of Case Managers should not be left on a desk or in a briefcase. They should be stored in a secure area when not being used. Filing cabinets and desk drawers containing sensitive records should be locked when unattended.

Security of Information Release and Transmittal

Before releasing any patient information to a third party, a prudent Case Manager should do the following:

- Check that a signed "release" or "waiver" has been received and filed.
- Ensure that only the information that was explicitly requested is being released. No other information should be released.
- When particularly "sensitive" information is requested, such as information concerning sexually transmitted diseases, HIV/AIDS, substance abuse, or cancer, consult the organization's corporate counsel/corporate security officer before release.

What Should Be Done When a Patient Has Been Discriminated Against Due to Violation of Medical Privacy?

The Case Manager can suggest the patient seek redress under the following laws:

- Title I and Title V of the Americans with Disabilities Act of 1990, which prohibit employment discrimination against qualified individuals with disabilities in the private sector and in state and local governments
- Sections 501 and 505 of the Rehabilitation Act of 1973, which prohibit discrimination against qualified individuals with disabilities who work in the federal government
- The Civil Rights Act of 1991, which, among other things, provides monetary damages in cases of intentional employment discrimination

According to the Americans with Disabilities Act of 1990,[1] in workplaces with more than 25 employees, employers may not ask job applicants about medical information or require a physical examination before offering employment. Similarly, after employment is offered, an employer can ask for a medical examination only if it is required of all employees holding similar jobs. Applicants can be denied a job based only on the results of a physical examination if this examination reveals the applicant is physically unable to perform the "essential functions" the job requires (e.g., poor eyesight, even with corrective lenses, in an applicant for a position as a commercial pilot).

Under the Rehabilitation and Civil Rights Acts an employee cannot be discharged from employment, fired, or made to retire solely because of age, race, sex, or disability. Complaints or charges can be filed with the Equal Employment Opportunity Commission, the federal agency with the power to investigate, mediate, and file lawsuits to end employment discrimination.

ETHICAL ISSUES IN CASE MANAGEMENT

Ethics are the rules or standards governing the conduct of a person or members of a profession. The word "ethics" comes from the Greek root *ethos*, meaning "character" or that combination of positive qualities or values that distinguishes one person from another.

Ethical and legal principles are closely related, because both are based on what a given society values as an appropriate standard of conduct. Legal duties are what a society describes as the minimum acceptable standards of conduct. A legal duty usually carries a punishment for those whose conduct falls below its standards. Ethical duties, on the other hand, represent a society's version of ideal conduct for an individual or a profession. Lapses in ethical behavior, to the extent the behavior is also not illegal, are usually not punishable outside a professional society. In general, the demands of ethical duties usually exceed those of legal duties. It is held by the American Medical Association (AMA) that in the rare instances when legal duties and ethical duties are in conflict, a professional's ethical duties should supersede his or her legal duties.[2]

Five Ethical Principles of Case Management

To aid the Case Manager in making these decisions, the Case Management Society of America (CMSA) developed a written, ethical position statement in 1996: The CMSA

1996 Statement Regarding Ethical Case Management Practices (see Appendix E). This code consists of five principles a Case Manager should follow:

1. *Autonomy:* The Case Manager should encourage the client to make his or her own well-informed decisions. The patient's freedom to choose or act on his or her own behalf is one of the fundamental liberties that a Case Manager should secure for the client. This includes informed consent, providing options for the patient to choose from, education and empowering the patient to be independent and self-directed. The Case Manager's goal is to promote the development of informed self-advocacy.
2. *Beneficence:* This is the state or quality of being kind, charitable, or beneficent and implies that the Case Manager has an obligation to "do good" for his or her patient, rather than for himself or herself, for the provider, or for the insurer.
3. *Nonmaleficence:* An amplification of the Case Manager's obligation of beneficence. Nonmaleficence implies that a Case Manager has an obligation not just to do good by doing "a good job" but to actively seek to prevent harm from coming to the patient. Therefore, the Case Manager cannot abnegate his or her responsibility of beneficence by stating the patient has made his or her own choice and, therefore, the injuries that come to him or her as a result of this decision are "his or her fault." Predictable harm that could come to the patient should be prevented through education and counseling.
4. *Justice:* Justice is the upholding of what is just or fair, in accordance with honor, standards, or law. Justice is derived from the Case Manager's sense of moral rightness and is manifest by ensuring equity of treatment for one's patients. Decision making is based on evidenced-based criteria and the same criteria is used for all patients. Often in case management, this means balancing what is just for one's patient versus what is just for the larger society. The following question illustrates the point: Should extraordinary measures (and resources) be taken to preserve a single patient in a vegetative state rather than spending the resources on preventive care for thousands?
5. *Veracity:* An adherence to the truth. It is the obligation of the Case Manager to conform, in his or her dealings with patients and families, to fact or truth, to accuracy and precision. Without veracity in dealings with the patient, a rapport or trusting relationship will never develop between the Case Manager and the patient. As a result the goal of patient self-advocacy can never be attained. A lack of truth and fair dealing not only undermines the credibility of the Case Manager but may be a source of legal liability.

In a situation in which two or more equally desirable outcomes are in conflict, an ethical dilemma exists. For example, protecting a patient's confidentiality is a desirable outcome, whereas notifying the spouse of the risk of contracting the patient's potentially lethal venereal disease is another desirable outcome. The resulting conflict is an ethical dilemma.

When an ethical dilemma is identified the Case Manager has the obligation to act in the best interest of the patient, the payer, and society at large. Balancing these sometimes competing obligations is one of the great challenges in the field of case management.

Laws of Ethical Decision Making

By their nature ethical dilemmas have no easy answer, and no answers are provided in this section. As stated previously, ethical dilemmas occur in a situation in which two or more equally desirable outcomes are in conflict but only one outcome is possible. That brings us to the four ineluctable laws of ethical decision making:

1. Case Managers must make decisions as to which of the equally desirable outcomes will occur.
2. Choosing one outcome logically implies the other desirable outcomes will not occur.
3. Those that stood to benefit from the outcome that was not chosen will be displeased and may feel alienated or betrayed by the Case Manager.
4. Effective ethical decision makers must be content with the realization that the decision made was the most fair and circumspect decision the situation allowed. Without this sense of "self-content" or "job satisfaction," the Case Manager, as an ethical decision maker, would suffer from self-doubt, equivocation, and decision paralysis.

Common Ethical Dilemmas in Case Management

The following examples are the three most common dilemmas encountered in case management.

1. *Focus of advocacy:* For whom is the Case Manager an advocate? For the patient? For the patient's family? For the insurer who employs the Case Manager? For society at large? The answer to all these questions should be yes. But the best interests of each of these parties are not always harmonious and may be in conflict. For example, the insurance company wants to limit its medical expenditures, the patient may need more benefits than he or she is entitled to under the strict limits of the policy, and the family may be impoverished by funding futile care for a dying patient. As unrestricted medical spending raises the cost of medical care beyond the reach of some members of society, where should medical spending be restricted and by whom? Experienced Case Managers have encountered all these scenarios, sometimes in the same case.
2. *Supremacy of values:* Values may be defined as a set of behaviors or characteristics held in high esteem by a person or group of people. Values are derived from education, personal experiences, cultural expectations or norms, and religious or social laws. What a Case Manager values affects decisions. A Case Manager will want to make decisions that are in accord with his or her own values. What occurs when the values of the patient are in conflict with those of the Case Manager? Some decisions made by the Case Manager will require him or her to violate the patient's values or his or her own values. Should they? Whose values will have supremacy? Whose should have? The patient's? The family's? The insurer's? Should a Case Manager surrender his or her values just to accommodate a paying client (or anyone)? Should he or she run roughshod over the values of the patient because the patient does not agree with the values the Case Manager holds dear? There is no right answer.

3. *Conflict of duties:* A Case Manager has a positive duty to put the best interests of the client first. What should the Case Manager do when the best interests of his or her client cause harm to another? Can a Case Manager ethically act in a way that will cause harm to the patient? Does a Case Manager's duty to the patient supersede his or her duties to others? What is the Case Manager's duty to others? Some common examples of this dilemma of conflict of duties involve the issue of the confidentiality of the patient's medical record and the privacy of information gained during medical interviews. For example, should a Case Manager inform a parent that her child (a minor) is in a physically abusive relationship or that her child is addicted to illegal drugs? Should a Case Manager inform the husband of her client that his wife has contracted HIV and does not intend to tell him? Should a Case Manager warn the authorities when he or she becomes aware the client intends to commit a homicide or a suicide? Should a Case Manager inform the insurer when he or she becomes aware the medical condition currently being covered was a "preexisting condition" and therefore not eligible for coverage under the policy? Some of these examples may seem like easy decisions, others less so. Each decision involves a potential "beneficence" to a third party, but it also involves a potential harm to the client. To whom does the Case Manager have a duty? What are the limits of that duty?

Ethical Considerations

Case Managers face many ethical challenges daily. Generally, when thinking of ethical challenges a Case Manager's thoughts revolve around how to attain the best outcome for a patient given the constraints of a limited benefit plan or resources. However, the challenges can be subtler and more complex than that. As long as the Case Manager is truly the patient's advocate, these dilemmas can be worked out with some assertiveness and creativity. For example, awareness of insurance limits, specialty programs such as charitable specific disease organizations, and other community resources allows case management plans to be put into place to meet a patient's needs without causing an ethical dilemma. Similarly, "flexing" benefits (asking payers to put alternate benefit plans into place) when they make financial and clinical sense are ethically appropriate and should be sought.

"Dual relationships"[3] are one of the least understood and one of the most serious ethical issues that Case Managers face today. A dual relationship is defined as a relationship in which a Case Manager has assumed more than one role with respect to a client, a subordinate, or a student. This concept may also extend to "multiple relationships." A Case Manager may have to balance his or her obligations to the patient, the patient's family, the patient's employer, his or her own employer, and the payer. This can occur when the employer expects the Case Manager to save benefit dollars, the patient and family want the best for the patient regardless of cost, and the payer wants to pay at the normal benefit level (not at 100% of a negotiated fee).

In some cases putting in services before they are needed will save benefit dollars later, but the employer or payer may not see the potential savings. This is an ethical dilemma the Case Manager has to face each and every day. It is only natural when managing a particular case to become close to the patient and his or her family. However, a Case Manager must remember that the patient, the employer, the vendor, the subordinate, and so on, do not exist to meet the Case Manager's needs. Avoiding dual relationships may not always be entirely possible; however, the Case Manager has an obligation to set appropriate boundaries and constantly reevaluate those relationships in an ethical context.

If the Case Manager believes his or her objectivity is threatened, he or she should set up a mechanism to consult with an impartial third party at regular intervals. Whether dealing with a patient or a subordinate, expectations should be clearly defined and ongoing feedback should occur regularly. If objectivity and professionalism become impossible, such as in the situation of being asked to manage a family member or close friend, the patient should be reassigned to another Case Manager.

The ethical Case Manager is accountable to everyone he or she deals with for his or her decisions and actions.

In the managed care environment the role of the Case Manager is to balance the best possible ethical outcome with the responsibility to the employer to be judicious with finances and to be certain that distribution is fair and equitable to all patients.[3]

INFORMED CONSENT

Informed consent is defined as a person's agreement to allow something to happen (such as surgery) that is based on a full disclosure of facts needed to make the decision intelligently. For a patient to give informed consent, several legal criteria must be filled. A statement of informed consent must have the following elements:

- Information given both verbally and in writing to the patient
- An opportunity for questions and answers to clarify the patient's understanding
- Disclosure of information that a reasonable medical practitioner would disclose under the same or similar circumstances
- Disclosure of background information needed to make the decision-making process meaningful
- Patient's written consent form with specific permission spelled out in the agreement
- Consent witnessed by a third party, preferably someone other than the Case Manager

LEGAL ASPECTS OF CASE MANAGEMENT

Today, Case Managers assume responsibilities in all care settings, from critical care and mental health to workers' compensation and HMOs. Although the Case Manager's role involves providing patient and family education, aiding communication, seeking new healthcare resources, and improving outcomes, even this positive an involvement projects legal liability. A Case Manager's autonomy and responsibility puts him or her at a higher risk for malpractice litigation. Common causes in malpractice litigation are as follows[4]:

- Discourteous behavior
- Communication failures
- Lack of patient understanding
- Lack of information given to the patient and/or family

For some, it is surprising the terms "bad clinical outcome" and "negligence" are absent from this list. Investigations into the cause of malpractice litigations[5,6] reveal the following surprising facts[7]:

- In the course of standard medical management, there is a substantial amount of injury to patients.
- Many of these injuries are the result of substandard care.
- Malpractice litigation infrequently compensates patients injured by medical negligence.
- Malpractice litigation rarely identifies or holds providers accountable for their substandard care

Said differently, malpractice suits don't necessarily occur because of negligence or even a bad outcome but because of bad relationships between providers and patients. One study documented that "poor relationships with providers before the injury"[8] were responsible for 53% of calls to plaintiff attorney's offices. Other important causes for calling an attorney mentioned in this article were explicit recommendations by healthcare providers to seek legal counsel and the impression, held by the patient, of not being kept informed by providers.

Managing the patient relationship, keeping the patient and family informed, and using prudence and circumspection when discussing litigation with patients are all areas in which the Case Manager exerts considerable control. Through this control, a Case Manager can prevent unnecessary litigation.

Liability Issues in Case Management

When examining instances of professional liability, several areas are noted for their high risk of litigation: premature discharge, bad faith claims denials, negligent patient assessment, negligent referral, invasion of privacy, breach of confidentiality, and lack of informed consent. These high-risk occurrences are explained in more detail below.

Premature Discharge

When a Case Manager encourages the discharge of a patient or refuses to approve payment for continued stay in a healthcare facility, he or she undertakes a grave responsibility. Discharging a patient before the patient is ready or discharging the patient to an outpatient setting inappropriate to meet that patient's needs can have disastrous results.

In the case of *Wickline v. State of California*, Lois Wickline's physician requested additional hospitalization for his patient. MediCal, the insurer in this case, refused. Medical complications, which may have been avoided if Ms. Wickline was hospitalized, necessitated the amputation of her leg. Ms. Wickline successfully sued MediCal. This settlement was later overturned. Some lessons derived from this case are that Case Managers and their employers can be held responsible for bad outcomes and that a Case Manager's input can affect the medical judgment of providers. Therefore, Case Managers should aggressively seek all data necessary to make an informed decision and exercise their influence with restraint—always in the best interests of the patient.

In the case of *Wilson v. Blue Cross of Southern California, Blue Cross Blue Shield of Alabama, and Western Medical Review*, a depressed patient was discharged from a psychiatric hospital against the recommendations of the treating physician. The patient subsequently committed suicide. The patient's estate sued the insurer and the utilization management company for wrongful death. During the trial it was revealed that the medical director had not adequately reviewed the medical record before denying continued hospitalization. The medical director of the insurer claimed it was the treating physician's responsibility to make him aware of all information necessary to substantiate continued stay in the hospital. Although the courts found Mr. Wilson's suicide could not be causally related to his early discharge, the case has been interpreted to support the position that insurers exercise "reasonable care" when denying coverage for services, even if the attending physician does not appeal the decision.

A Case Manager may decrease the risk associated with patient discharges by

- Reviewing the patient's complete medical record
- Discussing the intention to discharge the patient with the treating physician
- Confirming the adequacy of follow-up medical care for the patient
- Confirming the integrity of the patient's social support network

Bad Faith

Bad faith occurs when any of the following criteria are met:

- There is no reasonable basis for the denial of benefits. This often occurs because a procedure for determining medical necessity or appropriateness of proposed care does not exist.
- The insurer is aware that claims are denied without a reasonable basis but does nothing about it.
- An insurer's impenetrable bureaucracy, complicated or unnecessary claims procedures, or frank ineptitude in claims processing results in dangerous delays in approval. The courts view these inappropriate delays as de facto denials.

All insurers and their agents are contractually obligated to act in "good faith and fair dealing" in the administration of claims. Bad faith claims are often the result of the plaintiff's perception of an inappropriate denial of benefits.

A landmark case that demonstrates bad faith on the part of the insurer is *Fox v. Healthnet*.[9] In this case the courts awarded the estate of Nelene Fox $89.3 million based on the insurer's refusal to pay for a bone marrow transplant. Although Ms. Fox had met all benefit provisions for treatment of her metastatic breast cancer, Healthnet refused to pay. The managers in Healthnet even went so far as to coerce her treating physician to reverse his recommendation for the procedure. Ms. Fox was able to raise money and received her transplant after a delay of 2 months. She did not go into remission and died 8 months later. The jury was notified that bonuses were paid to the utilization executives based on the total dollars in medical care denied during the year. Healthnet evinced bad faith when it placed corporate earnings before the interests of its subscribers and actively conspired to deny them appropriate medical care.

Case Managers can decrease their risk of bad faith litigation by observing the following suggestions[10]:

- *Medical director decision making:* Only the medical director should issue claims denials.
- *Document everything:* The medical director and the Case Manager should extensively document denials and their rationale.
- *Review medical records:* Medical records may contain mitigating circumstances that could change a claims denial to an approval. Information gleaned from medical records should be communicated to the medical director. A Case Manager should

record the time, date, findings of his or her chart review, and any discussion with attending physicians in his or her notes.
- *Review benefit allowance and exclusions:* A full understanding of the benefit contract obviates many discussions of medical necessity and appropriateness. Consultation with legal counsel or medical experts may be necessary in some cases.
- *Determine medical necessity:* Many claims for services may be denied for lack of medical necessity. This decision is the province of the medical director and should be the product of a well-described and documented procedure.
- *Be aware of timelines:* Be aware of regulatory and contractual turnaround times for case review. These may range from a few days to more than a month. In emergent situations subscribers have the right to an expedited review, usually completed in 24 hours. If the evaluation of the case will take longer than the time allowed, the subscriber should be informed of the delay and given the reasons and the expected date of completion.
- *Prepare for the appeals process:* In most instances a subscriber is entitled to appeal adverse decisions made by the insurer. The courts have held that failure to inform the patient of his or her right to appeal is a violation of good faith. The prudent Case Manager should include information regarding a patient's right to appeal the adverse decision in the letter of denial. This information should include the name, address, or phone number of the appeals coordinator; the appropriate methods of appealing (phone, letter, through provider, etc.); timelines for appeal; and when a response can be expected.

Negligent Patient Assessment

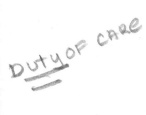

A Case Manager is expected to make recommendations based on an intimate understanding of the patient's condition and his or her individual care needs. In other words, a Case Manager has a duty of care to provide a comprehensive assessment of a case. This comprehensive assessment should include an appreciation of not only the patient's medical condition but also his or her intellectual, educational, psychological, social, religious, and financial conditions. Without this information a Case Manager's recommendations may lead to disastrous outcomes because of unrecognized barriers to care (e.g., the patient is precluded from a treatment because it violates a cultural or religious law, or a minor may not receive appropriate care because one or both parents are intellectually incapable of following a complex care plan). With these caveats in mind, a skillful patient assessment should include the following:

- Chief complaint
- Current diagnoses
- Current treatments (including medications) and treatment plan
- Past medical history
- Social history (including educational achievements, available family and community support system, sexual history and orientation, and history of substance abuse)
- Religious affiliations and involvement
- Insurance eligibility for private and federal programs and their benefits packages
- Expected outcomes

Careful attention to this list should limit a Case Manager's exposure to malpractice litigation.

Appropriate Referral

In the gatekeeper role a Case Manager often makes referrals to specific providers for a patient's care. Under the legal theory of ostensible agency, that provider becomes an "agent" of the Case Manager. The Case Manager may be held responsible for negligent actions taken by the provider within the scope of his or her practice. The Case Manager has an affirmative duty to ensure the care provided is of the highest quality available. It is therefore imperative for the Case Manager to be knowledgeable about the providers he or she recommends. This knowledge should include the status of the provider's licensure, accreditation, certifications, and relevant clinical experience as well as any history of patient complaints, negligence, malpractice, or criminal activity. Much of this information is available through the credentialing process of insurers and managed care organizations. The Case Manager should follow up with patients to review their experience with referred providers. Incidents of dissatisfaction, negligence, or misconduct should be reported to appropriate agencies. A Case Manager can decrease the risk of malpractice litigation by observing the following rules:

- Be aware of the criteria for credentialing providers in the network.
- Make no personal recommendations concerning a provider; when asked about the quality of a particular provider, refer only to the credentialing criteria he or she must meet to be on the provider panel.
- When possible, do not recommend a single provider but provide the patient with a list of providers in the appropriate specialty. Allow the patient to choose the provider.
- Notify the appropriate authorities immediately of any suspicion of illegal, unethical, irregular, or dangerous behavior in providers.

Breach of Confidentiality (Invasion of Privacy)

A breach of confidentiality is the purposeful or negligent release of the content of a privileged communication (e.g., doctor–patient) in which the publication of such information causes injury to the patient. Both professional ethics and statutory law (see HIPAA regulations) require medical information to be kept confidential. Therefore, disclosing confidential information to another, without the consent of the patient, puts the Case Manager at risk for litigation. The following suggestions can be used by the Case Manager to limit the risk of breach of confidentiality litigation:

- The Case Manager should be conversant with the applicable federal and state regulations on the disclosure of medical information.
- Medical information that pertains to HIV/AIDS, venereal diseases, abortion, mental illness, or substance abuse is particularly sensitive. All requests for this information should be discussed first with the patient and legal counsel before disclosure. The documentation of these discussions is essential for avoiding liability. Be aware that this information may require that its own specific consent form be signed before disclosure.
- Patients should be informed their medical information might be shared with others to provide appropriate medical care. A record of this discussion, including the patient's views, should be memorialized in the Case Manager's record.
- Patients should be informed of their right to refuse the disclosure of information but also that this refusal may affect the ability of providers to render effective medical treatment.

Lack of Informed Consent

A person's agreement to allow something to happen (such as surgery) should be based on a full disclosure of the facts needed to make the decision intelligently. In medicine, as in most other venues, every individual of adult years and sound mind has the right to determine what shall be done with his or her own body. This implicit right allows the patient to control the course of his or her own medical treatment.[11]

There are requirements for full disclosure. When obtaining consent for a procedure, treatment, or medical, surgical, or psychological intervention the provider should disclose the following:

- A description of the proposed treatment, therapy, or surgery (e.g., surgery, endoscopy, radiation therapy, intravenous medication)
- The projected or desired outcomes of the proposed treatment
- The likelihood of the treatment's success
- Reasonably foreseeable risks or hazards inherent in the proposed treatment or care (communicated in a manner that the patient can understand)
- Alternatives to the proposed care or treatment plan
- Consequences of forgoing the treatment

Informed consent to a medical procedure or treatment is required by law; it is derived from the theory that performing a procedure or treatment on a patient without full disclosure of risks and benefits and the patient's informed consent constitutes assault and battery. The following criteria[12] for obtaining informed consent have been developed for Case Managers and should be observed:

- The patient must consent voluntarily.
- The patient must have the capacity to give consent.
- The patient must be an adult (under existing state law).
- In the event the patient is a minor or an adult without capacity to consent, parents, attorneys, or legal guardians may give consent.
- The patient must have a full understanding of the scope of activities of the treatment plan, with all its attendant risks, benefits, and alternatives.
- The Case Manager must obtain informed consent before the beginning of the professional relationship.
- The Case Manager must document the consent. (A signed consent agreement is adequate.)

Malpractice Risk Management

Case Managers are at risk for malpractice litigation. These litigations can arise from acts of omission as well as commission. Failure to do something that should be done (omission) is a "breach of obligation" for the Case Manager, just as doing something that should not be done (an act of commission) is a "breach of obligation."[13] Both events can result in malpractice actions.

To perfect a malpractice suit, a plaintiff (the person who sues) must prove two points: (1) negligence on the part of the Case Manager and (2) injury resulting from the Case Manager's negligence. Negligence (by omission or commission) that occurs without injury does not constitute grounds for a malpractice incidence. For example, failure to recommend cardiac rehabilitation after a myocardial infarction is not a litigable offense if the patient does not have another heart attack (i.e., suffers no injury as a result of the negligence). Similarly, a suit based on an injury that does not arise from medical negligence cannot be litigated successfully. For example, if a patient developed aplastic anemia after an appropriately prescribed and delivered course of chemotherapy, he or she is not entitled to sue because no negligence was involved.

In sum then, patients must suffer an injury as a result of the Case Manager's breach of duty for the legal system to find that he or she "caused" the injury. To reduce the risk of liability, a Case Manager should take the following precautions:

- Use credentialed, reputable providers.
- Offer the patient several choices of providers, whenever possible.
- Develop written guidelines for as many decisions as possible.
- Be consistent in decision making.
- Document justification for varying from criteria.
- Document all contacts with the patient and with those associated with his or her care. Be especially careful in recording the patient's participation in the decision-making process.
- Document the patient's compliancy or lack of compliancy with the treatment plan.
- Establish quality assurance programs to monitor for consistency in decision-making and payment guidelines.
- Implement grievance procedures, following state guidelines for timeliness and specialty peer review.
- Always address the patient's concerns.
- Always contact and inform the patient's physician.

Negligent Referral

Although negligent referral is a common cause of litigation in physician malpractice cases, it is a relatively new term used within case management. Negligent referral occurs when a patient is referred to a healthcare provider who is known to be unqualified due to a lack of skill or judgment. In some cases the lack of skill or judgment may be due to a physical or mental impairment such as drug abuse, alcoholism, or systemic disease. In other cases it may simply be due to general carelessness or apathy on the part of the clinician. The Case Manager can incur liability even if he or she was completely unaware of any problem associated with the healthcare provider to whom he or she referred a patient. The Case Manager is expected, in this situation, to do what any other reasonably prudent and careful Case Manager would do in the same situation. In the case of a referral, it would be to make sure the healthcare provider to whom he or she is referring a patient is both professionally qualified and lacks any physical or mental impairment that might harm the patient.

Case Managers need to be aware of court cases that address the liability associated with Case Managers performing a utilization review. Case Managers are at risk for damages if their referral of patients to providers is negligently performed and harm comes to the patient as a result.[14] An example of this is *Wickline v. State of California* discussed earlier. Lois Wickline had surgery for a vascular disease followed by a number of complications. The Medicaid (MediCal) program stopped payment for inpatient hospital care. Ms. Wickline's physician asked for payment for 8 additional days of acute care. Medicaid agreed to pay for an additional 4 days. After 4 days the physician took no further action and the patient went home. Ms. Wickline developed additional complications, and her leg was amputated. She sued the Medicaid program, claiming she would not have lost her leg if she hadn't been discharged early due to termination of payment. The courts stated that physicians cannot shift their legal responsibility for the welfare of their patient to a third party by complying with a cost-containment program.[15] However, the courts also stated that providers can shift their liability to payers for adverse determination as long as they satisfy their "duty to protest" such decisions. The California Court of Appeals further stated that third-party payers of healthcare services can be held legally accountable when medically inappropriate decisions result from defects in the design or implementation of cost-containment mechanisms, as, for example, when appeals made on a patient's behalf for medical or hospital care are arbitrarily ignored or unreasonably disregarded or overridden.[16]

A prudent Case Manager discusses all denials of care with the treating physician and records the outcome of the conversation. Letters of denial should contain all the information the subscriber needs to appeal the decision, including an explanation of the appeals process and necessary timelines.

Legal Terms with Which a Case Manager Should Be Familiar

- Abandonment: The termination of a professional relationship (physician–patient) without reasonable notice to the patient and without an opportunity for the patient to acquire alternative care or services, thereby resulting in injury to the patient.
- Agency: The relationship between two or more persons by which one—the principal—consents that the other(s)—the agent(s)—shall act on his or her behalf. A principal–agent relationship exists between the Case Manager and his or her employer. Agency implies that an agent has legal obligations to the principal, including

  - Using care and skill
  - Acting in good faith
  - Staying within the limits of the agent's authority
  - Obeying the principal and carrying out all reasonable instructions
  - Advancing the interests of the principal
  - Acting solely for the principal's benefit

  These duties of agency imply a conflict of interest between the Case Manager's duties to his or her employer and the professional duties he or she owes the patient. This conflict is largely unresolved and has become an ethical sticking point for most Case Managers.
- Apparent authority (*see also* Ostensible agency): When a principal has taken such actions that would indicate to third parties that someone is his or her agent, the principal is held to have given "apparent authority" to the agent. The principal is held responsible for this agent's actions. Apparent authority is seen in the managed care setting when provider's names are placed in HMO network brochures or in a hospital setting when the hospital lists a physician as a member of the hospital staff, even though there is no employer–employee relationship.
- Bad faith (claims denial): An attempt to mislead or deceive another or a neglect or refusal to fulfill some duty or some contractual obligation. Bad faith is not

simply bad judgment or even negligence, but rather it implies a conscious doing of a wrong. Insurance companies, managed care organizations, and their agents owe a duty of "good faith and fair dealing" to their subscribers. This implies acting in the subscriber's best interest, within the limits of the insurance contract. A failure to follow through on this duty, especially when denying medical care, can result in a bad faith claim. A common example of bad faith can be seen when an insurance company purposely denies claims on frivolous or unfounded grounds to save money.

A "bad faith claims denial" has three components:

- The absence of a reasonable basis for the denial of benefits
- The insurer's (or its agent's) knowledge or reckless disregard of the lack of reasonable basis for denying a claim
- Misfeasance or maladministration in processing of claims for benefits

- Bill of particulars: An amplification of a legal complaint that supplies more information and detail, thereby giving the defendant a more specific picture of the claim(s) against him or her.
- Breach of confidentiality: A failure of a fiduciary duty or a refusal to hold secret a privileged communication entrusted by one party to another.
- Claim: A request for payment from an insurance company, by an insured, under the terms of an insurance contract, or a report by the insured provider of care to the insurance company based on notification from a patient or the patient's attorney of an event out of which malpractice has been alleged.
- Comparative negligence: A method of measuring negligence among the participants in a suit, both defense and plaintiff, in terms of percentages of culpability. Damages are then diminished in proportion to the amount of negligence attributable to the complaining party.
- Complaint: The document by which the plaintiff gives the court and the defendant notice of the transactions, occurrences, or series of transactions or occurrences intended to be proved and the material elements of each cause of action or defense.
- Confidentiality: The state or quality of being confidential; treated as private and not for publication.
- Corporate negligence: A term that encompasses the legal grounds for managed care organizations' liability based on the corporate activities of the managed care organization itself rather than on the care-related activities of participating healthcare professionals. Negligent credentialing and negligent supervision are examples of corporate negligence.
- Corporate practice of medicine: A legal doctrine that prohibits corporations from engaging in the practice of medicine, that is, the treatment of injuries, the discovery of the cause and nature of disease, and the administration of remedies or the prescribing of treatment. In states that recognize this doctrine, corporations, including hospitals, cannot employ physicians.
- Damages: A monetary compensation recovered by the courts for acts of tort. These recoveries or compensations are for both tangible injuries or torts (medical expenses, lost earnings) and intangible injuries (pain and suffering).
- Discovery: The ascertainment of what is not previously known; generally, the pretrial stage of a lawsuit beginning with the service of "summons and

complaint" and concluding with the filing of a "note of issue." During this time period, all evidence that is material and necessary in the prosecution or defense of action is produced and exchanged by the parties or as ordered by the court.

- Event (incident): A situation that is reported by the insured provider to his or her insurance company, which may lead to a formal claim or malpractice suit.
- Examination-before-trial: A method of obtaining disclosure of information that is material and necessary to the underlying lawsuit by way of sworn oral testimony. This usually occurs during the discovery phase of litigation.
- False Claims Act: A federal act providing for civil and criminal penalties against individuals who knowingly present false claims to the government. The criminal False Claims Act makes it illegal to present a claim upon or against the United States that the claimant knows to be false, fictitious, or fraudulent. The civil False Claims Act allows that any person who knowingly presents, or causes to be presented, to the U.S. government a false or fraudulent claim for payment approval, or who knowingly makes, uses, or causes to be made or used a false record or statement to get a false or fraudulent claim paid or approved by the government by getting a false or fraudulent claim allowed or paid violates the Act. The penalties for violation include substantial fines and imprisonment.
- Hold-harmless provision: A contractual arrangement between the insurer and the provider of service that is typically contained in a managed care contract. This provision specifies that the provider assumes the liability for covered services and cannot sue or assert any claims against enrollees for those covered services, even if the managed care organization becomes insolvent.
- Informed consent: A person's agreement to allow something to happen (such as surgery) that is based on a full disclosure of the facts needed to make the decision intelligently. In medicine, as in most other venues, every individual of adult years and sound mind has the right to determine what shall be done with his or her own body and to control the course of his or her own medical treatment.[17] As such, providers are required to disclose the following to the patient:

  - The nature of the proposed treatment (surgery, endoscopy, catheterization, etc.)
  - The projected or desired outcomes of the proposed treatment and the likelihood of success
  - Reasonably foreseeable risks or hazards inherent in the proposed treatment or care (communicated in a manner that the patient can understand)
  - Alternatives to the proposed care or treatment plan
  - Consequences of forgoing the treatment

  Informed consent is required by law and is derived from the theory that performing a procedure or treatment on a patient without full disclosure of risks and benefits and the patient's informed consent constitutes assault and battery.
- Inherent risk: A complication commonly associated with a procedure but not the result of the negligence of the operator (physician, nurse, or other provider performing the procedure or treatment). For example, excessive bleeding is an inherent risk of vascular surgery.
- Invasion of privacy: An unwarranted appropriation or exploitation of another's private affairs with which the public has no legitimate concern; a wrongful intrusion into one's private activities in such a manner as to cause mental

suffering, shame, or humiliation to a person of ordinary sensibilities. Such an invasion by an individual or government may constitute an actionable tort.
- Liability: A debt, responsibility, or obligation.
- Liability, joint and several: An obligation of a group as a whole and all its individual members. The harmed party can sue all liable parties as a group or any one of them individually. He or she may not, however, recover more compensation by suing each of them individually than by suing them as a group.
- Liability limits: A restriction or upper boundary on the amount of money an insurance company will pay to satisfy a claim against an insured. A claim for a sum beyond this limit is not protected by the insurance policy and is the responsibility of the defendant.
- Liable: A term that means bound by law or fairness; responsible; accountable.
- Malpractice: An act of professional negligence. It has two components: (1) negligence, a deviation from the approved and accepted standards of care, as defined within a given specialty, and (2) injury, which is damage to the patient as a result of the stated negligence or deviation from the standard of care.
- Most-favored-nation clause: A contractual arrangement between a purchaser and provider. In this arrangement the provider is obligated to render products or services to the purchaser at the same rate as his or her most-favored customer.
- Negligence: A failure to use the degree of care a reasonably prudent and careful person would use under similar circumstances. Acts of omission, commission, or both may constitute negligence.
- Negligent credentialing: A failure on the part of the managed care organization or hospital to exercise reasonable care in screening and selecting providers or staff members. Negligent credentialing can occur when a managed care organization selects a provider who negligently injures a patient and is found to have a history of doing the same or is found not to have the appropriate training, experience, skills, or licensure to care for the patient.
- Negligent referral: A failure to use such care in making a referral as a reasonable professional would use under similar circumstances. Referring a patient to a provider who does not possess the skills, experience, licensure, or certifications to care for that patient constitutes a negligent referral.
- Ombudsman: A person whose occupation consists of investigating customer complaints against his or her employer. These employees are often found in the appeals and grievance section of the quality management departments of HMOs.
- Ostensible agency (*see also* Apparent authority): An implied or presumptive agency that exists in which one, either intentionally or from want of ordinary care, induces another to believe that a third person is his or her agent, although that third person was never, in fact, employed by him or her. An example is a physician working in a hospital's emergency department. He or she is employed by a physician group that is contracted to the hospital. However, a patient entering the emergency department may reasonably assume the physician works for the hospital. In these cases the "principal" is responsible for the acts of her or his "agent" when she or he has given actual authority for that agent to act. Further, when a principal (e.g., insurance company) has taken such actions as would indicate to third parties (e.g., patients) that someone (e.g., Case Manager) is her or his agent, the principal is held to have given "apparent authority" to the agent

and will be liable for her or his acts. A Case Manager can be a real or ostensible agent of the insurer, physician, hospital, or healthcare facility. A Case Manager's actions can become the liability of her or his employer or principal.

- Out-of-court settlement: An agreement or transaction between two litigants to settle the matter privately, without being referred to the judge for authorization or approval, before the court has rendered its decision.
- Privacy: The quality or condition of being secluded from the presence or view of others; the state of being free from unsanctioned intrusion; the state of being concealed; secrecy.
- Privileged communications: The information that a person authorized to practice medicine, registered nursing, and so on acquires in attending to a patient in a professional capacity and that is necessary to enable him or her to act in that capacity. Such information shall not be disclosed unless the patient waives that privilege. Disclosure of such information may constitute an invasion of privacy, which is an actionable tort.
- *Res ipsa loquitor* (from the Latin: "The thing speaks for itself"): A doctrine of law with reference to cases in which mere proof that an occurrence took place is sufficient under the circumstances to shift the burden of proof upon the defendant to prove that it was not due to his or her negligence. Implied in this doctrine is that the instrumentality causing injury was in the defendant's exclusive control and that the accident was one that ordinarily does not happen in the absence of negligence. An example of res ipsa loquitor is when a patient is found to have a surgical instrument left in his or her abdomen after an appendectomy (assuming there was only one surgeon involved).
- *Respondeat superior* (from the Latin "Let the master answer"): A master is liable, in certain cases, for the wrongful acts of his or her servant (likewise, a principal for those of his or her agent). A master–servant or principle–agent relationship exists in which one person, for pay or other valuable consideration, enters into the service of another and devotes his or her personal labor for an agreed period (e.g., employee–employer). A hospital, for example, can be held liable for the negligent actions of doctors or nurses in its employ.
- Statute of limitations: The period of time in which a plaintiff may bring a lawsuit after an incident has occurred.
- Subpoena (from the Latin "under penalty"): A judicial process (or writ) requiring a witness to give relevant information or testimony "under penalty" of contempt for disobedience.
- Summons: A document issued by the plaintiff's attorney, which, when properly delivered, commences a legal action.
- Tort (from the Latin "to twist," implying injury): A damage, injury, or a wrongful act done willfully, negligently, or in circumstances involving strict liability; a legal wrong committed upon the person or property independent of contract. A tort may be
  - A direct invasion of some legal right of the individual
  - The infraction of some public duty by which special damage accrues to the individual
  - The violation of some private obligation by which like damage accrues to the individual

- Vicarious liability: The legal liability that a person may have for the action of someone else. For instance, in the employer–employee relationship, an insurer could be vicariously liable for the action of the Case Managers employed in its plan.

INTERSTATE COMPACT FOR NURSING

Multistate Nursing Practice

Nurses are licensed in the state in which they practice, and each state regulates the practice of those nurses who are licensed in that state. To provide direct patient care, a nurse would require a license in the state in which he or she provided care; however, the licensing requirement for "telenursing" was not as well understood.

In 1997 the National Council of State Boards of Nursing (NCSBN) issued a policy statement on telenursing, stating that telenursing is an activity included in the practice of nursing and therefore is regulated by the state boards of nursing (Box 3-1). They further opined that Case Managers who provide services either on site or telephonically/electronically outside their state of licensure are violating the law.

Failing to comply with this law has serious consequences. Punishment for violations of this law varies by state but consists of up to $1,000 in fines, permanent loss of the professional license, and up to 1 year in jail. Case Managers can also face disciplinary action from the Commission for Case Management Certification because they are required to "obey all laws and regulations."[18] Additionally, malpractice insurance carriers will not cover "improperly" licensed nurses if some untoward incident should occur to a patient under their care.

Case Managers are required to be licensed in the states in which their patients reside when Case Manager–patient interactions occur. This presents an enormous problem to Case Managers who interact with patients in more than one state, for example, those who work in large managed care organizations. These Case Managers would have to incur the costs and administrative difficulties associated with maintaining scores of licenses in different states. To address this issue the NCSBN developed the concept of an interstate nursing compact and adopted a model compact in December 1997 (Table 3-1).

> **BOX 3-1**
>
> **Telenursing:** This term refers to the use of telecommunications and information technology for providing nursing services whenever a large physical distance exists between patient and nurse, or between any number of nurses.

Nurse Licensure Compact

The compact is fashioned after the interstate compact used for driver's licenses. That interstate compact allows drivers licensed in one state the ability to drive in all the states that have entered into the compact. The mutual recognition of a nurse's licensure allows a nurse to have one license in the nurse's state of residency and to practice in other states.

If a nurse works in more than one state and those states participate in the compact, the nurse only has to hold a license in the state in which the nurse has a primary

TABLE 3-1 Interstate Nursing Compact

Advantages:

- Need only one state license
- Decrease financial outlay
- Decrease personal malpractice liability
- Decrease administrative costs of maintaining multiple state licenses
- Employer verification is easier
- Mobility

Disadvantages:

- Responsible to multiple state nursing boards
- Cannot practice out of state if you have a restricted license or are subject to disciplinary action by state nursing board

residence. The current requirements for scope of practice, disciplinary procedures, and advanced practice authorization, however, largely remain unchanged. Nurses who work in several states still have to comply with the scope of practice statutes and regulations in each state in which they practice. The following is the unique nomenclature of this arrangement:

- Party state: Party states are any states that adopt the nurse licensure compact. A nurse that is licensed in a party state may practice, either in person or electronically, in any of the other party states in the compact.
- Home state: Under the compact, the primary state of residence is known as the home state.
- Remote state: A remote state is a party state that is not the home state. A nurse is subject to the laws and disciplinary procedures of every state he or she practices in.

The only restriction in this compact is that the nurse who wishes to practice outside of his or her home state must have an unrestricted license to practice nursing. He or she cannot be under either a state-sponsored disciplinary action or a monitoring agreement that prohibits the nurse from practicing across state lines.

The benefits of the compact are clear. Nurses need only maintain one license in their state of residency. Employers need only verify licensure in that state. Malpractice insurance will cover nurses practicing legally under the interstate compact. Organizations can use nurses to perform case management in compact states without the sizable administrative task of verifying and tracking multiple licenses. Nurses have increased mobility, which is essential during times of disaster. Patients are better protected, as the authority and responsibilities of nurses are clearly defined and monitored and information is shared among the participating compact states.

January 1, 2000, marks the date that the first states passed the compact into law: Maryland, Texas, Utah, and Wisconsin. The compact included registered nurses, licensed practical nurses, and vocational nurses since 1998. On August 16, 2002, the NCSBN approved the model language for the inclusion of advanced practice registered nurses. In April 2005 Utah and Iowa agreed to mutually recognize advanced practice registered nurse licenses, but as of April 25, 2005, no implementation date has been set for the advanced practice registered nurse compact. As of March 31, 2006, 20 states have enacted registered nurse, licensed practical nurse, and vocational nurse licensure compact legislation, and three states are pending implementation. A current listing of participating states can be found at www.ncsbn.org.

REFERENCES

1. Americans with Disabilities Act of 1990. 42 U.S.C. §12101, et seq.
2. American Medical Association. (1997). *Code of medical ethics: Current opinions with annotations.* Chicago: American Medical Association.
3. Keffler, M. J. (1997). Ethical decisions with limited resources. How is that possible? *Nurse Case Manager, 2*(5), 196–200.
4. Cesta, T., Tahan, H., & Fink, L. (1998). *The Case Manager's survival guide: Winning strategies for clinical practice.* St. Louis: Mosby.
5. Localio, A. R., Lawthers, A. G., & Brennan, T. A. (1991). Relation between malpractice claims and adverse events due to negligence. Results of the Harvard Medical Practice Study III. *New England Journal of Medicine, 325*(4), 245–251.
6. Brennan, T. A., Leape, L. L., & Laird, N. M. (1991). Incidence of adverse events and negligence in hospitalized patients. Results of the Harvard Medical Practice Study I. *New England Journal of Medicine, 325*(5), 370–376.
7. Huycke, L. I., & Huycke, M. M. (1994). Characteristics of potential plaintiffs in malpractice litigation. *Annals of Internal Medicine, 120*(9), 792–798.
8. Ibid.
9. *Fox v. Healthnet,* No. 21692 (Cal Sup Ct. Riverside County, filed June 19, 1992: settled April 6, 1994).
10. Quinn, C. (1997). Avoiding bad faith denials of medical claims. *Managed Care, 6*(4), 79–80, 83–55.
11. *Schloendorff v. The Society of the New York Hospital,* 211 N.Y. 125, N.E. 92 (1914) [April 14, 1914]. 1914 N.Y. LEXIS 1028.
12. Hogue, E. (1998). Tips make CMSA standards work for you. *Advisor, 6*(5), 75–76.
13. Hogue, E. (1995). Are Case Managers liable? *Journal of Care Management, 1*(2), 35–38, 53.
14. *Schloendorff v. The Society of the New York Hospital,* 211 N.Y. 125, N.E. 92 (1914) [April 14, 1914]. 1914 N.Y. LEXIS 1028.
15. Powell, S. K. (1996). *Nursing case management: A practical guide to success in managed care.* New York: Lippincott.
16. Powers, Pyles, & Verville. (1994). Legal hazards on the case management highway, *NALP,* 102.
17. *Fox v. Healthnet,* No. 21692 (Cal Sup Ct. Riverside County, filed June 19, 1992: settled April 6, 1994).
18. Commission for Case Management Certification. (2004). *Code of professional conduct of Case Managers with standards, rules procedures and penalties.*

Appendix 3-A

Principles of Practice Questions

1) Disclosure of confidential information is mandatory when
   A. It is pursuant to judicial proceedings.
   B. It is government mandated.
   C. A professional has a duty to warn a third party about the illness of a patient.
   D. All of the above
   E. None of the above

2) Case Managers are committed to obtaining informed consent, providing options for the patient to choose from, and educating the patient to make independent decisions. This principle is known as
   A. Veracity
   B. Beneficence
   C. Autonomy
   D. Nonmaleficence

3) Which of the following is subject to state and federal mandates regarding medical record retention?
   A. Financial files
   B. HMO insurance information
   C. Case management files
   D. Insurance claims files

4) Of the following, which activity(ies) may increase the risk of allegations of breach of patient confidentiality?
   1. Understanding applicable federal and state regulations on the disclosure of medical information
   2. Quickly transferring information to any and all parties that request it, without bothering to notify the patient, attorneys, and so on
   3. Informing the patient of his or her right to refuse the disclosure of medical information to any or all parties
   4. Transferring patient information concerning abortions and venereal and psychiatric diseases to third parties, without first discussing with the patient and/or attorneys
      A. 1, 3
      B. 2, 4
      C. 1, 2, 3
      D. All of the above
      E. None of the above

5) Of the following, which activity(ies) may decrease the risk of allegations of breach of patient confidentiality?
   1. Understanding applicable federal and state regulations on the disclosure of medical information
   2. Quickly transferring information to any and all parties that request it, without bothering to notify the patient, attorneys, and so on
   3. Informing the patient of his or her right to refuse the disclosure of medical information to any or all parties
   4. Transferring patient information concerning abortions and venereal and psychiatric diseases to third parties, without discussing first with the patient and/or attorneys
      A. 1, 3
      B. 2, 4
      C. 1, 2, 3
      D. All of the above
      E. None of the above

6) Which of the following should be disclosed to the patient when a provider is obtaining consent for a medical, surgical, or psychological intervention?
   1. The projected or desired outcomes of the proposed treatment and the likelihood of success
   2. Reasonably foreseeable risks or hazards inherent in the proposed treatment or care (which must be done in a manner that the patient can understand)
   3. Alternatives to proposed care or treatment plan
   4. Consequences of forgoing the treatment
      A. 1, 3
      B. 2, 4
      C. 1, 2, 3
      D. All of the above
      E. None of the above

7) Which of the following need not be disclosed to the patient when a provider is obtaining consent for a medical, surgical, or psychological intervention?
   1. The projected or desired outcomes of the proposed treatment and the likelihood of success
   2. The mood of the provider and his or her staff
   3. Alternatives to proposed care or treatment plan
   4. The names of all the patients the provider has treated with this intervention in the past
      A. 1, 3
      B. 2, 4
      C. 1, 2, 3
      D. All of the above
      E. None of the above

8) Which of the following are requirements for obtaining informed consent?
   1. The patient must consent voluntarily.
   2. The patient must have the capacity to give consent.
   3. The patient must be an adult (under existing state law).
   4. In the event that the patient is a minor or an adult without capacity to consent, parents, attorneys, or legal guardians may give consent.
      A. 1, 3
      B. 2, 4
      C. 1, 2, 3
      D. All of the above
      E. None of the above

94 CHAPTER THREE

9) To decrease patient allegations of lack of informed consent, a Case Manager should ensure which of the following?
   1. The patient must have a full understanding of the scope of activities of the Case Manager, with all its attendant risks, benefits, and alternatives.
   2. The Case Manager must document the consent. (A signed consent agreement is adequate.)
   3. The Case Manager must obtain informed consent before the beginning of the professional relationship.
   4. The Case Manager must consult with an attorney before each consent for treatment is signed.
      A. 1, 3
      B. 2, 4
      C. 1, 2, 3
      D. All of the above
      E. None of the above

10) Which of the following are not requirements for obtaining informed consent?
    1. The attorney must sign an affirmation stating that the patient is competent.
    2. The patient must have the capacity to give consent.
    3. The patient must be at least 10 years of age.
    4. In the event the patient is a minor or an adult without capacity to consent, parents, attorneys, or legal guardians may give consent.
       A. 1, 3
       B. 2, 4
       C. 1, 2, 3
       D. All of the above
       E. None of the above

11) Which of the following are requirements for obtaining informed consent?
    1. The patient may consent voluntarily or may be coerced if uncooperative.
    2. The patient must have the capacity to give consent.
    3. The patient must be an adult; however, emancipated minors must have their parents' consent.
    4. In the event the patient is a minor or an adult without capacity to consent, parents, attorneys, or legal guardians may give consent.
       A. 1, 3
       B. 2, 4
       C. 1, 2, 3
       D. All of the above
       E. None of the above

12) A case management consent agreement provides for which of the following?
    1. Release of clinical information to the Case Manager
    2. Claims payment
    3. Permission to review the case information with the parties involved in the care of the patient or the payment of services
    4. Provision of durable medical equipment
       A. 1, 2
       B. 2, 3
       C. 1, 3
       D. 3, 4

13) In the case management process, the stage of "obtaining approval" refers to
   A. Permission from the patient to implement case management
   B. Permission from the payer to implement a care plan
   C. Permission from claims to negotiate fees
   D. None of the above

14) Informed consent must contain which of the following elements?
   1. Disclosure of all possible side effects
   2. Disclosure of meaningful background information
   3. A chance for the patient to ask questions
   4. Performed by a registered nurse
       A. 1, 2, 3
       B. 2, 3, 4
       C. 2, 3
       D. All of the above

15) Obtaining an accurate history is important to the case management process. Toward that end, the Case Manager should
   1. Obtain a signed consent agreement or release of medical information from the patient
   2. Obtain the history directly from the patient
   3. Interview the employer
   4. Request medical records for review
   5. Interview the physician
       A. 1, 2, 3
       B. 1, 2, 3, 4
       C. 1, 2, 4, 5
       D. All of the above
       E. None of the above

16) Case Managers must balance their obligations; which of the following should be their priority?
   A. Interacting with the patient's attorney
   B. Interests of the insurance carrier
   C. Their employer
   D. The patient

17) Of the following, which are common causes of malpractice litigation?
   1. Discourteous behavior by the professional
   2. Provider–patient miscommunication
   3. Lack of patient understanding
   4. Failure to inform a patient's family of pertinent issues
       A. 1, 3
       B. 2, 4
       C. 1, 2, 3
       D. All of the above
       E. None of the above

18) Of the following, which are not common causes of malpractice litigation?
   1. Discourteous behavior by the professional
   2. Poor clinical outcomes
   3. Lack of patient understanding
   4. Substandard medical care
      A. 1, 3
      B. 2, 4
      C. 1, 2, 3
      D. All of the above
      E. None of the above

19) Common causes of malpractice litigation include which of the following?
   1. Discourteous behavior by the professional
   2. Poor clinical outcomes
   3. Lack of patient understanding
   4. Substandard medical care
      A. 1, 3
      B. 2, 4
      C. 1, 2, 3
      D. All of the above
      E. None of the above

20) Case management activities that have the highest risk of malpractice associated with them include which of the following?
   1. Patient discharge
   2. Claims denials
   3. Patient assessment
   4. Referral to providers
      A. 1, 3
      B. 2, 4
      C. 1, 2, 3
      D. All of the above
      E. None of the above

21) Of the following case management activities, which do not have the highest risk of malpractice associated with them?
   1. Patient admissions
   2. Patient assessment
   3. Claims approvals
   4. Referral to providers
      A. 1, 3
      B. 2, 4
      C. 1, 2, 3
      D. All of the above
      E. None of the above

22) Case Managers may decrease the legal liability associated with patient discharges through which of the following activities?
   1. Decreasing the average length of stay of their clients
   2. Confirming the integrity of the patient's support network
   3. Reducing the per-member, per-month medical costs of their clients
   4. Confirming the adequacy of follow-up outpatient care

A. 1, 3
B. 2, 4
C. 1, 2, 3
D. All of the above
E. None of the above

23) Which of the following activities are not associated with a decrease in the legal liability associated with patient discharges?
1. Decreasing the average length of stay of their clients
2. Confirming the integrity of the patient's support network
3. Reducing the per-member, per-month medical costs of their clients
4. Confirming the adequacy of follow-up outpatient care
    A. 1, 3
    B. 2, 4
    C. 1, 2, 3
    D. All of the above
    E. None of the above

24) Which of the following activities are associated with a decrease in the legal liability associated with bad faith allegations?
1. Decreasing the average length of stay of their clients
2. Expediting claims adjudication
3. Reducing the per-member, per-month medical costs of their clients
4. Securing an independent medical examination of the patient
    A. 1, 3
    B. 2, 4
    C. 1, 2, 3
    D. All of the above
    E. None of the above

25) Which of the following activities are associated with an increase in the legal liability associated with bad faith allegations?
1. Decreasing the average length of stay of their clients
2. Unnecessarily delaying claims adjudication
3. Reducing the per-member, per-month medical costs of their clients
4. Refusing an independent medical examination of the patient
    A. 1, 3
    B. 2, 4
    C. 1, 2, 3
    D. All of the above
    E. None of the above

26) Malpractice is _____ that results in harm to another person.
    A. A professional's wrongful conduct
    B. A professional's failure to meet acceptable standards of care
    C. The improper discharge of a professional's duties
    D. All of the above
    E. None of the above

27) Negligence is
   A. An act of omission
   B. An act of commission
   C. Failing to use the degree of care a reasonably prudent and careful person would under similar circumstances
   D. None of the above
   E. All of the above

28) _____ is an unlawful, wrongful act.
   A. Negligence
   B. Liability
   C. Malpractice
   D. Malfeasance

29) A tort is
   A. A damage, injury, or wrongful act independent of a contractual relationship
   B. An agreement by the parties involved to a resolution of a particular issue
   C. A voluntary assignation of a known right to someone else
   D. None of the above

30) The court case of *Wickline v. State of California* found
   1. Medical doctors have a duty to protest adverse determinations by payers.
   2. Medical doctors can shift their liability to payers if they do protest adverse determinations.
   3. Case Managers are not liable for their roles in adverse determinations.
   4. Payers of health care can be held accountable if their adverse decisions are arbitrary, made for cost containment, and are not based on acceptable medical standards of practice in the community.
   A. 1, 2, 3
   B. 2, 3, 4
   C. 1, 2, 4
   D. None of the above

31) In a malpractice suit the plaintiff must prove two points:
   1. His or her compliance with the prescribed treatment plan
   2. Negligence on the part of the Case Manager
   3. Injury from the Case Manager's negligence
   4. Intent on the part of the Case Manager
   A. 1, 4
   B. 2, 3
   C. None of the above
   D. All of the above

32) Communication failures, lack of information given to the family, lack of patient understanding, and discourteous behavior are all causes of
   A. Lack of patient compliance
   B. Patient injuries
   C. Patient complaints
   D. Malpractice litigation

33) Which of the following statements best defines ethics, as they relate to case management?
   1. The rules of conduct that govern a person or members of a profession
   2. The thoughts that govern a person's conduct
   3. A society's ideal for a person's conduct
   4. The minimal acceptable standards for a person's conduct
      A. 1, 3
      B. 2, 4
      C. 1, 2, 3
      D. All of the above
      E. None of the above

34) Which of the following statements are not true regarding ethics as they relate to case management?
   1. They are rules of conduct that govern a person or members of a profession.
   2. They are thoughts that govern a person's conduct.
   3. They are a society's ideal for a person's conduct.
   4. They are the minimal acceptable standards for a person's conduct.
      A. 1, 3
      B. 2, 4
      C. 1, 2, 3
      D. All of the above
      E. None of the above

35) Which of the following statements can be said to be true, when distinguishing ethical from legal principles?
   1. Civil punishments usually exist for lapses in legal duties.
   2. Ethical duties usually exceed legal requirements.
   3. Legal duties describe society's minimum acceptable behaviors.
   4. Ethical obligations describe society's ideals for personal and professional behavior.
      A. 1, 3
      B. 2, 4
      C. 1, 2, 3
      D. All of the above
      E. None of the above

36) When distinguishing ethical from legal principles, which of the following statements are not considered to be true?
   1. Civil punishments usually exist for lapses in legal duties.
   2. Ethical duties usually exceed legal requirements.
   3. Legal duties describe society's minimum acceptable behaviors.
   4. Ethical obligations describe society's ideals for personal and professional behavior.
      A. 1, 3
      B. 2, 4
      C. 1, 2, 3
      D. All of the above
      E. None of the above

37) Which of the following statements is (are) true regarding an ethical dilemma?
1. It involves a decision between two or more possible outcomes.
2. It involves the breaking of an ethical principle.
3. The possible outcomes are in conflict.
4. Solving an ethical dilemma is usually illegal.
    A. 1, 3
    B. 2, 4
    C. 1, 2, 3
    D. All of the above
    E. None of the above

38) In regard to ethical dilemmas, which of the following statements is (are) not true?
1. It involves a decision between two or more possible outcomes.
2. It involves the breaking of an ethical principle.
3. The possible outcomes are in conflict.
4. Solving an ethical dilemma is usually illegal.
    A. 1, 3
    B. 2, 4
    C. 1, 2, 3
    D. All of the above
    E. None of the above

39) Which of the following are ethical principles promulgated by the CMSA?
1. Autonomy
2. Beneficence
3. Nonmaleficence
4. Justice
    A. 1, 3
    B. 2, 4
    C. 1, 2, 3
    D. All of the above
    E. None of the above

40) Which of the following attributes are not ethical principles promulgated by the CMSA?
1. Autonomy
2. Insouciance
3. Nonmaleficence
4. Diversity
    A. 1, 3
    B. 2, 4
    C. 1, 2, 3
    D. All of the above
    E. None of the above

41) The ethical principle of justice implies all except which of the following qualities or attributes?
1. Upholding what is just or fair
2. Kindness
3. Equity of treatment
4. Charity

A. 1, 3
B. 2, 4
C. 1, 2, 3
D. All of the above
E. None of the above

42) **The ethical principle of beneficence implies all except which of the following qualities or attributes?**
   1. Upholding what is just or fair
   2. Kindness
   3. Equity of treatment
   4. Charity
      A. 1, 3
      B. 2, 4
      C. 1, 2, 3
      D. All of the above
      E. None of the above

43) **The ethical principle of autonomy is associated with all except which of the following attributes?**
   1. Promoting a patient's freedom to choose
   2. Preventing harm to the patient
   3. Encouraging patient self-advocacy
   4. Encouraging patients to do what is right for the Case Manager
      A. 1, 3
      B. 2, 4
      C. 1, 2, 3
      D. All of the above
      E. None of the above

44) **The ethical principle of nonmaleficence is associated with all except which of the following attributes?**
   1. Promoting a patient's freedom to choose
   2. Preventing harm to the patient
   3. Encouraging patient self-advocacy
   4. Encouraging patients to do what is right for the Case Manager
      A. 1, 3, 4
      B. 2, 4
      C. 1, 2, 3
      D. All of the above
      E. None of the above

45) **The ethical principle of veracity implies all except which of the following qualities or attributes?**
   1. Upholding what is just or fair
   2. Adherence to the truth
   3. Equity of treatment
   4. Conforming in one's dealings with others to accuracy or precision
      A. 1, 3
      B. 2, 4
      C. 1, 2, 3
      D. All of the above
      E. None of the above

46) Which of the following qualities or attributes are associated with the ethical principle of veracity?
   1. Upholding what is just or fair
   2. Adherence to the truth
   3. Equity of treatment
   4. Conforming in one's dealings with others to accuracy or precision
      A. 1, 3
      B. 2, 4
      C. 1, 2, 3
      D. All of the above
      E. None of the above

47) The term "ethics" is best defined as
   A. Rules or standards that govern a person's behavior
   B. A set of religious laws that govern a person's behavior
   C. A set of juridical laws that govern a person's behavior
   D. Instinctual or inborn standards of behavior

48) Ethical rules are derived from
   A. A set of personal or professional behaviors that embody the highest ideals of society
   B. A set of personal or professional behaviors that embody the minimal standards set by society
   C. A set of personal or professional behaviors found in one religious group
   D. A set of personal or professional behaviors that result in personal success or positive clinical outcomes

49) The differences between ethics and law are
   1. Ethics represent the highest standards for personal behavior, and law represents the minimal acceptable standards.
   2. The law represents the highest standards for personal behavior, and ethics represents the minimal acceptable standards.
   3. Lapses in strictly ethical behavior rarely result in punishment outside professional circles, whereas strictly legal infractions will.
   4. Lapses in strictly legal behavior rarely result in punishment outside professional circles, whereas strictly ethical infractions will.
      A. 1, 2
      B. 1, 3
      C. 1, 4
      D. All of the above

50) The term "ethical dilemma" is best defined as
   A. A conflict between two or more equally desirable outcomes, when only one outcome is possible
   B. A conflict between two or more possible outcomes, in which a lack of knowledge as to which outcome will be best prevents adequate decision making
   C. A conflict between two or more possible outcomes that occurs because of the indecisiveness of the Case Manager
   D. A conflict between two or more possible outcomes that occurs because of financial constraints

51) **The solutions to ethical dilemmas usually can be found in**
    A. Textbooks on ethics
    B. Textbooks on medical care
    C. A more appropriately designed healthcare system
    D. An examination of the best interests of all parties involved in the dilemma
    E. There are no solutions to ethical dilemmas.

52) **According to the code of ethics promulgated by the CMSA, the five ethical principles of case management are**
    A. Autonomy, veracity, beneficence, nonmaleficence, and justice
    B. Autonomy, veracity, beneficence, charity, and justice
    C. Autonomy, veracity, malfeasance, charity, and justice
    D. Autonomy, veracity, empathy, virtue, and justice
    E. Autonomy, veracity, forbearance, virtue, and justice

53) **Which of the following activities is (are) associated with an increase in the legal liability associated with negligent patient assessment allegations?**
    1. Failing to inquire about a patient's educational background
    2. Failing to inquire about a patient's cultural background
    3. Failing to inquire about a patient's religious background
    4. Failing to inquire about a patient's social support system
        A. 1, 3
        B. 2, 4
        C. 1, 2, 3
        D. All of the above
        E. None of the above

54) **Which of the following activities is (are) associated with a decrease in legal liability associated with allegations of negligent patient assessment?**
    1. Understanding a patient's family and social support system
    2. Understanding a patient's highest educational achievements
    3. Understanding a patient's religious affiliations
    4. Understanding a patient's cultural background
        A. 1, 3
        B. 2, 4
        C. 1, 2, 3
        D. All of the above
        E. None of the above

55) **Which of the following activities is (are) associated with decreased risk of allegations of negligent referral?**
    1. Understanding the credentialing criteria of the provider network
    2. Making a personal recommendation for a single provider
    3. Providing patients with a list of providers rather than the name of a single provider
    4. Protecting a provider who provides irregular or suspicious medical treatments
        A. 1, 3
        B. 2, 4
        C. 1, 2, 3
        D. All of the above
        E. None of the above

104 CHAPTER THREE

56) Which of the following activities is (are) associated with increased risk of allegations of negligent referral?
   1. Understanding the credentialing criteria of the provider network
   2. Making a personal recommendation for a single provider
   3. Providing patients with a list of providers rather than the name of a single provider
   4. Protecting a provider who provides irregular or suspicious medical treatments
      A. 1, 3
      B. 2, 4
      C. 1, 2, 3
      D. All of the above
      E. None of the above

57) The legal definition of agency includes which of the following?
   1. It is a relationship between two or more parties.
   2. One party consents to act on the behalf of the other party.
   3. The relationship carries the obligation that the principal is responsible for the actions of the agent.
   4. The relationship carries no obligations for the agent to the principal.
      A. 1, 3
      B. 2, 4
      C. 1, 2, 3
      D. All of the above
      E. None of the above

58) Agents have which of the following legal obligations to their principals?
   1. Using care and skill in the performance of their duties
   2. Acting in good faith in the performance of their duties
   3. Remaining within the limits of their authority
   4. Advancing the interests of the agent
      A. 1, 3
      B. 2, 4
      C. 1, 2, 3
      D. All of the above
      E. None of the above

59) Apparent authority (or ostensible agency) occurs with which of the following?
   1. A principal has taken such actions that would indicate to third parties that someone is his or her agent.
   2. A principal assigns duties and authorities to an agent via a written contract.
   3. A principal, aware that a third party is acting as his or her agent, does nothing to stop it.
   4. A principal assigns duties and authorities to an agent via an oral contract.
      A. 1, 3
      B. 2, 4
      C. 1, 2, 3
      D. All of the above
      E. None of the above

60) Which of the following pairs are examples of principals and their agents?
   1. Hospitals and community physicians (not employed by hospital)
   2. Hospitals and the nurses who work on the wards
   3. Case Managers and patients
   4. Insurers and Case Managers (employed by the insurer)

A. 1, 3
B. 2, 4
C. 1, 2, 3
D. All of the above
E. None of the above

61) **Which of the following pairs are not examples of principals and their agents?**
1. Hospitals and community physicians (not employed by hospital)
2. Hospitals and its phlebotomists (employed by the hospital)
3. Case Managers and network physicians
4. Insurers and their utilization review departments (employed by the insurer)
    A. 1, 3
    B. 2, 4
    C. 1, 2, 3
    D. All of the above
    E. None of the above

62) **Which of the following statements describes the legal term abandonment?**
1. Termination of a professional relationship without reasonable notice to the patient
2. Termination of a professional relationship without payment of debts
3. Termination of a professional relationship without giving the patient an opportunity to acquire alternative care or services
4. Termination of a professional relationship because of a disagreement
    A. 1, 3
    B. 2, 4
    C. 1, 2, 3
    D. All of the above
    E. None of the above

63) **Which of the following statements does not describe the legal term abandonment?**
1. Termination of a professional relationship without reasonable notice to the patient
2. Termination of a professional relationship without payment of debts
3. Termination of a professional relationship without giving the patient an opportunity to acquire alternative care or services
4. Termination of a professional relationship because of a disagreement
    A. 1, 3
    B. 2, 4
    C. 1, 2, 3
    D. All of the above
    E. None of the above

64) **The legal term claim is best described by which of the following?**
A. The state or quality of being confidential; treated as private and not for publication
B. The document by which the plaintiff gives the court and the defendant notice of the transactions, occurrences, or series of transactions or occurrences intended to be proved and the material elements of each cause of action or defense
C. A method of measuring negligence among the participants in a suit, both defense and plaintiff, in terms of percentages of culpability; damages are then diminished in proportion to the amount of negligence attributable to the complaining party
D. A report by the insured to the insurance company based on notification by a patient or the patient's attorney of an event out of which malpractice has been alleged
E. A failure of a fiduciary duty; refusing to hold secret a privileged communication entrusted by one party to another

65) **The legal term breach of confidentiality is best described by which of the following?**
   A. The state or quality of being confidential; treated as private and not for publication
   B. The document by which the plaintiff gives the court and the defendant notice of the transactions, occurrences, or series of transactions or occurrences intended to be proved and the material elements of each cause of action or defense
   C. A method of measuring negligence among the participants in a suit, both defense and plaintiff, in terms of percentages of culpability; damages are then diminished in proportion to the amount of negligence attributable to the complaining party
   D. A report by the insured to the insurance company based on notification by a patient or the patient's attorney of an event out of which malpractice has been alleged
   E. A failure of a fiduciary duty; refusing to hold secret a privileged communication entrusted by one party to another

66) **The legal term comparative negligence is best described by which of the following?**
   A. The state or quality of being confidential; treated as private and not for publication
   B. The document by which the plaintiff gives the court and the defendant notice of the transactions, occurrences, or series of transactions or occurrences intended to be proved and the material elements of each cause of action or defense
   C. A method of measuring negligence among the participants in a suit, both defense and plaintiff, in terms of percentages of culpability; damages are then diminished in proportion to the amount of negligence attributable to the complaining party
   D. A report by the insured to the insurance company based on notification by a patient or the patient's attorney of an event out of which malpractice has been alleged
   E. A failure of a fiduciary duty; refusing to hold secret a privileged communication entrusted by one party to another

67) **The legal term complaint is best described by which of the following?**
   A. The state or quality of being confidential; treated as private and not for publication
   B. The document by which the plaintiff gives the court and the defendant notice of the transactions, occurrences, or series of transactions or occurrences intended to be proved and the material elements of each cause of action or defense
   C. A method of measuring negligence among the participants in a suit, both defense and plaintiff, in terms of percentages of culpability; damages are then diminished in proportion to the amount of negligence attributable to the complaining party
   D. A report by the insured to the insurance company based on notification by a patient or the patient's attorney of an event out of which malpractice has been alleged
   E. A failure of a fiduciary duty; refusing to hold secret a privileged communication entrusted by one party to another

68) **The legal term confidentiality is best described by which of the following?**
   A. The state or quality of being confidential; treated as private and not for publication
   B. The document by which the plaintiff gives the court and the defendant notice of the transactions, occurrences, or series of transactions or occurrences intended to be proved and the material elements of each cause of action or defense
   C. A method of measuring negligence among the participants in a suit, both defense and plaintiff, in terms of percentages of culpability; damages are then diminished in proportion to the amount of negligence attributable to the complaining party
   D. A report by the insured to the insurance company based on notification by a patient or the patient's attorney of an event out of which malpractice has been alleged
   E. A failure of a fiduciary duty; refusing to hold secret a privileged communication entrusted by one party to another

69) **Which of the following statements best defines the legal term corporate negligence?**
   A. A method of obtaining disclosure of information that is material and necessary to the underlying lawsuit by way of sworn oral testimony
   B. The ascertainment of what is not previously known; generally, the pretrial stage of a lawsuit beginning with the service of summons and complaint and concluding with the filing of a "note of issue"
   C. A pecuniary compensation recovered by the courts for acts of tort; these recoveries, or compensations, are for both tangible (medical expenses, lost earnings) and intangible (pain and suffering) injuries (torts)
   D. A legal doctrine that prohibits corporations from engaging in the practice of medicine, that is, the treatment of injuries, the discovery of the cause and nature of disease, and the administration of remedies or the prescribing of treatment
   E. A term that encompasses the legal grounds for managed care organizations' liability based on the corporate activities of the managed care organization itself rather than on the care-related activities of participating healthcare professionals

70) **Which of the following statements best defines the legal term corporate practice of medicine?**
   A. A method of obtaining disclosure of information that is material and necessary to the underlying lawsuit by way of sworn oral testimony
   B. The ascertainment of what is not previously known; generally, the pretrial stage of a lawsuit beginning with the service of summons and complaint and concluding with the filing of a "note of issue"
   C. A pecuniary compensation recovered by the courts for acts of tort; these recoveries, or compensations, are for both tangible (medical expenses, lost earnings) and intangible (pain and suffering) injuries (torts)
   D. A legal doctrine that prohibits corporations from engaging in the practice of medicine, that is, the treatment of injuries, the discovery of the cause and nature of disease, and the administration of remedies or the prescribing of treatment
   E. A term that encompasses the legal grounds for managed care organizations' liability based on the corporate activities of the managed care organization itself rather than on the care-related activities of participating healthcare professionals

71) **Which of the following statements best defines the legal term damages?**
   A. A method of obtaining disclosure of information that is material and necessary to the underlying lawsuit by way of sworn oral testimony
   B. The ascertainment of what is not previously known; generally, the pretrial stage of a lawsuit beginning with the service of summons and complaint and concluding with the filing of a "note of issue"
   C. A pecuniary compensation recovered by the courts for acts of tort; these recoveries, or compensations, are for both tangible (medical expenses, lost earnings) and intangible (pain and suffering) injuries (torts)
   D. A legal doctrine that prohibits corporations from engaging in the practice of medicine, that is, the treatment of injuries, the discovery of the cause and nature of disease, and the administration of remedies or the prescribing of treatment
   E. A term that encompasses the legal grounds for managed care organizations' liability based on the corporate activities of the managed care organization itself rather than on the care-related activities of participating healthcare professionals

72) **Which of the following statements best defines the legal term discovery?**
   A. A method of obtaining disclosure of information that is material and necessary to the underlying lawsuit by way of sworn oral testimony
   B. The ascertainment of what is not previously known; generally, the pretrial stage of a lawsuit beginning with the service of summons and complaint and concluding with the filing of a "note of issue"
   C. A pecuniary compensation recovered by the courts for acts of tort; these recoveries, or compensations, are for both tangible (medical expenses, lost earnings) and intangible (pain and suffering) injuries (torts)
   D. A legal doctrine that prohibits corporations from engaging in the practice of medicine, that is, the treatment of injuries, the discovery of the cause and nature of disease, and the administration of remedies or the prescribing of treatment
   E. A term that encompasses the legal grounds for managed care organizations' liability based on the corporate activities of the managed care organization itself rather than on the care-related activities of participating healthcare professionals

73) **Which of the following statements best defines the legal term examination before trial?**
   A. A method of obtaining disclosure of information that is material and necessary to the underlying lawsuit by way of sworn oral testimony
   B. The ascertainment of what is not previously known; generally, the pretrial stage of a lawsuit beginning with the service of summons and complaint and concluding with the filing of a "note of issue"
   C. A pecuniary compensation recovered by the courts for acts of tort; these recoveries, or compensations, are for both tangible (medical expenses, lost earnings) and intangible (pain and suffering) injuries (torts)
   D. A legal doctrine that prohibits corporations from engaging in the practice of medicine, that is, the treatment of injuries, the discovery of the cause and nature of disease, and the administration of remedies or the prescribing of treatment
   E. A term that encompasses the legal grounds for managed care organizations' liability based on the corporate activities of the managed care organization itself rather than on the care-related activities of participating healthcare professionals

74) **Which of the following statements best defines the legal term joint and several liability?**
   A. A debt, responsibility, or obligation.
   B. An unwarranted appropriation or exploitation of another's private affairs with which the public has no legitimate concern; a wrongful intrusion into one's private activities in such a manner as to cause mental suffering, shame, or humiliation to a person of ordinary sensibilities.
   C. A complication that is commonly associated with a procedure but is not the result of negligence of the operator (physician, nurse, or other provider performing the procedure or treatment).
   D. A contractual arrangement between the insurer and the provider of service; it is typically contained in a managed care contract. This provision specifies that the provider assumes the liability for covered services and cannot sue or assert any claims against enrollees for those covered services, even if the managed care organization becomes insolvent.
   E. An obligation of a group and its individual members. The party that has been harmed is able to sue all of the liable parties as a group, or any one of them individually. He or she may not, however, recover more compensation by suing each of them individually than by suing them as a group.

75) Which of the following statements best defines the legal term hold harmless provision?
A. A debt, responsibility, or obligation.
B. An unwarranted appropriation or exploitation of another's private affairs with which the public has no legitimate concern; a wrongful intrusion into one's private activities in such a manner as to cause mental suffering, shame, or humiliation to a person of ordinary sensibilities.
C. A complication that is commonly associated with a procedure but is not the result of negligence of the operator (physician, nurse, or other provider performing the procedure or treatment).
D. A contractual arrangement between the insurer and the provider of service; it is typically contained in a managed care contract. This provision specifies that the provider assumes the liability for covered services and cannot sue or assert any claims against enrollees for those covered services, even if the managed care organization becomes insolvent.
E. An obligation of a group and its individual members. The party that has been harmed is able to sue all of the liable parties as a group or any one of them individually. He or she may not, however, recover more compensation by suing each of them individually than by suing them as a group.

76) Which of the following statements best defines the legal term inherent risk?
A. A debt, responsibility, or obligation.
B. An unwarranted appropriation or exploitation of another's private affairs with which the public has no legitimate concern; a wrongful intrusion into one's private activities in such a manner as to cause mental suffering, shame, or humiliation to a person of ordinary sensibilities.
C. A complication that is commonly associated with a procedure but is not the result of negligence of the operator (physician, nurse, or other provider performing the procedure or treatment)
D. A contractual arrangement between the insurer and the provider of service; it is typically contained in a managed care contract. This provision specifies that the provider assumes the liability for covered services and cannot sue or assert any claims against enrollees for those covered services, even if the managed care organization becomes insolvent.
E. An obligation of a group and its individual members. The party that has been harmed is able to sue all of the liable parties as a group or any one of them individually. He or she may not, however, recover more compensation by suing each of them individually than by suing them as a group.

77) Which of the following statements best defines the legal term invasion of privacy?
A. A debt, responsibility, or obligation.
B. An unwarranted appropriation or exploitation of another's private affairs with which the public has no legitimate concern; a wrongful intrusion into one's private activities in such a manner as to cause mental suffering, shame, or humiliation to a person of ordinary sensibilities.
C. A complication that is commonly associated with a procedure but is not the result of negligence of the operator (physician, nurse, or other provider performing the procedure or treatment).
D. A contractual arrangement between the insurer and the provider of service; it is typically contained in a managed care contract. This provision specifies that the provider assumes the liability for covered services and cannot sue or assert any claims against enrollees for those covered services, even if the managed care organization becomes insolvent.
E. An obligation of a group and its individual members. The party that has been harmed is able to sue all of the liable parties as a group or any one of them individually. He or she may not, however, recover more compensation by suing each of them individually than by suing them as a group.

78) Which of the following statements best defines the legal term liability?
A. A debt, responsibility, or obligation.
B. An unwarranted appropriation or exploitation of another's private affairs with which the public has no legitimate concern; a wrongful intrusion into one's private activities in such a manner as to cause mental suffering, shame, or humiliation to a person of ordinary sensibilities.
C. A complication that is commonly associated with a procedure but is not the result of negligence of the operator (physician, nurse, or other provider performing the procedure or treatment).
D. A contractual arrangement between the insurer and the provider of service; it is typically contained in a managed care contract. This provision specifies that the provider assumes the liability for covered services and cannot sue or assert any claims against enrollees for those covered services, even if the managed care organization becomes insolvent.
E. An obligation of a group and its individual members. The party that has been harmed is able to sue all of the liable parties as a group or any one of them individually. He or she may not, however, recover more compensation by suing each of them individually than by suing them as a group.

79) Which of the following statements is (are) true, regarding the False Claims Act?
1. It has both civil and criminal penalties.
2. It prohibits the presentation of false claims to the U.S. government.
3. Penalties for violation include substantial fines and imprisonment.
4. The Act is targeted only at physicians.
    A. 1, 3
    B. 2, 4
    C. 1, 2, 3
    D. All of the above
    E. None of the above

80) Which of the following statements is (are) not true, regarding the False Claims Act?
1. It prohibits the presentation of false claims to the U.S. government.
2. Physical therapists are exempt from this Act.
3. Penalties for violation include substantial fines and imprisonment.
4. The Act is targeted only at physicians.
    A. 1, 3
    B. 2, 4
    C. 1, 2, 3
    D. All of the above
    E. None of the above

81) Which of the following statements best defines the legal term liable?
A. A failure on the part of the managed care organization to exercise reasonable care in screening and selecting providers
B. A failure to use such care in making a referral, as a reasonable professional would use under similar circumstances; referring a patient to a provider who does not possess the skills, experience, licensure, or certifications to care for that patient
C. A failure to use the degree of care a reasonably prudent and careful person would use under similar circumstances
D. A contractual arrangement between a purchaser and a provider; in this arrangement, the provider is obligated to render products or services to the purchaser at the same rate as his or her most favored customer
E. Bound by law or fairness; responsible; accountable

82) Which of the following statements best defines the legal term most favored nation clause?
   A. A failure on the part of the managed care organization to exercise reasonable care in screening and selecting providers
   B. A failure to use such care in making a referral, as a reasonable professional would use under similar circumstances; referring a patient to a provider who does not possess the skills, experience, licensure, or certifications to care for that patient
   C. A failure to use the degree of care a reasonably prudent and careful person would use under similar circumstances
   D. A contractual arrangement between a purchaser and a provider; in this arrangement, the provider is obligated to render products or services to the purchaser at the same rate as his or her most favored customer
   E. Bound by law or fairness; responsible; accountable

83) Which of the following statements best defines the legal term negligence?
   A. A failure on the part of the managed care organization to exercise reasonable care in screening and selecting providers
   B. A failure to use such care in making a referral, as a reasonable professional would use under similar circumstances; referring a patient to a provider who does not possess the skills, experience, licensure, or certifications to care for that patient
   C. A failure to use the degree of care a reasonably prudent and careful person would use under similar circumstances
   D. A contractual arrangement between a purchaser and a provider; in this arrangement, the provider is obligated to render products or services to the purchaser at the same rate as his or her most favored customer
   E. Bound by law or fairness; responsible; accountable

84) Which of the following statements best defines the legal term negligent referral?
   A. A failure on the part of the managed care organization to exercise reasonable care in screening and selecting providers
   B. A failure to use such care in making a referral, as a reasonable professional would use under similar circumstances; referring a patient to a provider who does not possess the skills, experience, licensure, or certifications to care for that patient
   C. A failure to use the degree of care a reasonably prudent and careful person would use under similar circumstances
   D. A contractual arrangement between a purchaser and a provider; in this arrangement, the provider is obligated to render products or services to the purchaser at the same rate as his or her most favored customer
   E. Bound by law or fairness; responsible; accountable

85) Which of the following statements best defines the legal term negligent credentialing?
   A. A failure on the part of the managed care organization to exercise reasonable care in screening and selecting providers
   B. A failure to use such care in making a referral, as a reasonable professional would use under similar circumstances; referring a patient to a provider who does not possess the skills, experience, licensure, or certifications to care for that patient
   C. A failure to use the degree of care a reasonably prudent and careful person would use under similar circumstances
   D. A contractual arrangement between a purchaser and a provider; in this arrangement, the provider is obligated to render products or services to the purchaser at the same rate as his or her most favored customer
   E. Bound by law or fairness; responsible; accountable

86) Which of the following components are necessary to constitute a malpractice incident?
1. A deviation from the approved and accepted standards of care
2. A violation of federal law
3. An injury to the patient that resulted from negligence
4. A violation of criminal law
    A. 1, 3
    B. 2, 4
    C. 1, 2, 3
    D. All of the above
    E. None of the above

87) Which of the following components are not necessary to constitute a malpractice incident?
1. A deviation from the approved and accepted standards of care
2. A violation of federal law
3. An injury to the patient that resulted from negligence
4. A violation of criminal law
    A. 1, 3
    B. 2, 4
    C. 1, 2, 3
    D. All of the above
    E. None of the above

88) Which of the following statements best describes the legal term ombudsman?
    A. A person whose occupation consists of investigating customer complaints against his or her employer
    B. An agreement between two litigants to settle the contested matter privately, without being referred to the judge for authorization or approval, before the court has rendered its decision
    C. The quality or condition of being secluded from the presence or view of others; the state of being free from unsanctioned intrusion
    D. Information that a person authorized to practice medicine, nursing, counseling, and so on acquires in attending to a patient in a professional capacity and which is necessary to enable him or her to act in that capacity
    E. A doctrine of law in which mere proof that an occurrence took place is sufficient under the circumstances to shift the burden of proof upon the defendant to prove that it was not due to his or her negligence

89) Which of the following statements best describes the legal expression out of court settlement?
    A. A person whose occupation consists of investigating customer complaints against his or her employer
    B. An agreement between two litigants to settle the contested matter privately, without being referred to the judge for authorization or approval, before the court has rendered its decision
    C. The quality or condition of being secluded from the presence or view of others; the state of being free from unsanctioned intrusion
    D. Information that a person authorized to practice medicine, nursing, counseling, and so on acquires in attending to a patient in a professional capacity and which is necessary to enable him or her to act in that capacity
    E. A doctrine of law in which mere proof that an occurrence took place is sufficient under the circumstances to shift the burden of proof upon the defendant to prove that it was not due to his or her negligence

90) **Which of the following statements best describes the legal term privacy?**
   A. A person whose occupation consists of investigating customer complaints against his or her employer
   B. An agreement between two litigants to settle the contested matter privately, without being referred to the judge for authorization or approval, before the court has rendered its decision
   C. The quality or condition of being secluded from the presence or view of others; the state of being free from unsanctioned intrusion
   D. Information that a person authorized to practice medicine, nursing, counseling, and so on acquires in attending to a patient in a professional capacity and which is necessary to enable him or her to act in that capacity
   E. A doctrine of law in which mere proof that an occurrence took place is sufficient under the circumstances to shift the burden of proof upon the defendant to prove that it was not due to his or her negligence

91) **Which of the following statements best describes the legal term privileged communication?**
   A. A person whose occupation consists of investigating customer complaints against his or her employer
   B. An agreement between two litigants to settle the contested matter privately, without being referred to the judge for authorization or approval, before the court has rendered its decision
   C. The quality or condition of being secluded from the presence or view of others; the state of being free from unsanctioned intrusion
   D. Information that a person authorized to practice medicine, nursing, counseling, and so on acquires in attending to a patient in a professional capacity and which is necessary to enable him or her to act in that capacity
   E. A doctrine of law in which mere proof that an occurrence took place is sufficient under the circumstances to shift the burden of proof upon the defendant to prove that it was not due to his or her negligence

92) **Which of the following statements best describes the legal expression res ipsa loquitor?**
   A. A person whose occupation consists of investigating customer complaints against his or her employer
   B. An agreement between two litigants to settle the contested matter privately, without being referred to the judge for authorization or approval, before the court has rendered its decision
   C. The quality or condition of being secluded from the presence or view of others; the state of being free from unsanctioned intrusion
   D. Information that a person authorized to practice medicine, nursing, counseling, and so on acquires in attending to a patient in a professional capacity and which is necessary to enable him or her to act in that capacity
   E. A doctrine of law in which mere proof that an occurrence took place is sufficient under the circumstances to shift the burden of proof upon the defendant to prove that it was not due to his or her negligence

93) **Which of the following statements are true concerning the legal term res ipsa loquitor?**
   1. It translates from Latin as "The thing speaks for itself."
   2. It proves that the defendant was negligent.
   3. It infers that the defendant was negligent.
   4. It translates from Latin as "Let the master answer."
      A. 1, 3
      B. 2, 4
      C. 1, 2, 3
      D. All of the above
      E. None of the above

94) **Which of the following statements are not true concerning the legal term res ipsa loquitor?**
   1. It translates from Latin as "The thing speaks for itself."
   2. It proves that the defendant was negligent.
   3. It infers that the defendant was negligent.
   4. It translates from Latin as "Let the master answer."
      A. 1, 3
      B. 2, 4
      C. 1, 2, 3
      D. All of the above
      E. None of the above

95) **Which of the following statements best describes the legal expression statute of limitations?**
   A. This maxim means that a master is liable, in certain cases, for the wrongful acts of his or her servant (and a principal for those of his or her agent). A master–servant or principal–agent relationship exists in which one person, for pay or other valuable consideration, enters into the service of another and devotes his or her personal labor for an agreed period.
   B. The period of time in which a plaintiff may bring lawsuit after an incident has occurred
   C. A judicial process requiring a witness to give relevant information or testimony "under penalty" of contempt for disobedience
   D. A document issued by the plaintiff's attorney which, when properly delivered, commences a legal action
   E. The legal liability that a person may have for the actions of someone else

96) **Which of the following statements best describes the legal expression respondeat superior?**
   A. This maxim means that a master is liable, in certain cases, for the wrongful acts of his or her servant (and a principal for those of his or her agent). A master–servant or principal–agent relationship exists in which one person, for pay or other valuable consideration, enters into the service of another and devotes his or her personal labor for an agreed period.
   B. The period of time in which a plaintiff may bring lawsuit after an incident has occurred
   C. A judicial process requiring a witness to give relevant information or testimony "under penalty" of contempt for disobedience
   D. A document issued by the plaintiff's attorney which, when properly delivered, commences a legal action
   E. The legal liability that a person may have for the actions of someone else

97) **Which of the following statements best describes the legal expression summons?**
   A. This maxim means that a master is liable, in certain cases, for the wrongful acts of his or her servant (and a principal for those of his or her agent). A master–servant or principal–agent relationship exists in which one person, for pay or other valuable consideration, enters into the service of another and devotes his or her personal labor for an agreed period.
   B. The period of time in which a plaintiff may bring lawsuit after an incident has occurred
   C. A judicial process requiring a witness to give relevant information or testimony "under penalty" of contempt for disobedience
   D. A document issued by the plaintiff's attorney which, when properly delivered, commences a legal action
   E. The legal liability that a person may have for the actions of someone else

98) **Which of the following statements best describes the legal expression vicarious liability?**
   A. This maxim means that a master is liable, in certain cases, for the wrongful acts of his or her servant (and a principal for those of his or her agent). A master–servant or principal–agent relationship exists in which one person, for pay or other valuable consideration, enters into the service of another and devotes his or her personal labor for an agreed period.
   B. The period of time in which a plaintiff may bring lawsuit after an incident has occurred
   C. A judicial process requiring a witness to give relevant information or testimony "under penalty" of contempt for disobedience
   D. A document issued by the plaintiff's attorney which, when properly delivered, commences a legal action
   E. The legal liability that a person may have for the actions of someone else

99) **Which of the following statements is (are) true regarding the legal term respondeat superior?**
   1. It translates as "Let the master answer."
   2. It proves negligence on the part of the defendant.
   3. It holds that in certain circumstances, the employer is responsible for wrongful acts committed by the employee.
   4. It translates as "The thing speaks for itself.""
      A. 1, 3
      B. 2, 4
      C. 1, 2, 3
      D. All of the above
      E. None of the above

100) **Which of the following statements is (are) not true regarding the legal term respondeat superior?**
   1. It translates as "Let the master answer."
   2. It proves negligence on the part of the defendant.
   3. It holds that in certain circumstances, the employer is responsible for wrongful acts committed by the employee.
   4. It translates as "The thing speaks for itself."
      A. 1, 3
      B. 2, 4
      C. 1, 2, 3
      D. All of the above
      E. None of the above

101) Which of the following statements is (are) true regarding the legal term tort?
1. It comes from a Latin word that means "twist."
2. It implies that testimony has been given falsely.
3. It refers to damage or injury that is done willfully or negligently.
4. It refers only to medical malpractice cases.
    A. 1, 3
    B. 2, 4
    C. 1, 2, 3
    D. All of the above
    E. None of the above

102) Which of the following statements is (are) not true regarding the legal term tort?
1. It comes from a Latin word that means "twist."
2. It implies that testimony has been given falsely.
3. It refers to damage or injury that is done willfully or negligently.
4. It refers only to medical malpractice cases.
    A. 1, 3
    B. 2, 4
    C. 1, 2, 3
    D. All of the above
    E. None of the above

103) A request by an insured or a provider to re-review a denial of a utilization review organization's decision is also known as
1. An appeal
2. A reconsideration
3. An expedited appeal
4. An IME
    A. 1, 2
    B. 1, 3
    C. 1, 4
    D. All of the above
    E. None of the above

104) As a result of the case of *Wickline v. State of California*, which of the following is true?
1. Providers can be held accountable for negative outcomes when they discharge patients solely at the request of the insurer or payer.
2. Case Managers can be held liable for negative outcomes as a consequence of their denials.
3. Insurers or utilization review firms can be held liable for negative outcomes as a consequence of their denials.
4. If a provider appeals an adverse determination and a negative outcome occurs, the liability may be passed to the insurer.
    A. 1, 2, 3
    B. 2, 3, 4
    C. All of the above
    D. None of the above

105) _____ refers to the Case Manager having a duty to promote good and to be the patient's advocate.
   A. Nonmaleficence
   B. Beneficence
   C. Advocacy
   D. None of the above

106) **Dual relationships refers to**
   A. The relationship between the Case Manager and the physician
   B. The relationship in which the Case Manager has more than one role in respect to a patient, subordinate, or student
   C. The relationship between the Case Manager and the patient and his or her family
   D. None of the above

107) **The court case of *Wickline v. State of California* found**
   1. Medical doctors have a duty to protest adverse determinations by payers.
   2. Medical doctors can shift their liability to payers if they do protest adverse determinations.
   3. Case Managers are not liable for their roles in adverse determinations.
   4. Payers of health care can be held accountable, if their adverse decisions are arbitrary, for cost containment, and are not based on acceptable medical standards of practice in the community.
      A. 1, 2, 3
      B. 2, 3, 4
      C. 1, 2, 4
      D. None of the above

108) **In a malpractice suit the plaintiff must prove two points:**
   1. His or her compliance with the prescribed treatment plan
   2. Negligence on the part of the Case Manager
   3. Injury from the Case Manager's negligence
   4. Intent on the part of the Case Manager
      A. 1, 4
      B. 2, 3
      C. None of the above
      D. All of the above

109) **The Case Manager can reduce his or her potential for liability by**
   1. Purchasing case management liability insurance
   2. Keeping the lines of communication open between the patient, family, provider, and him- or herself
   3. Educating the patient and family and testing for understanding
   4. Empowering the patient to participate in planning his or her care
   5. Documenting all discussions with the patient, family, and his or her caregivers
      A. 1, 2, 3, 4
      B. 2, 3, 4, 5
      C. All of the above
      D. None of the above

110) Which of the following is (are) true?
   1. Case Managers may use their nursing license in any state when managing cases telephonically, regardless of which state they are licensed in.
   2. Malpractice insurance does not cover Case Manager activities wherever the Case Manager performs them.
   3. The NCSBN has issued a policy stating that "telenursing" is not covered by the nurse's state board of nursing.
   4. Case Managers who provide case management services either on site or telephonically/electronically outside their state of licensure are violating the law.
      A. 1, 3
      B. 2, 4
      C. All of the above
      D. None of the above

111) The interstate compact does all the following except
   1. Limits a nurse's licensure requirements
   2. Prohibits her or him from practicing nursing in any state but her or his home state
   3. Is exactly like a driver's license, allowing the nurse to practice in any state
   4. Organizes the nurse's multistate licenses
      A. 1, 3
      B. 2, 4
      C. All of the above
      D. None of the above

112) Which of the following is (are) true of the interstate compact?
   1. Limits a nurse's licensure requirement to that of the state she or he resides in
   2. Allows the nurse to practice nursing in any participating compact state
   3. Is modeled after the driver's license, allowing the nurse to practice in participating compact states
   4. Decreases the administrative tasks for maintaining multistate licensure
      A. 1, 3
      B. 2, 4
      C. All of the above
      D. None of the above

113) Which of the following statements best describes the necessary components of medical record security?
   1. Creating policy and procedures that ensure only the Case Manager can view and manipulate a patient's medical record
   2. Providing an environment where patients' medical records can be stored securely when not in use (e.g., locking filing cabinets or a secure room used only by Case Managers)
   3. Making sure that unneeded or closed medical records are thoroughly destroyed (e.g., providing Case Managers with document shredders or employing a certified document destruction service)
   4. Backing up all electronic records daily, having an offsite storage facility and a well-designed document recovery plan in place
      A. 1, 3
      B. 2, 4
      C. 1, 2, 3
      D. All of the above
      E. None of the above

114) **Which of the following is (are) true regarding recommendations for the security of paper medical records?**
 1. Paper medical records should only be used in the case management office and should not be left unattended on a desk or kept in briefcases.
 2. Paper records should, as much as possible, have the patient's name, address, and diagnosis on every page.
 3. Paper medical records should be stored in a locked cabinet when not in use.
 4. Paper medical records can safely be disposed of by maintenance workers in the office trash bin.
    A. 1, 3
    B. 2, 4
    C. 1, 2, 3
    D. All of the above
    E. None of the above

115) **Of the following statements, which describe how a Case Manager should handle electronic medical records?**
 1. Electronic records should be accessed through a password known only to the Case Manager.
 2. All electronic records should be stored in an encrypted file format.
 3. Physical access to a Case Manager's computer should be limited by both a policy that restricts the area to Case Managers only and by having all Case Managers' computers in a separate room that can be locked when not in use.
 4. All electronic medical records should be backed up and stored safely on site, where the computers can be accessed and repaired easily.
    A. 1, 3
    B. 2, 4
    C. 1, 2, 3
    D. All of the above
    E. None of the above

NOTES

Appendix 3-B

Principles of Practice Answers

1) **ANSWER: D**

2) **ANSWER: C**

3) **ANSWER: C**
Case management files are the only files in the preceding list that are considered medical records.

4) **ANSWER: B**
A Case Manager can decrease the risk of allegations of breach of confidentiality by fully understanding the following: the implications of federal and state regulations on the disclosure of medical information; that venereal diseases, abortion, mental illness, and substance abuse are very sensitive topics and transferring such information should only be done after discussing it with the patients and attorneys; and that a patient has the right to refuse all information release.

5) **ANSWER: A**
A Case Manager can decrease the risk of allegations of breach of confidentiality by fully understanding the following: the implications of federal and state regulations on the disclosure of medical information; that venereal diseases, abortion, mental illness, and substance abuse are very sensitive topics and transferring such information should only be done after discussing it with the patients and attorneys; and that a patient has the right to refuse all information release.

6) **ANSWER: D**

7) **ANSWER: B**
When obtaining consent the provider is obligated to disclose the following: the desired outcome, all reasonably foreseeable risks and hazards of treatment, and all reasonable options for care, including the option not to treat, with its foreseeable consequences.

8) **ANSWER: D**

9) **ANSWER: C**
Although consulting with an attorney may be necessary in rare cases, it is unnecessary in every case.

10) **ANSWER: A**
Competence is assumed in most patients. In rare cases when the patient's competence is questioned, an affidavit from a physician attesting to competence will do. A patient must be an adult (under applicable state law) to give consent.

CHAPTER THREE

11) **ANSWER: B**
Emancipated minors are considered adults under most state laws. Consent must be given freely, without coercion.

12) **ANSWER: C**

13) **ANSWER: B**

14) **ANSWER: C**

15) **ANSWER: C**
Interviewing the employer for medical information is inappropriate.

16) **ANSWER: D**
Case Managers should not be dealing with patients' attorneys but should refer attorneys to their legal representative. Although the interests of the employer and insurance carrier are important, the first priority is the patient; the Case Manager is the patient's advocate.

17) **ANSWER: D**
Discourteous behaviors, communication failures, lack of patient understanding, and lack of family understanding are the most common causes of malpractice litigation. Malpractice litigation stems more commonly from poor relationships with patients than from negligent medical care.

18) **ANSWER: B**
For some, it is surprising that bad clinical outcomes and negligent medical care are not common causes of malpractice litigation. In fact, studies have demonstrated that patients rarely identify most substandard medical care, and most bad clinical outcomes are not litigated. Discourteous behaviors, communication failures, lack of patient understanding, and lack of family understanding are the most common causes of malpractice litigation. Malpractice litigation stems more commonly from poor relationships with patients than from negligent medical care.

19) **ANSWER: A**
For some, it is surprising that bad clinical outcomes and negligent medical care are not common causes of malpractice litigation. In fact, studies have demonstrated that patients rarely identify most substandard medical care, and most bad clinical outcomes are not litigated. Discourteous behaviors, communication failures, lack of patient understanding, and lack of family understanding are the most common causes of malpractice litigation. Malpractice litigation stems more commonly from poor relationships with patients than from negligent medical care.

20) **ANSWER: D**
When malpractice is alleged, the Case Manager is commonly accused of negligence in the following areas: premature discharge, bad faith claims denials, negligent patient assessment, negligent referral, invasion of privacy, breach of confidentiality, and treatment without informed consent.

21) **ANSWER: A**
When malpractice is alleged, the Case Manager is commonly accused of negligence in the following areas: premature discharge, bad faith claims denials, negligent patient assessment, negligent referral, invasion of privacy, breach of confidentiality, and treatment without informed consent. Approval of claims and admissions to hospitals do not carry a high malpractice risk.

Principles of Practice 123

22) **ANSWER: B**
The Case Manager has an obligation of "reasonable care" to the patient. Failing to ensure that the discharge is "safe" would be negligent on the part of the Case Manager. Reducing medical costs or utilization of services is not associated with decreased risk of litigation.

23) **ANSWER: A**
The Case Manager has an obligation of "reasonable care" to the patient. Failing to ensure that the discharge is "safe" would be negligent on the part of the Case Manager. Reducing medical costs or utilization of services is not associated with decreased risk of litigation.

24) **ANSWER: B**
Bad faith claims occur when there is no reasonable basis for denial of benefits or when long, purposeful delays in benefit adjudication result in de facto denials. Activities that decrease delays and increase communication with the client will decrease allegations of dealing in bad faith.

25) **ANSWER: B**
Bad faith claims occur when there is no reasonable basis for denial of benefits or when long, purposeful delays in benefit adjudication result in de facto denials. Activities that decrease delays and increase communication with the client will decrease allegations of dealing in bad faith.

26) **ANSWER: D**

27) **ANSWER: E**

28) **ANSWER: D**

29) **ANSWER: A**

30) **ANSWER: C**
Case Managers are liable for damages if their referral of patients to providers is negligently performed and harm comes to the patient as a direct result of that referral.

31) **ANSWER: B**

32) **ANSWER: D**
All these items are the common causes for malpractice litigation.

33) **ANSWER: A**
Ethics are the rules or standards that govern the conduct of a person or members of a profession. Ethical rules describe a society's ideal of how a person or professional should conduct himself or herself.

34) **ANSWER: B**
Ethics are the rules or standards that govern the conduct of a person or members of a profession. Ethical rules describe a society's ideal of how a person or a professional should conduct himself or herself. Thoughts that govern a person's conduct are not necessarily ethical or virtuous.

35) **ANSWER: D**
Ethical and legal principles are closely related because both are based on what a given society values as an appropriate standard of conduct. Legal duties are what a society describes as the minimum acceptable standards of conduct. A legal duty usually carries a punishment for those whose conduct falls below its standards. Ethical duties, on the other hand, represent a

society's conception of the ideal conduct for an individual or a profession. Lapses in ethical behavior, to the extent that the behavior is also not illegal, usually are not punishable outside of a professional society. In general, the demands of ethical duties usually exceed those of legal duties. For example, the AMA holds that in the rare instances when legal duties and ethical duties are in conflict, a professional's ethical duties should supersede his legal duties.

36) ANSWER: E

Ethical and legal principles are closely related because both are based on what a given society values as an appropriate standard of conduct. Legal duties are what a society describes as the minimum acceptable standards of conduct. A legal duty usually carries a punishment for those whose conduct falls below its standards. Ethical duties, on the other hand, represent a society's conception of the ideal conduct for an individual or a profession. Lapses in ethical behavior, to the extent that the behavior is also not illegal, usually are not punishable outside of a professional society. In general, the demands of ethical duties usually exceed those of legal duties. For example, the AMA holds that in the rare instances when legal duties and ethical duties are in conflict, a professional's ethical duties should supersede his legal duties.

37) ANSWER: A

An ethical dilemma exists where two or more equally desirable outcomes are in conflict.

38) ANSWER: B

An ethical dilemma exists when two or more equally desirable outcomes are in conflict.

39) ANSWER: D

40) ANSWER: B

41) ANSWER: B

The ethical principle of justice implies the upholding of what is just, in accordance with honor, standards, or law, and is derived from the Case Manager's sense of moral rightness. The qualities of kindness and charity are associated with the ethical principle of beneficence.

42) ANSWER: A

The ethical principle of justice implies the upholding of what is just or fair, in accordance with honor, standards, or law, and is derived from the Case Manager's sense of moral rightness. The qualities of kindness and charity are associated with the ethical principle of beneficence.

43) ANSWER: B

The ethical principal of autonomy asks the Case Manager to encourage the client to make his or her own well-informed decisions. Nonmaleficence is an amplification of beneficence, and this principle requires the Case Manager not only do good by doing a good job but also actively seek to prevent harm from coming to the patient. It requires the Case Manager to show the patient the course of action that will result in the best outcome.

44) ANSWER: A

The ethical principal of autonomy asks the Case Manager to encourage the client to make his or her own well-informed decisions. Nonmaleficence is an amplification of beneficence, and this principle requires the Case Manager not only do good by doing a good job but also actively seek to prevent harm from coming to the patient. It requires the Case Manager to show the patient the course of action that will result in the best outcome.

Principles of Practice   125

45) **ANSWER: A**
The ethical principle of justice implies the upholding of what is just or fair, in accordance with honor, standards, or law, and is derived from the Case Manager's sense of moral rightness. The qualities of accuracy, precision, and truth are associated with the ethical principle of veracity.

46) **ANSWER: B**
The ethical principle of justice implies the upholding of what is just or fair, in accordance with honor, standards, or law, and is derived from the Case Manager's sense of moral rightness. The qualities of accuracy, precision, and truth are associated with the ethical principle of veracity.

47) **ANSWER: A**

48) **ANSWER: A**
Ethical rules are meant to be a challenge to the individual or professional, and they represent the ideal behaviors toward which one should strive.

49) **ANSWER: B**
Ethics represent the highest standards of personal or professional behavior. Lapses in ethical behavior usually are not punishable outside of the professional society. Legal infractions, which represent lapses in the minimum standards for behavior, are punishable by society.

50) **ANSWER: A**
In a situation in which two or more equally desirable outcomes are in conflict, an ethical dilemma exists. By definition, ethical dilemmas do not depend on lack of knowledge, money, or skills of the decision maker.

51) **ANSWER: E**
Although being knowledgeable about ethics, medical care, and healthcare systems is helpful in avoiding violation of ethical principles and achieving the best results for one's clients, true ethical dilemmas, by definition, have no solution (a solution being defined here as a single answer that accommodates all equally deserving and conflicting outcomes). One may make a decision that accommodates one party and results in one desirable outcome. However, the other equally desirable outcomes do not occur, and the other deserving parties are disenfranchised. This is the inescapable result of decisions in ethical dilemmas.

52) **ANSWER: A**

53) **ANSWER: D**
The prudent Case Manager should be aware of a patient's intellectual, educational, psychological, social, religious, cultural, and financial status. Any of these may present barriers to the patient's medical care, compliance, and ability to follow up with providers as an outpatient.

54) **ANSWER: D**
The prudent Case Manager should understand a patient's intellectual, educational, psychological, social, religious, cultural, and financial status. Any of these may present barriers to the patient's medical care, compliance, and ability to follow up with providers as an outpatient.

55) **ANSWER: A**
A Case Manager can decrease the risk of allegations of negligent assessment by understanding the network's credentialing criteria; refusing to make personal recommendations for providers; providing the names of several providers rather than a single provider when

asked for a recommendation; and reporting all suspicious, illegal, or unethical provider behavior to the proper authorities.

56) **ANSWER: B**
A Case Manager can decrease the risk of allegations of negligent assessment by understanding the network's credentialing criteria; refusing to make personal recommendations for providers; providing the names of several providers rather than a single provider when asked for a recommendation; and reporting all suspicious, illegal, or unethical provider behavior to the proper authorities.

57) **ANSWER: C**
Agency is defined as the relationship between two or more persons by which one (the principal) consents that the other (the agent) shall act on his or her behalf. There are legal obligations for both the agent and the principal.

58) **ANSWER: C**
The agent has the following legal obligations to the principal: using care and skill, acting in good faith, staying within the limits of the agent's authority, obeying the principal and carrying out all reasonable instructions, advancing the interests of the principal, and acting solely for the principal's benefit. The agent should not act solely for his or her own benefit, nor should he or she assume authority not assigned him or her under the contract.

59) **ANSWER: A**
Apparent authority implies that a person or corporation has no direct assignment of authority or agency, such as occurs in a written or verbal contract. However, when the principal is held to have given "apparent authority" to the agent, the principal will be held responsible for the agent's actions.

60) **ANSWER: B**
Both the ward nurse and the Case Manager are employed by an entity that grants them authority to act in a certain capacity. They are both agents of the hospital and insurance company, respectively. The physician who works in the community and the patient of the Case Manager are independent agents, who work for their own best interests.

61) **ANSWER: A**
Both the utilization review departments and the phlebotomists are employed by an entity that grants them authority to act in a certain capacity. They are both, by definition, agents. The physician who works in the community and the network physician are independent agents, who work for their own best interests. A Case Manager must be wary of recommending specific network physicians to patients, as this may then be construed as a principal–agent relationship.

62) **ANSWER: A**
The termination of a professional relationship (physician–patient, Case Manager–patient) without reasonable notice to the patient and without an opportunity for the patient to acquire alternative care or services, thereby resulting in injury to the patient, constitutes the legal definition of abandonment.

63) **ANSWER: B**
The termination of a professional relationship (physician–patient, Case Manager–patient) without reasonable notice to the patient and without an opportunity for the patient to acquire alternative care or services, thereby resulting in injury to the patient, constitutes the legal definition of abandonment.

Principles of Practice 127

64) **ANSWER: D**
65) **ANSWER: E**
66) **ANSWER: C**
67) **ANSWER: B**
68) **ANSWER: A**
69) **ANSWER: E**
70) **ANSWER: D**
71) **ANSWER: C**
72) **ANSWER: B**
73) **ANSWER: A**
74) **ANSWER: E**
75) **ANSWER: D**
76) **ANSWER: C**
77) **ANSWER: B**
78) **ANSWER: A**
79) **ANSWER: C**
The False Claims Act is a federal act providing for civil and criminal penalties against individuals who knowingly present false claims to the government. The criminal False Claims Act makes it illegal to present a claim upon or against the United States the claimant knows to be false, fictitious, or fraudulent. The civil False Claims Act says that any person who knowingly presents, or causes to be presented, to the U.S. government a false or fraudulent claim for payment approval, or knowingly makes, uses, or causes to be made or used a false record or statement to get a false or fraudulent claim paid or approved by the government by getting a false or fraudulent claim allowed or paid, violates the Act. The penalties for violation include substantial fines and imprisonment. The Act does not exclude or exempt any party from prosecution or penalties.

80) **ANSWER: B**
The False Claims Act is a federal act providing for civil and criminal penalties against individuals who knowingly present false claims to the government. The criminal False Claims Act makes it illegal to present a claim upon or against the United States that the claimant knows to be false, fictitious, or fraudulent. The civil False Claims Act says that any person who knowingly presents, or causes to be presented, to the U.S. government a false or fraudulent claim for payment approval, or knowingly makes, uses, or causes to be made or used a false record or statement to get a false or fraudulent claim paid or approved by the government by getting a false or fraudulent claim allowed or paid, violates the Act. The penalties for violation include substantial fines and imprisonment. The Act does not exclude or exempt any party from prosecution or penalties.

81) **ANSWER: E**
82) **ANSWER: D**

83) **ANSWER: C**

84) **ANSWER: B**

85) **ANSWER: A**

86) **ANSWER: A**
Malpractice is a professional negligence that has two components. The first is negligence or a deviation from the approved and accepted standards of care, as defined within a given specialty. The second is injury or damage to the patient as a result of the stated negligence or deviation from the standard of care.

87) **ANSWER: B**
Malpractice is a professional negligence that has two components. The first is negligence or a deviation from the approved and accepted standards of care, as defined within a given specialty. The second is injury or damage to the patient as a result of the stated negligence or deviation from the standard of care. It does not require a violation of federal or criminal law.

88) **ANSWER: A**

89) **ANSWER: B**

90) **ANSWER: C**

91) **ANSWER: D**

92) **ANSWER: E**

93) **ANSWER: A**
A doctrine of law with reference to cases where mere proof that an occurrence took place is sufficient under the circumstances to shift the burden of proof upon the defendant to prove that it was not due to his or her negligence. Implied in this doctrine is that the instrumentality causing injury was in the defendant's exclusive control and that the accident was one that ordinarily does not happen in the absence of negligence. An example of res ipsa loquitor is when a patient is found to have a surgical instrument left in his or her abdomen after an appendectomy. (Assuming only one surgeon was involved, of course.)

94) **ANSWER: B**
A doctrine of law with reference to cases where mere proof that an occurrence took place is sufficient under the circumstances to shift the burden of proof upon the defendant to prove that it was not due to his or her negligence. Implied in this doctrine is that the instrumentality causing injury was in the defendant's exclusive control and that the accident was one that ordinarily does not happen in the absence of negligence. An example of res ipsa loquitor is when a patient is found to have a surgical instrument left in his or her abdomen after an appendectomy. (Assuming only one surgeon was involved, of course.) Respondeat superior translates as "Let the master answer."

95) **ANSWER: B**

96) **ANSWER: A**

97) **ANSWER: D**

98) **ANSWER: E**

99) **ANSWER: A**
This maxim holds that a master is liable, in certain cases, for the wrongful acts of his or her servant (and a principal for those of his or her agent). A master–servant or principal–agent relationship exists in which one person, for pay or other valuable consideration, enters into the service of another and devotes his or her personal labor for an agreed period (for example, employee–employer).

100) **ANSWER: B**
This maxim holds that a master is liable, in certain cases, for the wrongful acts of his or her servant (and a principal for those of his or her agent). A master–servant or principal–agent relationship exists in which one person, for pay or other valuable consideration, enters into the service of another and devotes his or her personal labor for an agreed period (for example, employee–employer).

101) **ANSWER: A**
The word tort comes from the Latin *torquêre*, to twist, and implies injury. In law, a tort is a damage, injury, or a wrongful act done willfully, negligently, or in circumstances involving strict liability—a legal wrong committed upon the person or property independent of contract. It may be either a direct invasion of some legal right of the individual, an infraction of some public duty by which special damage accrues to the individual, or the violation of some private obligation by which like damage accrues to the individual. Torts are not specific to medical malpractice cases.

102) **ANSWER: B**
The word tort comes from the Latin *torquêre*, to twist, and implies injury. In law, a tort is a damage, injury, or a wrongful act done willfully, negligently, or in circumstances involving strict liability—a legal wrong committed upon the person or property independent of contract. It may be either a direct invasion of some legal right of the individual, an infraction of some public duty by which special damage accrues to the individual, or the violation of some private obligation by which like damage accrues to the individual. Torts are not specific to medical malpractice cases.

103) **ANSWER: A**
An expedited appeal may be requested if an urgent need exists for a particular service or treatment. An IME is an independent medical exam and is most often used in workers' compensation or disability cases.

104) **ANSWER: C**
Case Managers should aggressively seek all data necessary to make an informed decision that is in the best interests of their patient.

105) **ANSWER: B**

106) **ANSWER: B**
Dual relationship is a term that reflects the conflict between the Case Manager and another individual due to the nature of having more than one role with the individual. An example of this is being the Case Manager and the mother of the patient.

107) **ANSWER: C**
Case Managers are liable for damages if their referral of patients to providers is negligently performed and harm comes to the patient as a direct result of that referral.

108) **ANSWER: B**

109) **ANSWER: B**

All these strategies will assist the Case Manager in building a positive relationship with the patient. Poor relationships are one of the foremost reasons for litigation. The first answer, purchasing case management liability insurance, is effective after one has a malpractice case but will not reduce one's potential for liability.

110) **ANSWER: B**

Nurse Case Managers must obey all laws. The practice of nursing is regulated on a state-by-state basis. Practicing outside the state of licensure is a violation punishable by law and not covered by malpractice insurance carriers.

111) **ANSWER: D**

The interstate compact limits licensure requirements to the nurse's state of residence and allows the nurse to practice in any participating compact state without additional licenses.

112) **ANSWER: C**

The interstate compact limits licensure requirements to the nurse's state of residence and allows the nurse to practice in any participating compact state without additional licenses. Presently, only 20 states participate, with three more states pending implementation.

113) **ANSWER: D**

114) **ANSWER: A**

Paper records in the possession of Case Managers should not be left on a desk or in a briefcase where they can be viewed by unauthorized personnel or lost. The Case Manager should limit the use of patient and provider names on paper records when possible. The use of file numbers and/or provider and patient code numbers is recommended. Access to the area in which paper records are stored should be limited. Only those who "need to know" should have this access. The area in which paper records are stored should be locked when not in use. They should be stored in a secure area when not being used. Filing cabinets and desk drawers containing sensitive records should be locked when unattended. Case Managers should personally destroy (not simply discard) paper records when they are no longer needed. Paper shredders should be readily available in the case management area, preferably at each Case Manager's work station. Alternatively, a certified document destruction service can be employed to handle these sensitive files.

115) **ANSWER: C**

Electronic medical records should be backed up and stored at a site distant from the place where Case Managers work to prevent loss of patient records due to fire, theft, or natural disaster.

CHAPTER 4

Psychosocial Aspects

PSYCHOSOCIAL AND NEUROLOGICAL ASSESSMENT

A complete medical evaluation should be performed before psychological testing to rule out underlying medical conditions that may cause behavioral symptoms (e.g., chronic subdural hematoma, frontal lobe tumors, Cushing's syndrome, hypothyroidism, neurosyphilis, and Parkinson's disease). After a physiological cause has been ruled out, a comprehensive psychological assessment should be performed. Comprehensive testing may use "self-report questionnaires." These questionnaires are standardized, validated tools that patients fill out by themselves. The Minnesota Multiphasic Personality Inventory (MMPI/MMPI-A) and cognitive and intellectual problem solving, such as the Wechsler Intelligence Scales, are common types of these tools. This type of psychological assessment is different from an assessment derived from an interview with a mental health professional in that the self-administered examination provides a different type of data and allows flexibility in the timing and geography of its administration.

An experienced professional will use the results from a variety of psychological tests to come to a diagnostic conclusion. A psychological diagnosis should be based on an array of data. These data should include the results of an independent medical evaluation, personal interviews, a detailed review of all available psychiatric records, and the administration of a comprehensive set of psychological tests to confirm or rule out a diagnosis. The review of such standardized psychological data allows others to examine the objective basis for the diagnosis and confirm or refute the conclusions.

BEHAVIORAL HEALTH AND PSYCHIATRIC DISABILITY CONCEPTS

The 1990 Americans with Disabilities Act (ADA) is a civil rights law that prohibits, under certain circumstances, discrimination against individuals with disabilities. The Act defines a disability as a "physical or mental impairment that substantially limits one or more major life activities." Among its other benefits, the enactment of ADA afforded protection to individuals with psychiatric disabilities in the workplace. The ADA also protects those who may not currently have a disabling impairment but have a history of such impairment or have an employer who believes that the employee has such impairment.

Because of widespread abuses, in 1999 the Supreme Court severely limited the number of people who can claim coverage under the ADA. The court narrowed the ADA's definition of disability, including who is covered and to what extent the limitation is covered that results from the person's physical or mental impairment. The Court held that these issues must be assessed while considering any mitigating measures, including medication. The State of California enacted legislation that further protects people with disabilities under the California Fair Employment and Housing Act (FEHA). When the Supreme Court narrowed its interpretation of the ADA definition of disability, California widened its definition under the FEHA to state that the impact of any limitations on major life activities due to physical or mental impairment is to be assessed without regard to mitigating measures. They also stated the limitation need only make achievement of a major life activity "difficult." Therefore, a person with a diagnosed major clinical syndrome who functions quite well while taking medication may not be covered under the ADA. However, the same person would be covered under the FEHA, as long as the major clinical syndrome alone, without medication, makes achievement of a major life activity difficult. When making a determination of mental disorder or defect, the courts generally rely on psychologists or psychiatrists.

The accepted standard criteria for psychiatric diagnoses are delineated in the *Diagnostic and Statistical Manual of Mental Disorders*, fourth edition (DSM-IV), published by the American Psychological Association. The DSM-IV is a compilation of common definitions and criteria sets for classifying mental disorders. It helps clinicians make consistent diagnoses of these disorders. The DSM-IV defines a mental disorder as involving a clinically significant behavioral or psychological pattern or syndrome occurring in an individual that is associated with one or more of the following conditions:

1. The individual experiences subjective distress, such as anxiety or depression.
2. The individual is impaired in one or more important areas of life functioning, such as the ability to work or care for oneself or one's family.
3. The individual may experience a significantly increased risk of disability, injury, or loss of freedom.
4. The behavioral syndrome is not an expected response to a normal stressful event, such as a brief episode of depression after the death of a loved one.

The DSM-IV further parses a diagnosis into five dimensions or axes that describe different aspects of that disorder or disability[1]:

Axis I: Clinical disorders, including major mental disorders, and learning disorders, substance use disorders. These disorders frequently require acute treatment.

Axis II: Personality disorders and developmental disorders, such as mental retardation.

Axis III: Acute medical conditions and physical disorders that may influence the psychiatric condition.

Axis IV: Psychosocial and environmental factors contributing to the disorder, such as loss of a job or the death of a family member.

Axis V: Global Assessment of Functioning. Axis V is usually recorded as a number on a scale of 0 to 100, where 100 is top level functioning.

The most frequent mental disorders that may find protection under the ADA and FEHA are the clinical syndromes of mood disorders, anxiety disorders, and psychotic disorders, including diagnoses such as panic disorder, posttraumatic stress disorder, major depression, and bipolar affective disorder. It also should be noted that some clinical syndromes are specifically not covered under the ADA, including illegal drug use, drinking at work, and criminal pathologies, such as compulsive stealing or setting fires (i.e., kleptomania and pyromania). These disorders are listed in the DSM-IV under Axis I, the major clinical syndromes. Axis II, personality disorders, are described as enduring and rigid patterns of behavior, thinking, and feeling that are maladaptive and may lead to distress of oneself and/or others, such as a paranoid or antisocial personality.

As is noted above, psychiatric diagnoses are organized on a matrix of five axes, and a patient may have overlapping diagnoses. Appendix G provides a brief overview of the axes, and Appendix F provides the Global Assessment of Functioning scale used in Axis V. Axis V is used for reporting the clinician's judgment of the overall level of the individual's functioning. This system of assessment is useful in creating a plan of care and measuring and evaluating its success.

FAMILY DYNAMICS

Experienced Case Managers realize their focus in a case rarely ends with the patient alone but extends to the patient's family. The patient's family becomes the primary caregiver and, in many cases, becomes the medical decision maker for patients who are minors or who are rendered incompetent by virtue of their injury or illness. The Case Manager needs to work with the family to provide better care for the patient. They need to understand the family and how it functions to reach their case management goals. Relating well to the family and empathizing with the stressful conditions that illness or injury bring are indispensable tools. This understanding will make communication easier and help the patient and family through their difficult period. The following section outlines some of the issues of family dynamics during a patient illness.

Adaptive and Maladaptive Families

Some families are remarkably adaptable in crisis situations. When a catastrophic illness affects a family member, families that successfully care for the patient and are able to weather the crisis intact have similar characteristics. Successful families are flexible in their roles within the family, are able to maintain the ability to solve problems, communicate with each other and outsiders effectively, seek out and accept help, and maintain their relationship with the community:

- *Flexible family roles:* Adaptive families appreciate that the sick family member cannot perform his or her own jobs in the home. Further, they realize the sick person creates new jobs within the family, which include taking care of the patient's activities of daily living and managing his or her medications, doctor's visits, and therapy sessions. Adaptive families share the new roles equally so as not to overburden one family member.
- *Problem solving:* Adaptive families are not passive. They do not wait for someone to tell them what to do to solve the problems that an ill family member creates. They quickly identify the problems and seek internal or external resources to solve them.

- *Communication:* When a family is able to openly discuss the problems they have identified, such as fears, unequal or unsustainable work burdens, or financial needs, they are able to share more of the work and have more people involved in finding solutions.
- *Seek and accept help:* Families may come to realize the problems encountered cannot be handled with the resources within the family. Adaptive families put aside reticence and a misplaced sense of pride and actively seek help from their community support network, from charities, support organizations, or paid professionals. When help is offered they accept it readily and incorporate it into their care plan.
- *Community relationships*: Both the patient and the family can become cut off from the community due to the demands of giving care or from grief or fatigue. The adaptive family realizes their community can be a source of physical, emotional, and financial support and as such needs to be engaged rather than avoided.

Maladaptive families, on the other hand, are unable to achieve a balance between meeting a patient's needs and maintaining their own functioning. These families may overindulge the patient and foster his or her dependency. In caring for the sick family member, maladaptive families may ignore or mistreat other family members. Conversely, maladaptive families may abandon or ignore the patient. They may deny the existence of the patient's illness or disability to the patient's detriment. In some cases one family member (such as a mother, wife, or husband) accepts all responsibility as the patient's caretaker. She or he performs all the work for the ill family member. Most frequently, this responsibility falls on a female member of the household. The other family members remain inflexible in their roles and do not, or cannot, help out.

An example is a family whose child is severely disabled and requires constant care. The mother of the child takes on all the additional work of caring for the child. This usually includes cleaning and changing the patient, preparing the patient's special diet, administering medications, and taking the patient to physicians and therapists. In this maladaptive family the husband does not relieve the caretaker of other duties to balance her workload, such as helping out with the chores at home, such as cooking, cleaning, shopping, or entertaining the other children. He views these chores as "women's work" and beneath his status. This caretaker (mother/wife) may find it difficult to perform all these duties and may become angry and bitter at the husband and other family members who are not "helping out." In this setting the caretaker and the patient become isolated, and both suffer in the process. Such maladaptive patterns stem from a family's inability to communicate effectively with each other, with care providers, or with support networks. Additionally, they fail to seek and accept help, to maintain flexibility in role relationships, and to retain relationships with the community.

The following questions can help the Case Manager determine how the family will deal with the catastrophically ill patient:

- Are there other sick family members at home?
- Have there been any in the past?
- How does the family treat these sick family members?
- How did the family function during this illness?

- How have other family crises (financial, social, political) been dealt with in the past?
- Who is available for caregiving?
- What are responsibilities for that potential caregiver now? (Does he or she have a job, other children, or elderly parents to care for?)
- What social or community resources can be brought to bear? Does the local senior center have a geriatric program to which that parent can attend? Can the local church provide a volunteer to help clean the house or do shopping for the family?
- What financial resources can be brought to bear?
- Is there a leader in the family? (Matriarch? Patriarch?)
- Are there any healthcare professionals in the family?
- What is the level of understanding about the disease or injury?
- What is the level of understanding about the course of treatment?
- What is the level of understanding about the prognosis?
- What is the level of understanding about possible limitations, disabilities, or handicaps the patient may experience?

MULTICULTURAL ISSUES AND HEALTH BEHAVIOR

It is important for the Case Manager to recognize that patients do not abandon their cultural and religious beliefs when they enter the healthcare system. Sometimes, these beliefs conflict with the treatment plan as outlined by the healthcare team. For the Case Manager to be successful in developing a trusting, effective relationship with the patient, the Case Manager needs to understand and respect the patient's beliefs.

According to the National Center for Cultural Competence, "Nowhere are the divisions of race, ethnicity and culture more strongly drawn than in the health of the people of the United States."[2] Data from the 2010 census showed that only 79.4% of U.S. households use English as the language spoken at home.[3] Approximately 13% speak Spanish and 3% speak Asian/Pacific languages.[3] The Census Bureau conducted a survey in 2010[3] that determined 12.5% of people in the United States are foreign-born. This trend is expected to continue.[4]

If treatment plans and case management interventions are to have favorable outcomes and increase patient participation and patient satisfaction, it is important for the Case Manager to understand the following:

- The patient's attitudes toward seeking help from healthcare providers
- Any culturally based belief systems of the etiology of illness and disease and those related to health and healing
- Culturally defined, health-related needs of individuals, families, and communities
- Beliefs, values, traditions, and practices of a culture, especially those that deal with treatment of illnesses

Knowledge of customs and healing traditions are indispensable to the creation of effective treatment plans and case management interventions. After all, healthcare services must be received and accepted to be successful.[5]

Although there are many resources on specific cultural beliefs, such as the National Center for Cultural Healing,[6] the Case Manager must not forget that each patient is an individual. Each individual has a unique intellect, education, and acculturation. Each brings his or her own experience and belief systems.

The following are some examples of cultural beliefs about disease and healing:

- For Americans of northern European extraction, treatment choices are influenced by their sense of empowerment and control. Typically, this type of patient prizes his autonomy and his right to be informed about his condition, its possible treatments, and his ability to choose or refuse life-prolonging medical care. They see advance directives for health care as a way to insure that their wishes concerning end-of-life care are enforced even when they are no longer able to speak for themselves. They are most likely to accept narcotic analgesics, request assisted death, and refuse life-sustaining care.[7]
- Self-identified Hispanic families tend to provide a great deal of emotional strength and social support to the patient. They will be very concerned over the effect of the illness or injury on the family. Because they generally hold physicians in high regard, they tend to defer to the physician's judgment and not challenge or dispute the treatment plan. The Case Manager has an advantage, as these families are more likely to inform the Case Manager than the physician of any problems with the treatment plan.
- Mexican Americans are more likely than other groups to attribute breast cancer to breast fondling and breast trauma. Other Hispanics believe sinful behaviors, such as the abuse of drugs and alcohol, are the cause of breast cancer. Latin immigrants believe that intercourse during menstruation contributes to cervical cancer.[8]
- African Americans may harbor a distrust of the medical profession and they do not readily seek professional medical care. Some blame this mistrust on a history of abuses that include slaves being used in medical research, deception, and mistreatment (such as in the Tuskegee syphilis study), abuses from sickle cell screening, and minority-focused sterilization in the 1970s.[8,9] African Americans tend to be more likely to believe physicians and other healthcare providers make treatment decisions based on personal profit motives rather than the best interests of their patients.
- Many Asian Pacific Americans believe the family should guide important medical decisions. Many Korean Americans believe the family should make all decisions about life support. Children, especially the eldest son, are charged with the duty to preserve their parents' lives by all means. How the family cares for the sick and elderly is a matter of family pride and given great scrutiny by relatives and the community. These cultural values can affect end-of-life care. For example, the children may refuse to stop life support even when it is deemed hopeless, or accept hospice care for a dying parent as it would appear to some in the community that they are shirking their "filial duty." Additionally, because some believe the spirit inhabits the site of death, a home death is desirable.
- Chinese custom forbids a person from forgoing aggressive medical treatment or seeking an assisted suicide. Children are thought to be rewarded in the present or next life for taking all life-extending measures for their parents. Taoism, Buddhism, and Confucianism, on the other hand, embrace death as a natural event, and those patients who forgo life-sustaining treatments so their families don't suffer are viewed as compassionate.

As one can see, culture influences treatment options, how people seek health care, and how they respond to healthcare providers. It is important for the Case Manager to be aware during each interaction with the patient of possible cultural challenges to see the entire picture and provide culturally competent care with good outcomes. As much as possible, it is helpful for the Case Manager to explore these beliefs and, when possible, work within the limits set by them.

PSYCHOLOGICAL ASPECTS OF CHRONIC ILLNESS AND DISABILITY

Case Managers know from firsthand experience what a "change agent" an episode of illness can be to a patient, not just in the physical sense but also psychologically. The illness does not need be as "catastrophic" as metastatic cancer to cause serious changes in a person's life. A carpenter who suffers from arthritis of the hands, a dancer who suffers from vertigo, and a professional athlete who injures a knee are examples of patients whose injuries, although not considered catastrophic by most, have serious effects beyond the physical realm and into the social and psychological spheres. These patients have not just suffered an illness or painful injury, they have also lost careers, hopes, dreams, social status, and income. As a further example, a father of three who because of illness is no longer the breadwinner for the family experiences more than the pain and disability of his illness; he also suffers the loss of self-respect, social status, and independence.

Case Managers who hope to intervene successfully in these situations must assess the effects of the illness or injury beyond the patient's physical self. The assessment must explore what limitations, disabilities, and effects on sense of self, relationships, employment, interests, hopes, and aspirations this illness brings. As a result of these life changes precipitated by major illness and injury, patients commonly experience

- Loss
- Anger
- Fear/anxiety
- Depression
- Dependency

If anticipated by the Case Manager, and noted early, these reactions can be treated with education, support, counseling, and, in some cases, medication. During the intake interview the Case Manager can ask questions that may help determine the patient's response to his or her current situation:

- Have you ever (personally) suffered from a serious injury or illness in the past?
- Have you ever had a serious illness in your family?
- How did you deal with these situations?
- Do you know anyone with this type of illness?
- How did they deal with it?
- What do you know about your current disease?
- What do you know about its treatments?
- What do you know about its prognosis?
- What do you know about possible limitations, disabilities, or handicaps that are sometimes associated with it?
- How do you feel about these?
- What do you believe will happen to you?
- Do you believe you'll be limited, handicapped, or disabled?
- What are your plans for dealing with these disabilities and limitations?

Effects of a Patient's Illness and Injury on Family and Caregivers

A holistic approach to the care of a patient dictates the Case Manager examine the environment the patient is in and how this environment can be used to support and heal the patient during his or her illness. Catastrophic illness and injuries have "ripple effects" that extend outward from the patient and exert their profound effects on his or her environment. The environment, in turn, has effects on the patient. Those closest to the patient and those most dependent on the patient are likely to suffer the greatest amount of turmoil. For example, let us examine the hypothetical case of Mr. Green.

Mr. Green is a 32-year-old partner in a business. He is a husband and father of four children. While vacationing with his family at a ski resort, he collides with a tree and sustains a fracture of his cervical spine. After several days his spinal cord injury stabilizes, and he is diagnosed with quadriplegia. The neurosurgeons and rehabilitation specialists report that after a long period of rehabilitation, he may be able to return home and, perhaps, even work. During his inpatient stay at the rehabilitation hospital, the following questions may be asked by the patient's family and friends:

Questions asked by his wife:
- Will my husband's disabilities diminish or grow worse?
- Will he suffer?
- Will he die?
- Will I have to live alone the rest of my life?
- What will we do for income?
- Who will pay the bills?
- Will I have to go to work?
- What can I do to earn an income?
- Will I ever be able to match my husband's income?
- Do we have enough insurance?
- What does his disability policy allow?
- If I go to work, who will watch the children?
- Will the children have to come out of private schools?
- What about contributions to their college funds?
- If I go to work, who will do the shopping, cleaning, and household chores?
- Can we still afford the house mortgage and taxes?
- Will we have to move?
- Can we afford the payments on the cars?
- Will we have to sell the cars?
- What will I do for transportation?
- Will we have to purchase a specialized van to transport my husband?
- With all the attention on my husband, will the children feel neglected?

Questions asked by his children:
- Will Daddy die?
- Will Mommy remarry?
- Will he ever come home?
- Will he have to stay in the wheelchair?
- If I hug him, will it hurt him?
- Will he ever be happy again?
- Will he ever be able to play with me?

- Will we have to move from our home?
- Will we have to leave school?
- Who will rake the leaves and take out the garbage?
- Who will play with the little kids in the family?
- What if something happens to Mommy?
- Could Mommy get sick and die?
- What will happen to us?

Questions asked by his business partners:
- Will he ever return to work?
- What will we do without his expertise?
- Can the business survive?
- What happens if we replace him, and he wants to come back to work?
- What if he wants to sell his share of the business? Can we afford to buy him out?
- Can we afford to pay him while he rehabilitates? Do we have to?
- What will happen to the clients who depend on Green's critical skills for their business to go forward?
- What will happen to the suppliers who depend on Green for businesses to go forward?

Questions asked by his parents:
- What can we do to help our son and his family?
- Can we afford to pay their expenses?
- Do we have enough room for them to live with us?
- Can we live comfortably with his wife and children?
- What if our son dies?
- What about our retirement and our "golden years"?
- Is there any end in sight to these responsibilities?
- Will our helping out our son's family jeopardize or deplete our retirement savings?
- What happens to us when our money's gone? What will happen to our son's family?
- Who will help us? (We were hoping that our son could help us out in our retirement.)
- Who will help out our daughter? (We were hoping that our son could care for his handicapped, dependent sister who lives with us, when we are gone.)

These types of questions can go on and on. The number of people affected by a catastrophic illness is surprisingly large. The family (or caretakers) may also suffer from the symptoms of loss, anger, anxiety, fear, depression, and dependency. The well-tempered Case Manager should be aware of the impact of catastrophic illness on the family and friends of the patient. These are the same people who may be asked to lend the patient financial, social, and psychological support in the future.

Chronic Disease

The Centers for Disease Control and Prevention (CDC) reports[10] 7 of 10 deaths among Americans each year are from chronic diseases. In 2005, 133 million Americans—almost one of every two adults—had at least one chronic disease.

Diabetes

The incidence of diabetes in the U.S. is staggering. Approximately 25 million people in the United States have diabetes.[11] Seven million of these people are undiagnosed. In 2010 approximately 1.9 million new cases were diagnosed in people age 20 or younger. Diabetes was the seventh leading cause of death listed on U.S. death certificates in 2007. If this continues one of three adults in the United States will have diabetes by 2050. Among adults, diabetes is the leading cause of new cases of blindness, kidney failure, and amputations not related to accidents or injury. Diabetics have a shorter life expectancy and about twice the risk of dying on any given day as a person of similar age without diabetes. Financially, the total cost of diabetes (direct and indirect) in 2007 was $174 billion.

Heart Disease and Stroke

Heart disease and stroke are the leading killers in the United States. They are the first leading cause of death for men and third for women. Cardiovascular diseases account for more than one-third of U.S. deaths.[12] More than 83 million U.S. adults currently live with one or more types of cardiovascular disease. An estimated 935,000 heart attacks and 795,000 strokes occur each year. Nearly 68 million adults have high blood pressure, and about half are not well controlled. An estimated 71 million adults have high cholesterol, and two of three do not have this under control.

Chronic Obstructive Pulmonary Disease

In 2005 chronic obstructive pulmonary disease caused an estimated 126,005 U.S. deaths in people older than 25 years.[13] This was an increase of 10,000 from the year 2000. In the United States the key factor in the development and progression of chronic obstructive pulmonary disease is tobacco use. Asthma, air pollutants, obesity, genetic factors, and respiratory infections also play a role.

Implications

These are just some of the statistics that are driving our healthcare costs up, our patients' quality of life down, and a growing trend in legislation to address chronic disease population management. Modifiable behaviors can help reduce chronic disease. Per the CDC, more than one-third of adults do not meet the recommendations for aerobic exercise, less than 24% of adults and 22% of high school students do not get the recommended five or more servings of fruit and vegetables per day, and 20% of high school students smoke tobacco.

Today more than ever there is a growing focus on chronic disease management. Case Managers are positioned and ready for this challenge. Case Managers are already serving patients with chronic illnesses, especially when their disease processes put them in need of hospitalizations, equipment, home care, and so on. Case Managers need to use their skills cooperatively with the patient, family, and provider to assist the patient to self-management with the goal of controlling and/or slowing down the progression of the disease process and improving the patients' life. This will lead to improved outcomes, increased patient satisfaction, and reduced healthcare costs.

Hypothetical Case of Mrs. Rodriguez

Mrs. Rodriguez is an 82-year-old Hispanic woman who has lived alone since her husband died 10 years ago. She has three grown children who live in the local area. She sees one daughter, Maria, every few days. Mrs. Rodriguez speaks and reads both English and Spanish but prefers Spanish. She is alert and oriented but does not make decisions easily. She never worked outside her home and has a Medicare card because her husband worked. She also participates in the state's Medicaid program. She has about $500 in savings and lives on her Supplemental Security Income check with some assistance from her children. She lives in a very small second-floor apartment and has resisted moving to a first-floor apartment as suggested by her daughter.

Her diagnoses are as follows:

    Diabetes type 2 for 25 years
    Hypertension for 34 years
    Coronary artery disease for 14 years
    Heart failure for 12 years
    Depression for 9 years
    Osteoarthritis for 16 years
    Retinopathy

Despite the fact that Mrs. Rodriguez has multiple disease processes and medications to take on a daily basis, she has always considered herself in good health but recently is rating her health as "fair." She has few outside contacts. She reports that most of her friends have died, are too ill to visit, or have moved away to live with relatives. Her parish priest visits weekly because she is having trouble getting out of her apartment to church.

The Case Manager receives a referral from Mrs. Rodriguez's primary care provider after a hospital admission for a change in mental status. She was diagnosed as having a delirium caused by hypoglycemia, constipation, and dehydration. Mrs. Rodriguez couldn't remember whether she ate lunch or dinner. She stated she felt bloated for a few days and hadn't felt like eating but believes she took her medications as prescribed. In the hospital she was hydrated, given an enema, fed, and observed overnight. She was released the next morning to the care of her daughter Maria.

The Case Manager contacts Mrs. Rodriguez and learns that Mrs. Rodriguez keeps all her medications in one shoebox. In this shoebox Mrs. Rodriguez has kept every medication she has ever been prescribed so that if she needs it again it hasn't been "wasted." She monitors her blood glucose twice a day but doesn't write it down. She has been having increased knee pain and taking Percocet two to three times every day for about 2 weeks. She is not taking any fiber or stool softeners with the pain medication. The vegetables she prefers are mostly starches. She doesn't really like fruit. She has a blood pressure cuff but rarely monitors her blood pressure as the doctor does it on her regular visits to him. She has a scale but hasn't weighed herself in months. She says that "it's too depressing. I can't exercise anyway so what's the point?" She is agreeable to calls from the Case Manager and is receptive to working on some health-related goals "if they help me feel better."

The two main concerns for Mrs. Rodriguez are constipation and pain. With approval from her primary care provider, the Case Manager discusses dietary changes with her. Mrs. Rodriguez agrees to try alternating oatmeal and bran for breakfast. The primary care provider has also advised her to take a stool softener (Colace) daily. She arranges for the local pharmacy to deliver it. Mrs. Rodriguez is in the habit of waiting until her pain is not manageable before she will take her Percocet. The primary care provider orders a nonsteroidal anti-inflammatory medication that she is to take twice a day regularly. She is instructed to take the Percocet as needed for pain, when the pain interferes with her ability to function. At the same time the Case Manager talks to her about an over-the-counter topical analgesic cream she can apply to her knees. Mrs. Rodriguez is doubtful and afraid it will cost too much. After discussion she agrees to ask one of her children if they can buy it for her to try. Mrs. Rodriguez promises to call if she feels bloated or her pain is unmanageable. They agree to talk again in 1 week.

The Case Manager calls Mrs. Rodriguez in 1 week to get an update. Mrs. Rodriguez states she didn't eat the bran because she didn't like it. She did try it but prefers the oatmeal and has been eating that every morning. She states that next time Maria does her shopping she will buy a small box of raisins and try it in the cereal. She states her son bought the topical ointment that contains capsaicin and she has been using it before she goes to bed. She states it helps her to fall asleep faster. She has been taking the stool softener and states she has been moving her bowels regularly every other day. Her knee pain is still present but after taking the nonsteroidal anti-inflammatory medication for 1 week the pain is decreased and she is taking less Percocet: one to two a day at most.

The Case Manager has had a successful beginning with this patient. She began by addressing the patient's most important health issues. She developed rapport and credibility with the patient by doing so. The Case Manager can now work with the patient on her other identified needs: reconciling her medications, keeping a log of her blood glucoses, keeping a log of her blood pressures, weighing herself regularly, discussing symptom triggers that she should use to call the physician or Case Manager, and so on. Regular contact among the Case Manager, the patient, and physician can minimize emergency department visits, hospitalizations, and exacerbations.

HEALTH COACHING

Health coaching has shifted from a traditional education approach to a team approach using motivational interviewing to bring forth behavior changes, such as with patients with multiple health conditions. Dr. Karen Lawson, the program director for the health coaching track at the Center for Spirituality and Healing, University of Minnesota, uses the mnemonic RULE to summarize the guiding principles in motivational interviewing[14]:

R	Resist the righting reflex
U	Understand your patient's motivation
L	Listen
E	Empower

Healthcare professionals tend to be proscriptive, that is, they tell patients what they need to do in order to achieve their health goals. In coaching Case Managers need to assist patients in achieving their own healthcare goals. Patients should be encouraged to choose the goals that mean the most to them. It is the Case Manager's job as a healthcare coach to support, encourage, and empower the patient to grow and take steps to achieve the health goals. Case Managers need to foster a positive environment, assist the patient in recognizing that he or she has choices in how to achieve health goals, and praise the patient along the way toward them.

Health coaching works best with regular face to face meetings or telephone calls. The time, date, and goals for each contact should be mutually agreed on. Meetings or calls should be agreed on by all participants. At the beginning of the session the patient should always confirm that the time is still okay before proceeding.

During coaching sessions the Case Manager should listen more than he or she speaks. The patient should be encouraged to present the issues that concern him or her the most. This will convey to the patient that you are listening, will engender a sense of control, and will put the patient at ease. The Case Manager can use the patient's concerns as a starting place and guide the conversation later on to the provider's or Case Manager's concerns.

Case Managers can be effective as healthcare coaches when managing chronic disease state populations. The goals are the same: self-management, patient satisfaction, and improved outcomes.

Case Managers are trained to think of themselves as the "fixers" of patients. This is especially true in experienced professionals. This can prevent them from empathizing with the patient. Case Managers cannot expect their patients to want a healthier behavior just because everyone should want to be healthier. Case Managers need to understand what motivates their patients. This can only be achieved by listening to what they say. Sometimes patients do not know what truly motivates them or that their behaviors are not in sync with their values. Only through an open discussion can a Case Manager assist patients in seeing these discrepancies and guiding them to appropriate behavioral changes to move them toward their health goals.

SPIRITUALITY AS IT RELATES TO HEALTH BEHAVIOR

Spirituality is a part of most people's lives. In the context of their coping with a chronic or serious illness, spirituality takes on an increased importance. Serious illnesses bring about fears and uncertainties in the patient and can raise some fundamental questions:

- Has my life had meaning and purpose?
- Will my life have meaning and purpose with this new disability?
- What may I hope for in this life?
- Why am I suffering?
- Does my suffering have meaning?
- What happens after I die?

Spirituality can offer comfort and meaning to a patient's life and provide a coping mechanism for his or her suffering. A patient's spirituality can affect his or her quality of life, medical decision making, and medical outcomes. Therefore, spirituality has a bearing on clinical care and case management. Case Managers should be aware of the effects of spirituality on the patient's health and healthcare decisions. They should be responsive to their patients' spiritual needs and observe the appropriate ethical boundaries.

What Is Spirituality?

Spirituality is an individual's experience with the transcendent rather than the material world. Spiritual beliefs are concerned with matters of the spirit, the supernatural, and the eternal, as well as with the meaning and purpose of life. Spirituality may be an aspiration for an understanding of life that is higher, more complex, or more integrated with one's worldview, as contrasted with a life understood only through the experience of the senses.

Is Spirituality Religiosity?

Spirituality is <u>not</u> the same as religiosity or religiousness. Although religiosity today often carries the pejorative connotation of an exaggerated or affected piety and religious zeal, it can also be defined as a belief in, and practice of, the tenets of an organized religion. This latter definition is the one used in this text.

Although spirituality is not religiosity, it is one of the dimensions of religiosity. Other dimensions of religiosity include a belief in the precepts of the religion (e.g., belief in the truthfulness of the Bible) and the practice of the rites and obligations of the religion (e.g., attending services, fasting, or giving to charity).

A spiritual person operating within a religion can be said to experience his or her creator in the world around him or her. For a religious person this experience occurs within the context of orthodox religious beliefs. Although spiritual people can be adherents to traditional and orthodox religions, it does not follow that all spiritual people are religious. A person can have a rich spiritual life and yet exist outside of a formal religion. This spiritual dimension of his or her life can form the basis of a personal belief system that sustains him or her and gives comfort and meaning during his or her life's challenges.

Is Spirituality Important to Patients?

Surveys of primary care physicians and seriously ill patients about their attitudes on spirituality have demonstrated that a majority of both groups considered spirituality important. Further, both groups believe it is important that physicians attend to patients' spiritual concerns. However, few patients in these surveys reported receiving such care. Physicians have been reluctant to engage in spiritual discussions for multiple reasons:

- Lack of time
- Lack of training in this area
- Fear of offending the patient
- Feeling that it is the hospital chaplain's responsibility
- Fear of facing their own existential doubts or religious inadequacies

Physician reluctance to engage the patient in a spiritual discussion provides the Case Manager with an opportunity to address an important unmet need and make an appropriate referral. Appropriate provision of spiritual care within a diverse population of seriously ill outpatients is a complex task that requires sensitive and methodical screening.

Spirituality and Health Outcomes

Spirituality can affect health outcomes. In studies of terminal cancer patients, spiritual well-being was found to offer some protection against end-of-life despair in those for whom death is imminent. When surveyed, those cancer patients who reported a high degree of spiritual well-being were at a decreased risk of a desire for a hastened death, hopelessness, and suicidal ideation. When results were controlled for disease duration, disease severity, and pain, low spiritual well-being was still the strongest predictor of each outcome variable. Additionally, depression was highly correlated with desire for hastened death in participants low in spiritual well-being but not in those high in spiritual well-being. Other studies of depressed patients with chronic illness have shown that a greater intrinsic spirituality independently predicted shorter duration of depressive symptoms in chronically ill patients. Alternatively, certain forms of spirituality may increase the risk of death. According to a medical study of hospitalized elderly men and women, those who held beliefs that their illnesses were the result of divine punishment, work of the devil or demons, or abandonment by God appear to be at increased risk of death, even after controlling for baseline health, mental health status, and demographic factors.

Spirituality and Medical Decision Making

Spirituality and religious beliefs can affect a patient's medical decision making. These beliefs may prohibit certain medical procedures (e.g., Jehovah's Witnesses and blood transfusions, Catholics and abortion). The spiritual concept of life's meaning and purpose can affect a patient's choice of therapy. Take, for example, a decision to undergo a lifesaving surgery whose likely outcome is a life of disability. If this patient's concept of the purpose of life is to provide for his family and contribute to society, how will that affect his decision to undergo a therapy that will leave him bed-bound and unable to work? Will he be willing to accept a life of dependence? Will this affect his choice of therapy?

Another spiritual concept that can affect medical decision making is the meaning of suffering. Does the patient believe that suffering is ennobling and should be tolerated at all costs? Or is suffering merely an epiphenomenon of the disease process and therefore should be avoided? Should procedures that promote or prolong suffering be avoided, even if they might save the patient's life?

Neglecting the spiritual needs of patients can have a deleterious effect on medical decision making and outcomes. Many patients may be driven away from effective medical treatment when their spiritual issues are ignored or derided by clinical personnel. This tendency is exemplified by a review of the medical records of seriously ill pediatric patients by Asser and Swan.[15] These investigators described the cases of 172 children who died after their parents relied on faith healing instead of standard medicine and found that most of the children would have survived if they had received medical care. Clearly, for some patients spirituality is important in their choice of care, more so than even the efficacy of treatment. If spirituality plays an important role in how some patients decide on treatment and caregivers do not account for it, the decision-making process may be unsatisfactory to all involved.

Spirituality and Role of the Case Manager

The previous discussion demonstrates the importance of spirituality to some patients. A Case Manager, therefore, must be concerned with significant effects on quality of life and health outcomes that result from a patient's spirituality. The Case Manager manifests these concerns by evaluating his or her patient's spirituality and asking about spiritual concerns. With this information in hand, the Case Manager can offer resources for spiritual counseling. The Case Manager who hopes to maximize therapeutic efficacy and improve patient outcomes must respect his or her patients in this manner, especially when the patients' spirituality is a critical life factor.

Taking a Spiritual History

A Case Manager working with a terminally ill patient inevitably plays a role in supporting the patient's inquiry into spiritual questions. A tool created to help this exploration is called a spiritual history. A spiritual history is an inquiry into what gives meaning to a person's life and is one way to understand a patient more fully. It is not a substitute for chaplains or religious counselors. In fact, integral to the spiritual history is an assessment of the need for a referral to chaplains and other spiritual care providers. In addition, it addresses a patient's specific preferences or needs regarding medical care, death, and dying that are based on the patient's religious beliefs.

The key element of the spiritual history is listening to what is important to the patient and being available to the patient while you both explore these issues. This is at the root of compassionate caregiving. Although several versions of the spiritual history exist, they all include specific questions about religious background, beliefs, and desires. An excellent example by Bruce Ambuel[16] is on the following page.

Ethical Boundaries

Although many patients express interest in discussing the spiritual dimensions of their care, not all do. Further, most patients surveyed stated that having caregivers proselytize their own faith would make them uncomfortable. Case Managers should observe boundaries when discussing spirituality:

- Avoid being judgmental of the patient's clinical decisions based on his or her spirituality. This can destroy a relationship that might otherwise survive to offer suggestions and therapeutic alternatives that work within the patient's spiritual beliefs.
- Do not force your religious beliefs on patients. Studies show that patients are neither appreciative of it nor receptive to it. Proselytizing or prescribing religious activities for patients is not recommended or encouraged. Case Managers need to honor the trust patients give them by respecting their patients' autonomy.
- Do not blur the boundaries between case management and spiritual counseling. Although patients with life-altering illnesses may request such counseling, it is best referred to religious professionals. This protects the clinical relationship the Case Manager has established and precludes accusations of a Case Manager using coercion to ensure clinical compliance by dint of an assumed spiritual authority.
- Praying with patients. Studies have shown that many patients with catastrophic illnesses will request that clinicians and other caregivers pray with them. This is a controversial area with bioethicists and others. On the one hand, it is a simple request that may offer solace to the patient and strengthen a caring relationship. On the other hand, some believe it crosses the line between secular caregiver and spiritual counselor. Guidelines

> **BOX 4-1**
>
> **Proselytize:** To convert to some religion, system, opinion, or the like; to bring or cause to come over

TITLE: Taking a Spiritual History
FIRST AUTHOR: Bruce Ambuel, PhD

Taking a Spiritual History

S—spiritual belief system
- Do you have a formal religious affiliation? Can you describe this?
- Do you have a spiritual life that is important to you?
- What is your clearest sense of the meaning of your life at this time?

P—personal spirituality
- Describe the beliefs and practices of your religion that you personally accept. Describe those beliefs and practices that you do not accept or follow.
- In what ways is your spirituality/religion meaningful for you?
- How is your spirituality/religion important to you in daily life?

I—integration with a spiritual community
- Do you belong to any religious or spiritual groups or communities?
- How do you participate in this group/community? What is your role?
- What importance does this group have for you?
- In what ways is this group a source of support for you?
- What types of support and help does or could this group provide for you in dealing with health issues?

R—ritualized practices and restrictions
- What specific practices do you carry out as part of your religious and spiritual life (e.g., prayer, meditation, service)?
- What lifestyle activities or practices does your religion encourage, discourage, or forbid?
- What meaning do these practices and restrictions have for you? To what extent have you followed these guidelines?

I—implications for medical care
- Are there specific elements of medical care that your religion discourages or forbids?
- To what extent have you followed these guidelines?
- What aspects of your religion/spirituality would you like the doctors or nurses to keep in mind as they care for you?
- What knowledge or understanding would strengthen our relationship?
- Are there barriers to our relationship based upon religious or spiritual issues?
- Would you like to discuss religious or spiritual implications of health care?

T—terminal events planning
- Are there particular aspects of medical care that you wish to forgo or have withheld because of your religion/spirituality?
- Are there religious or spiritual practices or rituals that you would like to have available in the hospital or at home?
- Are there religious or spiritual practices that you wish to plan for at the time of death, or following death?
- From what sources do you draw strength in order to cope with this illness?
- For what in your life do you still feel gratitude even though ill?
- When you are afraid or in pain, how do you find comfort?
- As we plan for your medical care near the end of life, in what ways will your religion and spirituality influence your decisions?

have been offered for the middle road and state that praying with patients may occur when

- The patient has initiated the request
- After referral to an appropriate religious counselor has been made
- When other religious personnel are not available

REFERENCES

1. Allpsych (n.d.). From the *Diagnostic and Statistical Manual,* Fourth Edition. Retrieved from http://www.psych.org/mainmenu/research/dsmiv.aspx
2. National Center for Cultural Competence.
3. U.S. Census. Retrieved November 27, 2011, from http://www.census.gov/compendia/statab/2012/tables/12s0041.pdf
4. National Center for Cultural Competence, Georgetown University Center for Child and Human Development, Washington, DC.
5. Ibid.
6. Cultural Healing. Retrieved November 27, 2011, from www.culturalhealing.com/resourcesmain.htm/statab/2012/tables/12s0041.pdf
7. Caralis, P. V., Davis, B., Wright, K., & Marcial, E. (1993). The influence of ethnicity and race on attitude toward advance directives, life prolonging treatments and euthanasia. *Journal of Clinical Ethics, 4,* 155–165.
8. Berger, J. T. (1998). Cultural and ethnicity in clinical care. *Archives of Internal Medicine, 158,* 2085–2090.
9. Dula, A. (1994). African American suspicion of the healthcare system is justified: What do we do about it? *Cambridge Quarterly of Healthcare Ethics, 3,* 347–357.
10. Centers for Disease Control and Prevention. Chronic disease and health promotion. Retrieved October 30, 2011, from http://www.cdc.gov/chronicdisease/overview/index.htm
11. Centers for Disease Control and Prevention. Diabetes. Retrieved October 30, 2011, from http://www.cdc.gov/diabetes/
12. Centers for Disease Control and Prevention. Heart disease and stroke. Retrieved October 30, 2011, from http://www.cdc.gov/dhdsp/
13. Centers for Disease Control and Prevention. COPD. Retrieved October 30, 2011, from http://www.cdc.gov/copd/
14. Lawson, K., & Wolever, R. (2009). *Health coaching for behavior change: Motivational interviewing methods and practice.* Sea Girth, NJ: The Healthcare Intelligence Network, eBook.
15. Asser, S. M., & Swan, R. (1998). Child fatalities from religion-motivated medical neglect. *Pediatrics, 101,* 625–629.
16. Ambuel, B. (2003). Taking a spiritual history #19. *Journal of Palliative Medicine, 6*(6), 932–933.

Appendix 4-A

Psychosocial Aspects Questions

1) Which of the following statements is (are) true regarding the psychological aspects of chronic disease and disability?
   1. Only catastrophic illnesses such as cancer and spinal cord injuries have psychological ramifications.
   2. Even injuries that are usually considered minor can have severe social and psychological ramifications.
   3. Psychological reactions such as euphoria and mania are common in catastrophic illnesses.
   4. Psychological reactions such as depression and dependency are common in catastrophic illnesses.
      A. 1, 3
      B. 2, 4
      C. 1, 2, 3
      D. All of the above
      E. None of the above

2) Which of the following statements is (are) not true regarding the psychological aspects of chronic disease and disability?
   1. Only catastrophic illnesses such as closed head injuries or lymphoma have psychological ramifications.
   2. Even injuries that are usually considered minor can have severe social and psychological ramifications.
   3. Psychological reactions such as euphoria and complacency are common in catastrophic illnesses.
   4. Psychological reactions such as depression and dependency are common in catastrophic illnesses.
      A. 1, 3
      B. 2, 4
      C. 1, 2, 3
      D. All of the above
      E. None of the above

3) Which of the following characteristics is (are) commonly associated with maladaptive families?
   1. An inability to communicate with each other, healthcare providers, and support networks
   2. Fostering dependency in the patient through overindulgence
   3. An inability to maintain flexibility in role relationships
   4. Ignoring or mistreating other family members to accommodate the sick family member
      A. 1, 3
      B. 2, 4
      C. 1, 2, 3
      D. All of the above
      E. None of the above

4) Which of the following statements is (are) true regarding the psychological aspects of catastrophic illness or injury?
   1. Certain illnesses have the same or similar effects on all patients.
   2. Minor illnesses may cause catastrophic physiological reactions in some patients.
   3. Major illnesses and grave prognoses will cause depression in all patients.
   4. A patient's reactions to illness may extend beyond the illnesses' pain and disability and can affect the patient's self-respect and social status.
      A. 1, 3
      B. 2, 4
      C. 1, 2, 3
      D. All of the above
      E. None of the above

5) Which of the following statements is (are) not true regarding the psychological aspects of catastrophic illness or injury?
   1. Certain illnesses have the same or similar effects on all patients.
   2. Minor illnesses may cause catastrophic physiological reactions in some patients.
   3. Major illnesses and grave prognoses will cause depression in all patients.
   4. A patient's reactions to illness may extend beyond the illnesses' pain and disability and can affect the patient's self-respect and social status.
      A. 1, 3
      B. 2, 4
      C. 1, 2, 3
      D. All of the above
      E. None of the above

6) Which of the following reactions do patients with major illness or injury commonly experience?
   1. Loss
   2. Anger
   3. Fear and anxiety
   4. Depression
      A. 1, 3
      B. 2, 4
      C. 1, 2, 3
      D. All of the above
      E. None of the above

7) Which of the following reactions do patients with major illness or injury commonly experience?
   1. Loss
   2. Euphoria
   3. Fear and anxiety
   4. Contentment
      A. 1, 3
      B. 2, 4
      C. 1, 2, 3
      D. All of the above
      E. None of the above

8) Which of the following reactions do patients with major illness or injury not experience?
   1. Loss
   2. Happiness
   3. Fear and anxiety
   4. Peace
      A. 1, 3
      B. 2, 4
      C. 1, 2, 3
      D. All of the above
      E. None of the above

9) Which of the following statements is (are) true regarding how Case Managers deal with patients with catastrophic illness and injury?
   1. Anxiety may be treated with education and counseling.
   2. Severe depression may respond to appropriate antidepressant medication and should be recommended.
   3. Diagnosing depression may require skillful interviewing.
   4. Case Managers should avoid dealing with the psychological aspects of major illnesses.
      A. 1, 3
      B. 2, 4
      C. 1, 2, 3
      D. All of the above
      E. None of the above

10) Which of the following characteristics is (are) commonly associated with maladaptive families?
    1. An inability to communicate with each other, healthcare providers, and support networks
    2. Abandoning the patient
    3. An inability to maintain flexibility in role relationships
    4. Denying the existence of the family member's illness or disability
       A. 1, 3
       B. 2, 4
       C. 1, 2, 3
       D. All of the above
       E. None of the above

152 CHAPTER FOUR

11) Which of the following statements is (are) true regarding how Case Managers deal with patients with catastrophic illness and injury?
    1. Anxiety may be treated with education and counseling.
    2. Severe depression will never respond to antidepressant medication.
    3. Diagnosing depression may require skillful interviewing.
    4. Case Managers should avoid dealing with the psychological aspects of major illnesses.
        A. 1, 3
        B. 2, 4
        C. 1, 2, 3
        D. All of the above
        E. None of the above

12) Which of the following statements is (are) not true regarding how Case Managers deal with patients with catastrophic illness and injury?
    1. Anxiety may be treated with education and counseling.
    2. Severe depression responds only to electroconvulsive therapy, and it should be recommended.
    3. Diagnosing depression may require skillful interviewing.
    4. Case Managers should avoid dealing with the psychological aspects of major illnesses.
        A. 1, 3
        B. 2, 4
        C. 1, 2, 3
        D. All of the above
        E. None of the above

13) Which of the following statements is (are) true regarding patients with catastrophic injuries and illnesses?
    1. The negative effects are felt only by the patient.
    2. The spouse is never affected by the patient's injury.
    3. The Case Manager should restrict his or her inquiries to the patient's reactions, mood, and coping abilities.
    4. A history of adequately coping with major illness is a negative predictor for a patient's future coping ability.
        A. 1, 3
        B. 2, 4
        C. 1, 2, 3
        D. All of the above
        E. None of the above

14) Which of the following statements is (are) true regarding patients with catastrophic injuries and illnesses?
    1. The negative effects are felt by the patient and his or her family, friends, and coworkers, among others.
    2. The spouse is never affected by the patient's injury.
    3. The Case Manager should expand his or her inquiries beyond the patient's reactions, mood, and coping abilities to those of the family, friends, and caretakers.
    4. A history of adequately coping with major illness is a negative predictor for a patient's future coping ability.

A. 1, 3
   B. 2, 4
   C. 1, 2, 3
   D. All of the above
   E. None of the above

15) Which of the following statements is (are) not true regarding patients with catastrophic injuries and illnesses?
    1. The negative effects are felt by the patient and his or her family, friends, and coworkers, among others.
    2. The spouse is never affected by the patient's injury.
    3. The Case Manager should expand his or her inquiries beyond the patient's reactions, mood, and coping abilities to those of the family, friends, and caretakers.
    4. A history of adequately coping with major illness is a negative predictor for a patient's future coping ability.
       A. 1, 3
       B. 2, 4
       C. 1, 2, 3
       D. All of the above
       E. None of the above

16) Which of the following characteristics is (are) commonly associated with maladaptive families?
    1. An inability to communicate with each other, healthcare providers, and support networks
    2. An inability to seek and accept help
    3. An inability to maintain flexibility in role relationships
    4. An inability to retain relationships with the community
       A. 1, 3
       B. 2, 4
       C. 1, 2, 3
       D. All of the above
       E. None of the above

17) Which of the following characteristics is (are) common to the adaptable family?
    1. The family maintains flexibility in its role relationships.
    2. The family maintains its ability to solve problems within the family.
    3. The family communicates with each other and outsiders.
    4. The family seeks and accepts help willingly.
       A. 1, 3
       B. 2, 4
       C. 1, 2, 3
       D. All of the above
       E. None of the above

18) Which of the following characteristics is (are) common to the adaptable family?
    1. The family is inflexible in its role relationships.
    2. The family maintains its ability to solve problems within the family.
    3. The family communicates poorly with each other and outsiders.
    4. The family seeks and accepts help willingly.
        A. 1, 3
        B. 2, 4
        C. 1, 2, 3
        D. All of the above
        E. None of the above

19) Which of the following characteristics is (are) not common to the adaptable family?
    1. The family is inflexible in its role relationships.
    2. The family maintains its ability to solve problems within the family.
    3. The family communicates poorly with each other and outsiders.
    4. The family seeks and accepts help willingly.
        A. 1, 3
        B. 2, 4
        C. 1, 2, 3
        D. All of the above
        E. None of the above

20) Which of the following spiritual questions might a patient with a catastrophic illness ask him- or herself?
    1. Has my life had meaning?
    2. Why is this happening to me?
    3. What is the purpose of my life?
    4. Is this a punishment from God?
        A. 1, 3
        B. 2, 4
        C. 1, 2, 3
        D. All of the above
        E. None of the above

21) Which of the following spiritual questions might a patient with a catastrophic illness ask him- or herself?
    1. Has my life had meaning?
    2. How much will my care cost?
    3. What is the purpose of my life?
    4. Will I be entitled to disability?
        A. 1, 3
        B. 2, 4
        C. 1, 2, 3
        D. All of the above
        E. None of the above

22) Which of the following is (are) true regarding spirituality in patients suffering severe illness or disability?
    1. Spiritual concerns are rarely important to these patients.
    2. Spiritual concerns are regularly addressed by doctors and nurses caring for them.
    3. These patients are always receptive to religious proselytizing.
    4. Spiritual concerns are the same as religious concerns.

A. 1, 3
B. 2, 4
C. 1, 2, 3
D. All of the above
E. None of the above

23) **Ethical boundaries on spiritual discussion include all of the following except**
   1. Avoid being judgmental of clinical decisions based on spiritual beliefs.
   2. Religious proselytizing is appropriate for a Case Manager in this setting.
   3. Case Managers should avoid spiritual counseling while acting as a patient's case manager.
   4. Praying with his or her patient is always appropriate for a Case Manager.
      A. 1, 3
      B. 2, 4
      C. 1, 2, 3
      D. All of the above
      E. None of the above

24) **Ethical boundaries on spiritual discussion include all of the following except**
   1. Being judgmental of clinical decisions based on spiritual beliefs is appropriate in that it may encourage the patient to make a better clinical decision.
   2. Religious proselytizing is inappropriate for a Case Manager in this setting.
   3. Case Managers should provide spiritual counseling while acting as a patient's Case Manager.
   4. Praying with his or her patient is appropriate for a Case Manager only under limited conditions.
      A. 1, 3
      B. 2, 4
      C. 1, 2, 3
      D. All of the above
      E. None of the above

25) **It is appropriate for a Case Manager to pray with her or his patients under which of the following conditions?**
   1. When the patient initiates the request
   2. After an appropriate referral to a chaplain or spiritual counselor has been made
   3. When a chaplain or spiritual counselor is not available
   4. Only when the Case Manager is also a trained religious or spiritual counselor
      A. 1, 3
      B. 2, 4
      C. 1, 2, 3
      D. All of the above
      E. None of the above

26) **It is inappropriate for a Case Manager to pray with her or his patients under which of the following conditions?**
   1. When the Case Manager initiates the request
   2. After an appropriate referral to a chaplain or spiritual counselor has been made
   3. When a chaplain or spiritual counselor is not available
   4. Only when the Case Manager is also a trained religious or spiritual counselor
      A. 1
      B. 2, 4
      C. 1, 2, 3
      D. All of the above
      E. None of the above

27) **Which of the following statements is (are) true regarding a spiritual history?**
    1. Patients are rarely interested in discussing their spiritual issues, so a spiritual history is always inappropriate.
    2. It is an exploration in the meaning and purpose of a patient's life.
    3. It should be administered only by a trained religious or spiritual counselor.
    4. It addresses a patient's specific preferences or needs regarding medical care, death, and dying that are based on his or her religious beliefs.
        A. 1, 3
        B. 2, 4
        C. 1, 2, 3
        D. All of the above
        E. None of the above

28) **Which of the following statements is (are) true regarding a spiritual history?**
    1. Patients are rarely interested in discussing their spiritual issues, so a spiritual history is always inappropriate.
    2. It is an exploration of the patient's finances and ability to pay for medical care.
    3. It should be administered only by a trained religious or spiritual counselor.
    4. It addresses a Case Manager's religious beliefs.
        A. 1, 3
        B. 2, 4
        C. 1, 2, 3
        D. All of the above
        E. None of the above

29) **Which of the following is (are) true regarding spirituality in patients suffering severe illness or disability?**
    1. Spiritual concerns are commonly important to these patients.
    2. Spiritual concerns are rarely addressed by doctors and nurses caring for them.
    3. These patients are rarely receptive to religious proselytizing.
    4. Spiritual concerns are the same as religious concerns.
        A. 1, 3
        B. 2, 4
        C. 1, 2, 3
        D. All of the above
        E. None of the above

30) **A Case Manager is told by a paraplegic, "I feel like half a person." The Case Manager's response should be to**
    A. Distract the patient from self-pity
    B. Help the patient explore personal feelings
    C. Ignore the comment
    D. Actively discourage negative comments

31) **The Case Manager has a patient with a recent amputation. The patient expresses concern that his wife will no longer find him attractive. The Case Manager should realize that**
    A. The patient is in a grieving stage.
    B. The patient is experiencing self-pity, which will pass.
    C. Many patients have a distorted body image when they have an amputation.
    D. All of the above
    E. None of the above

32) A patient has had successful surgery for his or her condition, yet he or she remains anxious and uncertain. The Case Manager should
   A. Explore the patient's concerns and feelings with him or her
   B. Reassure the patient that everything will be fine
   C. Provide recommendations regarding rest and relaxation
   D. A, B
   E. None of the above

33) A variety of cognitive techniques may be used for pain control. Which of the following are examples of these techniques?
   1. Distraction
   2. Pain medication
   3. Relaxation training
   4. Biofeedback
       A. 3, 4
       B. 1, 2, 3
       C. 1, 3, 4
       D. All of the above
       E. None of the above

NOTES

Appendix 4-B

Psychosocial Aspects Answers

1) **ANSWER: B**
The illness does not need to be as "catastrophic" as a closed head injury, a cervical spinal injury, or cancer to cause serious changes in a person's life. A carpenter who loses the use of a hand, a dancer who suffers from vertigo, or a professional athlete who injures a knee are examples of patients whose injuries, although not considered catastrophic by most, have serious effects beyond the physical realm and into the social and psychological spheres. These patients have not just suffered a serious and painful injury but also have lost careers, hopes, dreams, social status, and income. As a result of the life changes precipitated by major illness and injury, patients commonly experience loss, anger, fear and anxiety, depression, and dependency.

2) **ANSWER: A**
The illness does not need to be as "catastrophic" as a closed head injury, a cervical spinal injury, or cancer to cause serious changes in a person's life. A carpenter who loses the use of a hand, a dancer who suffers from vertigo, or a professional athlete who injures a knee are examples of patients whose injuries, although not considered catastrophic by most, have serious effects beyond the physical realm and into the social and psychological spheres. These patients have not just suffered a serious and painful injury but also have lost careers, hopes, dreams, social status, and income. As a result of the life changes precipitated by major illness and injury, patients commonly experience loss, anger, fear and anxiety, depression, and dependency.

3) **ANSWER: D**
Maladaptive families are unable to achieve a balance between meeting a patient's needs and maintaining their own functioning. These families may overindulge the patient and foster dependency. Other family members may be ignored or mistreated in an effort to meet the needs of the sick member. Conversely, maladaptive families may abandon or ignore the patient. They may deny the existence of illness or disability to the detriment of the patient. These patterns stem from a family's inability to communicate effectively with each other, with care providers, or with support networks; seek and accept help; maintain flexibility in role relationships; and retain relationships with the community.

4) **ANSWER: B**
The illness does not need to be as "catastrophic" as a closed head injury, a cervical spinal injury, or cancer to cause serious changes in a person's life. A carpenter who loses the use of a hand, a dancer who suffers from vertigo, or a professional athlete who injures a knee are examples of patients whose injuries, although not considered catastrophic by most, have

serious effects beyond the physical realm and into the social and psychological spheres. These patients have not just suffered a serious and painful injury but also have lost careers, hopes, dreams, social status, and income. Others with the same injury would not necessarily be so profoundly affected. For example, a 90-year-old man who is told that he has prostate carcinoma, which may kill him in 10 years, will not have the same reaction as a 30-year-old man with the same diagnosis. Not every patient has the same reaction to illness or injuries, whether they are minor or catastrophic.

5) **ANSWER: A**
The illness does not need to be as "catastrophic" as a closed head injury, a cervical spinal injury, or cancer to cause serious changes in a person's life. A carpenter who loses the use of a hand, a dancer who suffers from vertigo, or a professional athlete who injures a knee are examples of patients whose injuries, although not considered catastrophic by most, have serious effects beyond the physical realm and into the social and psychological spheres. These patients have not just suffered a serious and painful injury but also have lost careers, hopes, dreams, social status, and income. Others with the same injury would not necessarily be so profoundly affected. For example, a 90-year-old man who is told that he has prostate carcinoma, which may kill him in 10 years, will not have the same reaction as a 30-year-old man with the same diagnosis. Not every patient has the same reaction to illness or injuries, whether they are minor or catastrophic.

6) **ANSWER: D**

7) **ANSWER: A**
As a result of changes precipitated by major illness and injury, patients commonly experience loss, fear and anxiety, depression, dependency, and anger.

8) **ANSWER: B**

9) **ANSWER: C**
As a result of changes precipitated by major illness and injury, patients commonly experience loss, anger, fear and anxiety, depression, and dependency. If anticipated by the Case Manager and noted early, these reactions can be treated with education, support, counseling, and, in some cases, medication. During the intake interview the Case Manager can ask some questions that may help determine the patient's response to his or her current situation.

10) **ANSWER: D**
Maladaptive families are unable to achieve a balance between meeting a patient's needs and maintaining their own functioning. These families may overindulge the patient and foster dependency. Other family members may be ignored or mistreated in an effort to meet the needs of the sick member. Conversely, maladaptive families may abandon or ignore the patient. They may deny the existence of illness or disability to the detriment of the patient. These patterns stem from a family's inability to communicate effectively with each other, with care providers, or with support networks; seek and accept help; maintain flexibility in role relationships; and retain relationships with the community.

11) **ANSWER: A**
As a result of changes precipitated by major illness and injury, patients commonly experience loss, anger, fear and anxiety, depression, and dependency. If anticipated by the Case Manager and noted early, these reactions can be treated with education, support, counseling, and, in some cases, medication. During the intake interview the Case Manager can ask some questions that may help determine the patient's response to his or her current situation.

12) **ANSWER: B**
As a result of changes precipitated by major illness and injury, patients commonly experience loss, anger, fear and anxiety, depression, and dependency. If anticipated by the Case Manager and noted early, these reactions can be treated with education, support, counseling, and, in some cases, medication. During the intake interview the Case Manager can ask some questions that may help determine the patient's response to his or her current situation.

13) **ANSWER: E**
A patient's injury has "ripple effects" that impact family, friends, and coworkers. Because of these ripple effects, the Case Manager must be aware of what is going on in the patient's environment, make what interventions she or he can, and recommend more extensive counseling and education when appropriate. A personal history of effectively coping with a major illness in the past is a positive predictor for a patient's future coping abilities.

14) **ANSWER: A**
A patient's injury has "ripple effects" that impact family, friends, and coworkers. Because of these ripple effects, the Case Manager must be aware of what is going on in the patient's environment, make what interventions she or he can, and recommend more extensive counseling and education when appropriate. A personal history of effectively coping with a major illness in the past is a positive predictor for a patient's future coping abilities.

15) **ANSWER: B**
A patient's injury has "ripple effects" that impact family, friends, and coworkers. Because of these ripple effects, the Case Manager must be aware of what is going on in the patient's environment, make what interventions she or he can, and recommend more extensive counseling and education when appropriate. A personal history of effectively coping with a major illness in the past is a positive predictor for a patient's future coping abilities.

16) **ANSWER: D**
Maladaptive families are unable to achieve a balance between meeting a patient's needs and maintaining their own functioning. These families may overindulge the patient and foster dependency. Other family members may be ignored or mistreated in an effort to meet the needs of the sick member. Conversely, maladaptive families may abandon or ignore the patient. They may deny the existence of illness or disability to the detriment of the patient. These patterns stem from a family's inability to communicate effectively with each other, with care providers, or with support networks; seek and accept help; maintain flexibility in role relationships; and retain relationships with the community.

17) **ANSWER: D**
Some families are remarkably adaptable to these crisis situations. In a crisis situation such as with a catastrophic illness in a family member, successful families are flexible in their roles within the family, maintain the ability to solve problems, communicate with each other and outsiders effectively, accept help, and maintain their relationship with the community. This type of family is able to meet the new needs of a sick member without a loss of balance and functioning.

18) **ANSWER: B**
Some families are remarkably adaptable to these crisis situations. In a crisis situation such as with a catastrophic illness in a family member, successful families are flexible in their roles within the family, maintain the ability to solve problems, communicate with each other and outsiders effectively, accept help, and maintain their relationship with the community.

162 CHAPTER FOUR

This type of family is able to meet the new needs of a sick member without a loss of balance and functioning.

19) **ANSWER: A**
Some families are remarkably adaptable to these crisis situations. In a crisis situation such as with a catastrophic illness in a family member, successful families are flexible in their roles within the family, maintain the ability to solve problems, communicate with each other and outsiders effectively, accept help, and maintain their relationship with the community. This type of family is able to meet the new needs of a sick member without a loss of balance and functioning.

20) **ANSWER: D**

21) **ANSWER: A**
Choices 2 and 4 are financial concerns, and choices 1 and 3 concern spiritual issues.

22) **ANSWER: E**
During episodes of severe or terminal illness, patients often are concerned with spiritual as well as temporal issues. Although most patients are interested in having these issues addressed and believe physicians and nurses should at least discuss their needs, this rarely happens. Patients are rarely receptive to religious proselytizing, no matter how well intentioned. Spirituality and religiosity are not the same. Spirituality can exist outside of organized religions.

23) **ANSWER: B**
Case Managers should avoid being judgmental regarding clinical decisions made as the result of spiritual beliefs. Patients are rarely receptive to religious proselytizing. Spiritual counseling should be performed by professionals trained in that discipline. Case Managers should avoid blurring the lines between their clinical role and a spiritual counseling role. This is the reason praying with patients should be done only in limited conditions.

24) **ANSWER: A**
Case Managers should avoid being judgmental regarding clinical decisions made as the result of spiritual beliefs. Patients are rarely receptive to religious proselytizing. Spiritual counseling should be performed by professionals trained in that discipline. Case Managers should avoid blurring the lines between their clinical role and a spiritual counseling role. This is the reason praying with patients should be done in limited conditions.

25) **ANSWER: C**
Although praying with a seriously ill patient can give a patient solace and strengthen a therapeutic relationship, it can also blur the lines between a clinical relationship and religious coercion. Therefore, it should be encouraged in limited situations, such as when the patient requests it, when a chaplain or other spiritual advisor is not available, and after the Case Manager has made an appropriate referral to same.

26) **ANSWER: A**
Although praying with a seriously ill patient can give a patient solace and strengthen a therapeutic relationship, it can also blur the lines between a clinical relationship and religious coercion. Therefore, it should be encouraged in limited situations, such as when the patient requests it, when a chaplain or other spiritual advisor is not available, and after the Case Manager has made an appropriate referral to same.

27) **ANSWER: B**

28) **ANSWER: E**

29) **ANSWER: C**
During episodes of severe or terminal illness, patients often are concerned with spiritual as well as temporal issues. Although most patients are interested in having these issues addressed and believe physicians and nurses should at least discuss their needs, this rarely happens. Patients are rarely receptive to religious proselytizing, no matter how well intentioned. Spirituality and religiosity are not the same. Spirituality can exist outside of organized religions.

30) **ANSWER: B**
The Case Manager should permit and encourage the patient to explore his or her feelings without judgment, punishment, or rejection.

31) **ANSWER: C**
Many patients are embarrassed or ashamed when their body image changes due to illness or injury.

32) **ANSWER: A**
Communicating openly is always important in relieving anxiety and stress. If this is not done, the patient's anxiety could interfere with his or her recovery.

33) **ANSWER: C**
Pain medication is not a cognitive technique.

CHAPTER 5

Healthcare Management and Delivery

SERVICES AND AVAILABLE RESOURCES

Levels of Care

The Case Manager needs to have a comprehensive understanding of the various types and levels of healthcare services available in the community. This allows him or her to communicate the full range of options available to the patient who requires these services. The various levels of healthcare services represent increasing degrees of worker specialization and technical sophisticated care. The following are some of the different levels of care, other than acute care hospital admission.

Long-Term Care

Long-term care[1] is a level of care for patients (1) who require complex care and extensive convalescence, such as major trauma victims, and (2) with chronic and multiple medical, mental health, and social problems who are unable to take care of themselves. Skilled care of patients over a long period of time is expensive, and the Case Manager should be aware of how this care is financed. When the long-term care is medically necessary and not custodial, private health insurance bears the costs. When insurance limits are reached or the care required is custodial, the primary payer for long-term care is Medicaid. Medicare covers a limited amount of long-term care costs if the care is medically necessary and not considered custodial. Medicare pays 100% of the first 20 days in a skilled nursing facility (SNF) and then 80% up to a total of 100 inpatient days.

Custodial Care

Custodial care is defined by the Centers for Medicare & Medicaid Services as care that is primarily for the purpose of helping clients with their home personal care needs, such as activities of daily living (ADLs); this care could safely and reasonably be supplied by persons without professional skills or training. This type of care can be rendered at many out-of-hospital venues, including in the home, a SNF, a group home, a foster home, a convalescence home, a health-related facility, or an assisted living or senior complex.

Intermediate Care

Intermediate care is a level of care for the patient requiring slightly more assistance than one requiring custodial care. Such patients often need moderate assistance with ADLs and some restorative nursing supervision. Most facilities and insurers make little distinction between this and custodial care unless true skilled care is required.

Skilled Nursing and Subacute Care

Skilled nursing and subacute care[2] is one step down from acute hospital care. The criteria for admission into such a facility are that the patient must be medically stable and that the care required is subacute rather than acute. For an insurer to pay for care at this level, the required care must

- Need to be performed by a skilled, licensed professional
- Be required on a daily basis
- Take place at the SNF for reasons of patient safety and economy. In other words, if the care can be provided at a lesser level (e.g., the patient's home) safely and at a lesser cost, that is where the services should be provided.

Some of the most common reasons for skilled nursing care are frequent or complex wound care, rehabilitation (where the patient cannot participate long enough to qualify for an acute program), complex intravenous (IV) therapy, ventilator weaning, and combination therapies.

Nursing homes, intermediate care facilities, and SNFs all offer a level of care below acute care hospitalization in which the patient requires daily skilled care from licensed personnel. These facilities are known collectively as extended care facilities. It is important for the Case Manager to know the specific policy benefit the patient may have as it relates to extended care. Many insurance policies will not coordinate benefits with Medicare. That is, if the patient is in an extended care facility where Medicare is the primary payer, the private healthcare insurance will not cover the 20% that Medicare does not cover.

Inpatient Rehabilitation

Inpatient rehabilitation is an intense inpatient program for a patient who has a recent functional loss, such as an amputation or a stroke, and is a process aimed at enabling a patient with disabilities to reach and maintain his or her optimal physical, sensory, intellectual, psychiatric, and/or social functioning levels. The goal is for the patient to achieve independence in both living and functioning.

Medicare has strict admission criteria to an inpatient rehabilitation center, and many insurers model their criteria after the Medicare guidelines. Medicare has four main criteria for admittance to an inpatient rehabilitation center[3]:

1. Admitting diagnosis must include one of the following:
    - Amputation
    - Arthritis
    - Cardiac conditions

- Cerebral vascular disorder
- Chronic pain
- Congenital disorder
- Diabetes mellitus
- Fracture
- Head trauma/brain injury
- Multiple traumas
- Musculoskeletal disorder
- Neurological disorder
- Orthopedic condition
- Pulmonary condition
- Spinal cord injury

2. The primary reason for admission must be a recent functional loss. The patient has to have been independent in that function before the injury or illness and must now be dependent on someone else to carry out that function. If a patient had a cerebral vascular accident (CVA) 5 years ago and was totally dependent on others for his ADLs and had a second CVA now, he would not qualify for inpatient rehabilitation at this time. Assuming he had been independent before the first CVA, he would have met the criteria for inpatient rehabilitation 5 years ago.
3. The physician must document the expectation of significant improvement in the functional deficit in a reasonable time frame.
4. If a patient was previously in a rehabilitative program with an unsuccessful outcome, the patient must have some change in his or her condition that would indicate that progress is now possible.

It is important to note that some patients will not go directly from the acute care setting to the rehabilitation center. They do not make this transition because they are unable to endure the intensity of the program. These patients may go to a subacute or SNF setting, where their physical and psychological condition can be improved slowly. For example, they may begin with a half hour of therapy three times a day and increase their participation as their stamina increases. Depending on the amount of therapy available at the subacute facility they may continue there, or, if a more intense program is required, they can be transferred to an inpatient rehabilitation center. Often, unless special programs are necessary, patients such as elderly patients who have suffered a stroke will remain in the subacute setting until they are ready for discharge home. Generally, patients with brain trauma, spinal cord injuries, and multiple traumatic injuries need to slowly progress to an intense rehabilitation program. However, each patient needs to be individually assessed and monitored for progress.

Transitional Hospitals

Transitional hospitals[4] are acute care facilities for medically stable patients with long rehabilitation needs and care that is too complex for extended care facilities. Because these hospitals have only basic or disease-specific equipment and specialists, they are able to provide medically complex care at a lower cost than traditional hospitals. The following are examples of the types of care delivered in transitional hospitals:

- Burn care
- Extensive wound care
- Hemodialysis

- Hospice
- Infectious disease management
- IV medication therapies
- Neurobehavioral rehabilitation
- Pain control therapies
- Rehabilitation
- Total parenteral nutrition
- Ventilator care/weaning from ventilators

Alternate Care Facilities

Assisted Living Facilities

An assisted living facility provides its residents with help in ADLs. They differ from nursing homes in that they do not provide medical or skilled nursing care. The typical resident of an assisted living facility is a senior who has suffered a decline in health or cognition and who requires help with the ADLs. For example, assisted living communities typically offer their residents prepared meals three times a day and help with light housekeeping and laundry. They may also offer amenities such as a health club, pool, beauty parlor, and post office.

Assisted living is regulated by the individual states; as such, each state has their own requirements that assisted living communities must meet. These facilities are paid for by private funds, although in some cases long-term care insurance may pay for a licensed facility.

Group Home

A group home is a relatively new concept in caring for those who are incapable of caring for themselves. Before the 1970s this function was served by private or state-run institutions such as poor houses, orphanages, or psychiatric hospitals. However, a series of well-publicized cases of abuse and neglect in orphanages and asylums led states to seek alternative forms of care.

Group homes are small, typically with less than 10 residents who share facilities such as laundry, bathroom, kitchen, and common living areas. The homes have a resident manager, who organizes the residents' activities, supervises their chores, and ensures their safety. Depending on the abilities of the residents, they may do house maintenance chores themselves or have a service staff that cooks or cleans for them.

Although some group homes are privately funded, most are state funded. Each requires a state license and approval by the local community board.

Residential Care Facility

A residential care facility provides custodial care to persons who, because of physical, mental, or emotional disorders, are not able to live independently.

Home Care Services

Returning home is, by far, the preference of most hospitalized patients. Given the expense associated with inpatient care, early and appropriate discharge is the preference for payers. Home healthcare programs, consisting primarily of home visits by nurses and health aides, were conceived as a means to facilitate hospital discharge. To that end they have been extremely effective. In fact, home care was the fastest growing component of health care in the 1990s.

Home health care offers a wide range of healthcare services that can be provided to the patient at home. Home health care is usually less expensive, more convenient, and equally effective as that care available in a hospital or SNF.

In general, home health care includes intermittent skilled nursing care and other services, such as physical therapy, occupational therapy, and speech-language pathology (therapy) services. Services may also include medical social services or assistance from a home health aide.

Although common service providers such as nurses, home health aides, and physical, occupational, and speech therapists have been available through home care agencies for many years, now infusion care, ventilators, respiratory equipment, total parenteral nutrition, and complex wound care are regularly available. Much of this newer availability gained its impetus from managed care programs, which encouraged the early discharge of stable patients from hospital to home.

Because of its manifest success in maintaining quality and decreasing costs, even Medicare has entered this arena through Medicare risk contracts with health maintenance organizations (HMOs). Medicare patients enrolled in HMOs may have different benefits from those under the traditional Medicare model. As opposed to Medicare, managed care organizations frequently cover IV therapies at home, hearing aids, and prescription medications. Each health insurance policy needs to be carefully evaluated when planning a patient's care.

The traditional Medicare model allows for home health visits only if all four of the following criteria are met[5]:

1. The patient is homebound, which means he or she is confined to the home or it would be a great physical hardship to go to an outpatient treatment facility such as a rehabilitation center or a laboratory.
2. The care required includes intermittent skilled nursing services and possibly physical, occupational, and speech therapies.
3. The care must be requested by a licensed physician, who oversees the patient's care and reviews the patient's care plan at least every 60 days. The care plan has to be reasonable and medically necessary.
4. The home healthcare agency must be Medicare certified.

If the previously listed criteria are met, Medicare covers the following home care services:

- *Skilled nursing care:* This is covered on a very limited basis. The Case Manager must stress to the patient that an average skilled nursing visit is 45 minutes to 1 hour. Only in very rare situations are 8 hours deemed medically necessary. To qualify, the services the patient requires must call for the skill and training of a nurse.
- *Physical therapy or speech therapy:* If skilled nursing is deemed to be medically necessary, physical therapy or speech therapy is allowed if medically necessary. If these services are deemed medically necessary, then Medicare may also authorize occupational therapy.
- *Home health aides:* Intermittent home health aides may be authorized if medically necessary and skilled services such as nursing or therapies are in place. They are generally allowed up to three times per week for assistance in ADLs.

- *Home social services:* If skilled services are deemed medically necessary and the patient has social service needs, an assessment and subsequent visits may be authorized.
- *Medical supplies:* These are covered if the patient's nurse requires them to perform the patient's care (e.g., dressings for wound care or Foley catheters for incontinent patients).
- *Durable medical equipment:* All durable medical equipment must be ordered by a treating physician and authorized by Medicare. Not all equipment is a covered benefit, and some equipment such as oxygen has strict criteria for approval. The patient pays a 20% coinsurance on the equipment.

Home Oxygen

The following are the Medicare parameters for home oxygen use.[6] Home oxygen therapy is covered only if all of the following conditions are met:

- The treating physician has determined the patient has a severe lung disease or hypoxia-related symptoms that might be expected to improve with oxygen therapy.
- The patient's blood gas study meets the criteria stated below.
- The qualifying blood gas study was performed by a physician or by a qualified provider or supplier of laboratory services.
- The qualifying blood gas study was obtained under the following conditions (a or b):
  a. If the qualifying blood gas study is performed during an inpatient hospital stay, the reported test must be the one obtained closest to, but no earlier than, 2 days before the hospital discharge date, or
  b. If the qualifying blood gas study is not performed during an inpatient hospital stay, the reported test must be performed while the patient is in a chronic stable state (i.e., not during a period of acute illness or an exacerbation of his or her underlying disease).
- Alternative treatment measures have been tried or considered and deemed clinically ineffective.

Home Medications

In 1993, traditional Medicare approved a limited number of IV medications for home administration.[7] This change occurred because otherwise-independent patients were being admitted to nursing homes for administration of IV medications. The criteria for home IV medications include the use of an infusion pump and a prolonged infusion of at least 8 hours or infusion of the drug at a controlled rate to avoid toxicity. The following is a list of some of the approved medications that meet the previous criteria:

- Acyclovir
- Foscarnet
- Amphotericin B
- Vancomycin
- Ganciclovir
- Selected analgesics such as morphine sulfate
- Some chemotherapeutic agents when administered by continuous infusion over at least 24 hours

Medicare-certified home health agencies will have the latest list of approved medications.

Hospice

Hospice is a healthcare program whose goal is to provide supportive care and comfort to terminally ill patients and their families during the final stages of life. Ideally, this care is provided with dignity, at home, with the patient surrounded by his or her family and friends. For Medicare to pay a hospice benefit, all of the following criteria must be met[8]:

1. The patient must be entitled to Part A benefits of Medicare.
2. A physician certifies, in writing, that the patient is terminally ill after a face-to-face encounter. The term "terminally ill" in this context means the individual's prognosis is for a life expectancy of 6 months or less if the terminal illness runs its normal course.
3. The patient or family elects the hospice benefit.
4. The hospice provider must be Medicare certified.

A hospice referral can be made from home or the hospital setting; however, it requires a physician's referral. A hospice representative will interview the patient and his or her family. The hospice patient must waive standard Medicare benefits in lieu of the hospice benefit. The patient can receive standard Medicare benefits for unrelated medical problems. For example, if the patient has an inoperable brain tumor and has elected hospice care, treatments of the brain tumor would not be covered by standard Medicare benefits but treatment for a wound infection or complex pain management would be covered. Medicare pays this benefit out of Part A benefits. Part A pays for two 90-day benefit periods and one 30-day benefit period (210 days/7 months). In cases with a long duration of a terminal illness, indefinite extensions are available to the patient. Table 5-1 highlights the differences between the Medicare hospice benefit and the standard benefit.

Transportation

When patients are so infirm that transportation to and from healthcare facilities is impossible without assistance, the Case Manager can arrange for their transportation. The successful Case Manager will be informed about all the issues involved in this highly contentious benefit.

Ground Ambulance

A ground ambulance is of two general types: (1) basic life support, which includes a basic life support–certified paramedic and limited monitoring, and (2) advanced life support, which includes an advanced cardiac life support–certified paramedic, cardiac monitoring, and a drug box. Patients requiring oxygen must use advanced life support or basic life support ambulances.

Air Ambulance

An air ambulance provides cardiac monitoring, a medication box, and advanced cardiac life support–trained personnel, including a registered nurse. Many plans exclude air ambulance as a benefit. However, when medically necessary transportation is arranged and negotiated by a Case Manager, it may be approved. Scenarios in which an air ambulance may be approved when the benefit does not ordinarily exist include a patient with a traumatic injury in an inaccessible region (such as a mountaintop) or

TABLE 5-1 Standard Medicare Benefits versus Hospice Benefits

Service	Standard Benefit	Hospice
Skilled nursing services	Covered on an intermittent basis	Covered on a 24-hour, 7-day-a-week, on-call basis
Unskilled services	Nurses aides; maximum of two to three 1-hour visits per week	Personal care aides can be provided for 12 to 16 hours per day; also some homemaking services are included
Physician's services	A physician must order services	A physician must order services
Bereavement counseling	Not covered	Available during the terminal stages and for several months afterward
Social services and volunteers	Social services are very limited	These services are part of the hospice agencies' multidisciplinary staff
Homebound requirement	Mandatory	Not mandatory
Prescription drugs for symptom management and pain control	Rarely paid for	A covered benefit, with a 5% or $5 fee per prescription, whichever is less
Durable medical equipment and oxygen	Covered under strict criteria	Criteria are more lax under hospice and can be for the comfort of the patient
Respite care	Not covered	Limited respite (5 consecutive days per quarter) is allowed in an ECF
Physical, occupational, and speech therapies	Covered	Covered
Continuous care during periods of medical crisis	Not covered	Covered
Deductibles	20% for durable medical equipment	No deductible

for speeding an approved hospitalized transplant candidate to the hospital where the transplant organ awaits.

There are other issues involved in transporting patients that a Case Manager arranging for transportation of critically ill patients should recognize. The first issue is whether a transportation benefit exists under the patient's insurance plan. Not all insurance plans offer this benefit. Another issue is IV lines and peripheral tubes. When arranging transportation for patients with IV lines, a Case Manager should call for advanced life support transportation. If the patient has tubes (such as gastrostomy or percutaneous endoscopic gastronomy tubes) and lines that can be capped off, they should be capped and a less complex (and less expensive) mode of transportation can then be used.

When transportation is a covered benefit, the criteria for authorization usually include that only medically necessary transportation is covered and only if that transportation is to a healthcare facility. This commonly means transportation between two hospitals, between a hospital and an acute care rehabilitation facility, or after a traumatic injury from the site of the injury to the hospital. Transportation from a healthcare facility to the patient's home generally is not a covered benefit.

Wheelchair vans[9] or ambulette services generally are used for stable patients and for routine healthcare needs such as doctors' appointments. Wheelchair vans will accommodate a person with his or her own oxygen tank, but the personnel are not medically skilled or licensed to regulate it in any way. Because wheelchair vans, by their very nature, do not transport the critically ill, the medical necessity for their use is often difficult to establish. Without medical necessity, wheelchair vans are not a covered benefit under most insurance plans.

Durable Medical Equipment

There is an ever-increasing range of products available today to meet the patient's needs at home. These products can effectively treat and maintain a patient in his or her home environment. The following are criteria for meeting the designation of durable medical equipment:

- It has a medical/therapeutic purpose.
- It can withstand repeated use.
- It can be sterilized/disinfected between uses.
- It is not useful to a person in the absence of illness or injury.
- It is appropriate for use in the home.

Durable medical equipment can be divided into the following categories:

- *Basic mobility devices:* Walkers, crutches, and canes
- *Assistive devices for ADLs:* Bathroom equipment, ostomy, incontinence, wound care, dressing, feeding, and kitchen aids
- *Extensive mobility equipment:* Wheelchairs, motorized scooters, and hospital beds
- *Advanced high-tech equipment:* Oxygen, ventilators, infusion pumps, apnea monitors, and so on

The Case Manager needs to have a thorough understanding of the basic durable medical equipment that is available. Developing a working relationship with multiple equipment providers is essential for several reasons. One supplier cannot meet the need for all types of equipment available. Also, the patient should be offered a choice of vendors when setting up his or her care plan, because the vendor will work with the patient to satisfy his or her needs. In addition, a reliable vendor can be invaluable when special or emergency needs arise. A good vendor should work closely with the Case Manager, patient, family, physician, and other healthcare professionals to

- Perform an assessment when equipment is ordered and delivered
- Select and set up appropriate equipment
- Educate patients and their caregivers in the proper use of the equipment
- Inform the Case Manager if the equipment ordered by the physician is unsafe or not suitable and offer a reason for that determination
- Recommend more suitable equipment when necessary

- Service and maintain the equipment as needed[10]
- Loan equipment or replace equipment when lengthy repairs are required
- Clean and disinfect equipment between uses
- Complete insurance paperwork for the patient
- Be included in team conferences when planning for the patient's needs

CREDENTIALS

Quality Medical Services

The Case Manager has a dual responsibility in arranging for medically necessary services and for providing cost-effective care and quality services. The Case Manager has several options to ensure quality providers. He or she can use an established network of providers that has been credentialed by the insurer, or he or she can look for board-certified providers; institutions accredited by the Joint Commission (formerly the Joint Commission on Accreditation of Healthcare Organizations [JCAHO]), Centers of Excellence; and facilities accredited by the Rehabilitation Accreditation Commission (CARF), or specialty centers. By using well-established or credentialed providers, the risk for a poor outcome is minimized.

Rehabilitation Credentials

Case Managers have a responsibility to their patients to recommend qualified, credentialed providers. This is especially true in rehabilitation services, when patients are often unable to evaluate quality or advocate for themselves. The following three things are sought when referring patients:

1. Is the vendor accredited by the Joint Commission?
2. Is the facility accredited by CARF?
3. Is the physician board certified?

Joint Commission

The Joint Commission, formerly the Joint Commission on Accreditation of Healthcare Organizations (JCAHO), is an independent, not-for-profit organization established in 1951. The Joint Commission accredits and certifies more than 19,000 healthcare organizations and programs in the United States. Its sole purpose is to improve the quality of care provided to the public through the provision of healthcare accreditation and related services. These services support performance improvement in healthcare organizations.

Case Managers should look for accreditation of a healthcare provider by the Joint Commission when arranging for the following services:

- General, psychiatric, children's, and rehabilitation hospitals
- Healthcare networks, including health plans, integrated delivery networks, and preferred provider organizations
- Home care organizations, including those that provide home health services, personal care and support services, home infusion, and other pharmacy services
- Nursing homes and other long-term care facilities, including subacute care programs, dementia programs, and long-term care pharmacies

- Behavioral healthcare organizations—including those that provide mental health, chemical dependency, and mental retardation/developmental disabilities services for patients of various ages in various organized service settings—and managed behavioral healthcare organizations
- Ambulatory care providers, including outpatient surgical facilities, rehabilitation centers, infusion centers, group practices, and others
- Clinical laboratories

Accreditation by the Joint Commission is nationally recognized as a symbol of quality. It indicates the organization meets certain quality performance standards. Healthcare organizations strive to meet Joint Commission standards, because accreditation accomplishes several goals. A majority of state governments have come to recognize Joint Commission accreditation as a condition of licensure and the receipt of Medicaid reimbursement. Accreditation

- Assists the organizations in improving their quality of care
- May be used to meet certain Medicare certification requirements
- May be used to waive certain licensure requirements
- Enhances community confidence in the organization
- Enhances staff recruitment
- Provides an educational tool for the staff
- Expedites third-party reimbursement
- Often fulfills state licensure requirements
- May favorably influence liability insurance premiums
- Enhances access to managed care contracts
- May favorably influence bond ratings and access to financial markets

Rehabilitation Accreditation Commission

The Commission on Accreditation of Rehabilitation Facilities (CARF) is a private, not-for-profit organization that promotes quality rehabilitation services. CARF provides accreditation services worldwide at the request of health and human service providers. Established in 1966, CARF's mission is to promote the quality, value, and optimal outcomes of services through a consultative accreditation process that centers on enhancing the lives of the persons served. CARF establishes standards of quality for organizations to use as guidelines in developing and offering their programs or services to consumers. CARF standards are developed with input from consumers, rehabilitation professionals, state and national organizations, and funders. Every year the standards are reviewed and new ones are developed to keep current with the needs of the environment.

CARF believes in the following core values:

1. All people have the right to be treated with respect and dignity.
2. All people should have access to needed services that achieve optimal outcomes.
3. All people should be empowered to make informed choices.

When the Case Manager selects an accredited CARF facility, she or he can be assured of the following:

- The programs or services actively involve consumers in selecting, planning, and using services.
- The organization's programs and services have met consumer-focused, state-of-the-art national standards of performance.

- These standards were developed with the involvement and input of consumers.
- The organization is focused on assisting each consumer in achieving his or her chosen goals and outcomes.

Board Certification

The American Board of Medical Specialties and the American Medical Association recognize 24 specialty boards, which certify that physicians have met certain published standards. The intent of the certification process is to provide assurance to the public that a certified medical specialist has successfully completed an approved educational program and an evaluation, including an examination process designed to assess the knowledge, experience, and skills needed to provide high-quality patient care in that specialty. To be certified as a medical specialist by one of these boards, a medical doctor must complete the following requirements:

- Complete a course of study leading to the MD or DO degree from a recognized school of medicine.
- Complete 3 to 7 years of full-time training in an accredited residency program designed to train specialists in the field.
- Some specialty boards require assessments of individual performance and competence from the residency training director or from the chief of service in the hospital where the specialty is practiced.
- Most specialty boards require the person who seeks certification has an unrestricted license to practice medicine before he or she is allowed to sit for the certification exam.
- Some boards require the doctor have a period of experience in full-time practice in the specialty before taking the certification exam, usually 2 years after his or her training period. For specialties that require surgery, there are also minimum requirements regarding the hours spent in surgery.
- Finally, each candidate must pass a written examination given by the specialty board. Fifteen specialty boards also require an oral exam conducted by senior specialists in the same field.

Most boards issue certificates for a limited period of time (i.e., 7–10 years) with requirements of continuing education and review of credentials to be recertified.

The Case Manager should use these credentials as a baseline for evaluation. He or she must also obtain feedback from patients regarding their experiences with these providers and observe for outcomes. Whenever an irregularity is detected or suspected, he or she has a duty to investigate and to report to the appropriate credentialing body or to the National Physician's Database when appropriate.

MEDICAL HOME MODEL

The idea of a medical home, introduced by the American Academy of Pediatrics (AAP) in 1967, originally referred to a central location where a child's medical record could be stored for later retrieval. The AAP then expanded this idea to include an approach to providing comprehensive primary care for a child and his or her family. The AAP reported in a recent policy statement that the medical home should have the following characteristics: accessible, continuous, comprehensive, family-centered, coordinated, compassionate, and culturally effective care.[11]

Since the concept of the medical home was first promulgated, many other primary care organizations have become interested in it. They each have developed their own, slightly different model of the medical home. In March 2007 the AAP joined with the American Academy of Family Physicians, American College of Physicians, and the American Osteopathic Association to publish the Joint Principles of the Patient-Centered Medical Home. They collectively defined the medical home as "an approach to providing comprehensive primary care . . . that facilitates partnerships between individual patients, and their personal providers, and when appropriate, the patient's family."[12]

This consensus statement describes seven principles of a medical home: personal physician, physician-directed medical practice, whole-person orientation, coordinated care, quality and safety, enhanced access, and appropriate payment.[13] The medical home, like accountable care organizations (ACOs) and other new medical care delivery models, primarily exists in the form of demonstration projects and pilots.

ACCOUNTABLE CARE ORGANIZATION

Section 3022 of the Patient Protection and Affordable Care Act outlines the creation of many new healthcare delivery systems. One of these delivery systems is the ACO. According to the Centers for Medicare & Medicaid Services an ACO can be defined as "an organization of health care providers that agrees to be accountable for the quality, cost, and overall care of Medicare beneficiaries who are enrolled in the traditional fee-for-service program who are assigned to it."[14] Therefore, an ACO is a legal entity, recognized under state law, which provides healthcare services to a defined population.

An ACO is analogous to an HMO. The HMO is focused on improving medical quality and decreasing costs associated with a covered population by linking measures of medical quality and utilization to provider reimbursement. The ACO delivery model attempts to do the same. Like the HMO, the ACO can use different payment models, such as capitation, shared risk, or fee-for-service. Although HMOs traditionally contract with private insurers to manage their covered populations, ACOs contract with Medicare to manage services under Parts A and B in Medicare recipients.

Both HMOs and ACOs are shared savings programs. That is, they both depend on increasing clinical efficiency and reducing waste to provide higher quality medical services at costs lower than the premiums the payer (i.e., Medicare) pays them.

ACOs can have various forms and payment models; however, they all should have the same three core principles[15]:

1. Provider-led organizations with a strong base of primary care that are collectively accountable for quality and total per capita costs across the full continuum of care for a population of patients
2. Payments linked to quality improvements that also reduce overall costs
3. Reliable and progressively more sophisticated performance measurement, to support improvement and provide confidence that savings are achieved through improvements in care

Requirements for an ACO

To establish an ACO, the organization must adhere to certain requirements. Outlined in Section 3022 of the Patient Protection and Affordable Care Act are the following requirements for ACOs:

- The ACO shall be willing to become accountable for the quality, cost, and overall care of the Medicare fee-for-service beneficiaries assigned to it.
- The ACO shall enter into an agreement with the Secretary to participate in the program for not less than a 3-year period.
- The ACO shall have a formal legal structure that would allow the organization to receive and distribute payments for shared savings to participating providers of services and suppliers.
- The ACO shall include primary care ACO professionals that are sufficient for the number of Medicare fee-for-service beneficiaries assigned to the ACO.
- At a minimum, the ACO shall have at least 5,000 such beneficiaries assigned to it to be eligible to participate in the ACO program.
- The ACO shall provide the Secretary with such information regarding ACO professionals participating in the ACO as the Secretary determines necessary to support the assignment of Medicare fee-for-service beneficiaries to an ACO, the implementation of quality and other reporting requirements under paragraph (3), and the determination of payments for shared savings under subsection (d)(2).
- The ACO shall have in place a leadership and management structure that includes clinical and administrative systems.
- The ACO shall define processes to promote evidence-based medicine and patient engagement, report on quality and cost measures, and coordinate care, such as through the use of telehealth, remote patient monitoring, and other such enabling technologies.
- The ACO shall demonstrate to the Secretary that it meets patient-centeredness criteria specified by the Secretary, such as the use of patient and caregiver assessments or the use of individualized care plans.
- The ACO participant cannot participate in other Medicare shared savings programs.
- The ACO entity is responsible for distributing savings to participating entities.
- The ACO must have a process for evaluating the health needs of the population it serves.

Currently, ACOs exist only as pilot programs. Most practitioner groups and hospitals systems do not have the organization, integration, and sophisticated information systems needed to comply with ACO requirements. Those "leading edge" healthcare systems that do have the sophistication to become ACOs have balked at what they deem as too much administrative oversight, vague reporting requirements, and questions about their ability to reduce medical costs in already tightly managed systems.[16]

TRANSITIONS OF CARE

A transition of care can be defined as the movement of a patient from one healthcare environment to another or from one healthcare provider to another. Examples of transitions of care between healthcare providers include the transit of a patient between a primary care physician and a specialist or between a nurse practitioner and a patient's family. Transitions can occur within a hospital between the medical ward and the intensive care unit. They can also occur between healthcare facilities, such as from a nursing home to hospital or from an extended care facility to a hospice.

In the not too distant past a typical physician would examine and treat a patient in his or her office. If a patient needed to be admitted to the hospital, that same physician admitted the patient and treated the patient while in the hospital and supervised all consultants. When the patient left the hospital, that physician orchestrated the discharge and the patient was seen in his or her office for follow-up. In this model of medical treatment there were no "gaps" in the patient's care and the treating physician was always aware of the patient's full clinical picture.

Today, things are often vastly different. A patient may be cared for by a number of physicians, including a primary care physician and any number of specialists. The patient may or may not be admitted to the hospital by his or her primary care physician. Alternatively, the patient may be admitted by a consulting specialist, a nurse practitioner, or physician in an urgent care facility. If the primary care physician does not admit the patient, critical information about the patient's past medical history, allergies, current medications, and diagnostic plans may not be transferred to the next treating physician in the continuum of care. In the hospital the patient is likely to be cared for by a team of hospitalist physicians who have no prior experience with the patient. Every 8-hour shift brings a new physician to care for the patient and with that care come gaps in knowledge. When the patient is discharged, he or she may be discharged to a nursing home, rehabilitation hospital, or hospice, where he or she is cared for by new teams of physicians and nurses. Communication between the hospitalist who discharges the patient and the community physician are infrequent. Discharge summaries are rarely available to the community physician in time for the patient's first post-hospital visit. Therefore, the primary care physician may not have been informed about the patient's hospitalization, the tests performed, or the treatments given. He or she may not have been apprised of the discontinuation of old medications, the prescribing of new medications, new self-care regimens, or the patient's need for follow-up testing or treatment.

These scenarios demonstrate that when a patient transitions between healthcare providers, especially those patients with complex medical needs, he or she is at risk for adverse outcomes. The adverse outcomes can include continuation or recurrence of symptoms, temporary or permanent disability, and death.

These adverse outcomes are often due to medication errors or failures to follow prescribed treatments, therapies, and testing that were planned at hospital discharge.

In a study published by in the *Journal of General Internal Medicine* in 2003, Moore, Wisnivesky, Williams, and McGinn reported that after hospital discharge nearly half (49%) of hospitalized patients experience at least one medical error in medication continuity, diagnostic workup, or test follow-up.[17] Another study reported that 19% to 23% of patients suffer an adverse event, most frequently an adverse drug event.[18] In addition, a survey by the Agency for Healthcare Research and Quality found that 42% of the hospitals surveyed reported that "things fall between the cracks when transferring patients from one unit to another" and "problems often occur in the exchange of information across hospital units."[19]

From a healthcare management perspective, adverse clinical outcomes can result in avoidable emergency department visits or readmissions to the hospital. Research on Medicare fee-for-service beneficiaries who have been discharged from the hospital showed that, on average, 19.6% were readmitted to the hospital within 30 days and 34% were readmitted within 90 days.[20] These readmissions are not cheap. The costs of hospital readmissions within 30 days accounted for $15 billion of Medicare spending.[21] (This type of avoidable medical utilization burdens an already overburdened healthcare system and brings the "transition of care" issue to the attention of government health policymakers and insurers.)

The causes of transitional care errors include a lack of communication between groups of caregivers and the lack of clear boundaries of responsibility for the patient caused by the fragmented healthcare system. Communication does not occur for many reasons, including a lack of time, the demands of other patients, lack of full clinical information at the point of care transfer, and inability to speak with the patient or family members due to differences in culture, language, education, or cognitive ability.

Clinical responsibility was the traditional province of the primary care physician who had total responsibility for the care of the patient in and out of the hospital. Today, a cultural change has occurred in medicine, and "team-based" care is now the growing care model. However, with more caregivers, the responsibility for the patient's care is distributed among a group. Each member of this group is responsible for a unique clinical goal. For example, the surgeon is concerned with removing a patient's gallbladder safely; the intensive care nurse is responsible for getting the patient well enough to be transferred to the medical ward. The hospitalist is responsible for getting the patient well enough to be discharged to the community. However, almost no one is responsible for the patient's overall health and well-being.

Avoiding transitional care errors is difficult, because it requires all clinical information to be communicated at the time of patient transfer to a person who is able to understand and act on it. Current information systems do not provide this data, and current medical culture does not encourage physician to physician communication.[22] Additionally, the transfer of patient responsibility to the next provider in the clinical continuum is fraught with problems of clearly defining the responsibility and transferring it to the appropriate person. For example, the patient's next provider may not have the ability to care for all the patient's needs because of lack of understanding, training, or resources. This occurs when a physician discharges a patient home, giving a complicated care regimen to a patient's family member who do not have the intellectual or cultural understanding to follow it.

Despite these inherent difficulties, simple steps can decrease transitional care errors. To that end, the Joint Commission has committed itself to promoting more effective care transitions. As of 2006 accredited facilities are required to "accurately and completely reconcile medications across the continuum of care."

The Joint Commission defines medication reconciliation as the process of comparing the patient's current medication orders to all medications the patient has been taking. The reconciliation is performed by the doctor who prescribes the medications and should occur at every transition of care in which new medications are ordered or existing orders are rewritten. The reconciliation process involves developing a list of the patient's current medications and then comparing that list to a list of new medications to be prescribed. The doctor must then make a clinical decision as to which medications should stay and which should be eliminated. Finally, these changes need to be clearly communicated to the patient or his or her caregivers. By using this process the most common medication errors, such as medication omissions, duplications, dosing errors, or drug–drug interactions, can be reduced or eliminated. Other policy groups, such as the National Transitions of Care Coalition, have created "transition checklists" that not only list the patient's medications but clearly outline the plan of care and accountability after hospital discharge.[23]

In summary, to improve effective transitions of care and avoid adverse medical events, there needs to be better communication between groups of caregivers. This includes a need for an effective reconciliation of all prescribed medications as well as a need for hospitalist physicians to communicate more effectively with community-based physicians. Physicians, Case Managers, nurses, and pharmacists need to adequately educate the patient or his or her caregiver about medication use, encourage closer medical follow-up, and engage the patient's social support systems.

REFERENCES

1. Powell, S. K. (1996). *Nursing case management: A practical guide to success in managed care*. New York: Lippincott.
2. Ibid.
3. Ibid.
4. Ibid.
5. Retrieved November 2, 2011, from http://www.medicare.gov/Publications/Pubs/pdf/10969.pdf
6. Retrieved from https://www.cms.gov/MLNProducts/downloads/OxgnThrpy_DocCvg_FactSheet_ICN904883.pdf
7. Powell, S. K., & Wekell, P. M. (June,1996). *Nursing case management: A practical guide to success in managed care*. New York: Lippincott.
8. Retrieved November 2, 2011, from The National Archives and Records Administration. http://ecfr.gpoaccess.gov/cgi/t/text/text-idx?c=ecfr&sid=009d7a8f47e1232ab64f843034cf7275&rgn=div5&view=text&node=42:3.0.1.1.5&idno=42#42:3.0.1.1.5.2.3.1
9. Health Care Financing Administration. (1994). *The Medicare 1994 handbook*. Washington, DC: U.S. Government Printing Office.
10. Ibid.
11. Retrieved from http://www.medicalhomeinfo.org/downloads/pdfs/jointstatement.pdf
12. Retrieved from http://www.acponline.org/advocacy/where_we_stand/medical_home/approve_jp.pdf
13. Retrieved from http://www.medicalhomeinfo.org/about/medical_home
14. Retrieved from https://www.cms.gov/sharedsavingsprogram/
15. McClellan, M., McKethan, A. N., Lewis, J. L., Roski, J., & Fisher, E. S. (2010). A national strategy to put accountable care into practice. *Health Affairs, 29*(5), 982–990.
16. Retrieved from http://www.commonwealthfund.org/Newsletters/Washington-Health-Policy-in-Review/2011/May/May-9-2011/Model-ACO-Health-Centers-Skeptical.aspx
17. Moore, C., Wisnivesky, J., Williams, S., & McGinn, T. (2003). Medical errors related to discontinuity of care from an inpatient to an outpatient setting. *Journal of General Internal Medicine, 18*, 646–651.
18. Kripalani, S., Jackson, A. T., Schnipper, J. L., & Coleman, E. A. (2003). Promoting effective transitions of care at hospital discharge: A review of key issues for hospitalists. *Journal of Hospital Medicine, 2*(5), 314–323.
19. Agency for Healthcare Research and Quality. (2007). Hospital survey on patient safety culture: 2007 comparative database report. Retrieved from http://www.ahrq.gov/qual/hospsurveydb/
20. Jencks, S. F., Williams, M. V., & Coleman, E. A. (2009). Rehospitalizations among patients in the Medicare fee for service program. *New England Journal of Medicine, 360*, 1418–1428.
21. Medicare Payment Advisory Commission. (2007). Report to Congress: Promoting greater efficiency in Medicare.
22. Kripalani, S., et al. (2007). Deficits in communication and information transfer between hospital based and primary care physicians: Implications for patient safety and continuity of care. *Journal of the American Medical Association, 297*(8), 831–841. Retrieved from http://www.ntocc.org/Portals/0/TOC_Checklist.pdf

Appendix 5-A

Healthcare Management and Delivery Questions

1) Case Managers should complete a provider and service comparison to
   A. Obtain cost information for the insurer and the Case Manager's own files
   B. Ensure the quality of the services arranged
   C. Choose the most cost-effective provider available
   D. B, C
   E. All of the above

2) The Case Manager needs to be knowledgeable regarding charitable and not-for-profit programs and services available in the community because
   A. They are qualitatively superior to those that can be purchased privately.
   B. Personal Injury Protection (PIP) policy limits may restrict the range of options available to the client.
   C. A higher quality-of-life index is associated with these programs.
   D. All of the above
   E. None of the above

3) Healthcare needs provided over a period of time to patients who do not require acute hospital care but still require nursing, medical, and other healthcare services are covered under
   A. Group health
   B. Disability
   C. Workers' compensation
   D. Long-term care

4) When the Case Manager is arranging for discharge to a traumatic brain injury rehabilitation facility, he or she should
   1. Confirm that the facility can provide the therapies, by credentialed providers, the patient requires
   2. Verify that there is a board-certified medical director at the facility
   3. Ensure the facility is accredited by the Joint Commission and CARF
   4. Certify an unlimited length of stay to ensure the patient gets the care he or she needs

A. 1, 2, 3
   B. 2, 3, 4
   C. All of the above
   D. None of the above

5) When the Case Manager is arranging for transfer from the acute care setting to a traumatic brain injury rehabilitation facility, he or she needs to verify that the facility
   A. Can provide the therapies required by the patient
   B. Is directed by a board-certified medical director
   C. Is accredited by the Joint Commission and CARF
   D. A, C
   E. All of the above

6) The Case Manager should maintain her or his own referral file of facilities and providers that
   1. Have accredited expertise
   2. Have specialized programs
   3. Have subacute hospitals
   4. Have experimental protocols
      A. 1, 2
      B. 3, 4
      C. All of the above
      D. None of the above

7) When a patient has a spinal cord injury, the Case Manager should
   A. Leave the rehabilitation plans up to the patient and his or her family to plan
   B. Begin planning for the rehabilitation stay early in the hospitalization
   C. Not worry about rehabilitation, because the patient will probably not be able to work again and therefore will not need resources that can be used for someone else
   D. Not worry about rehabilitation, because the patient will probably return to his or her former activity level upon discharge

8) Which of the following statements is not true?
   A. The insurances governed by state regulations include disability, auto, and workers' compensation.
   B. The Case Manager must know the medical policy framework of the injured individual before beginning the case management process.
   C. A Case Manager working on an auto policy case needs to know the dollars available, the medical coverage, the lost wages, and the covered years.
   D. Plan flexibility is not an influencing factor in the Case Manager's ability to affect the case.

9) Excellent case management services delivered in an appropriate and timely fashion promote which of the following?
   A. Return to Work (RTW) outcomes
   B. Quality healthcare services
   C. Cost-effective healthcare services
   D. All of the above
   E. None of the above

10) Which of the following are not associated with adverse patient outcomes after a transition from one healthcare environment to another?
   1. Timely and complete communication of medical information from one provider to the next
   2. Unclear plans for patient follow-up
   3. The transfer of up-to-date medication list
   4. Failure to establish clear boundaries of clinical responsibility
      A. 1, 3
      B. 2, 4
      C. All of the above
      D. None of the above

11) Which of the following is a common side effect of nonsteroidal, anti-inflammatory medication?
   A. Impaired kidney function
   B. Impaired coordination
   C. Gastrointestinal irritation
   D. All of the above
   E. None of the above

12) Which of the following is the most common problem encountered by patients after a transfer of care?
   A. Missed follow-up appointment
   B. Duplicated clinical testing
   C. Postsurgical hemorrhage
   D. Adverse drug event

13) The clinical consequences of poorly executed transition of care include all of the following except
   A. Continuation or recurrence of symptoms
   B. Temporary or permanent disability
   C. Increased healthcare costs
   D. Death

14) Which of the following is (are) a core principle(s) of accountable care organizations?
   1. Provider-led organizations with a strong base of primary care that are collectively accountable for quality and total per capita costs across the full continuum of care for a population of patients; that savings are achieved through improvements in care
   2. Payments linked to quality improvements that also reduce overall costs
   3. Reliable and progressively more sophisticated performance measurement, to support improvement and provide confidence
   4. Utilization that depends on the Medicare enrollee's ability to pay additional copays and deductibles.

A. 1, 3
B. 2, 4
C. 1, 2, 3
D. All of the above

15) According to the Centers for Medicare & Medicaid Services, which of the following statements can be used to define an ACO?
    1. It is an organization of healthcare providers.
    2. They are accountable for clinical quality, cost, and care of enrolled patients.
    3. They care for Medicare beneficiaries who are assigned to the ACO.
    4. They earn profits by billing both Medicare and private insurers.
       A. 1, 3
       B. 2, 4
       C. 1, 2, 3
       D. None of the above

16) Which of the following is (are) true statements concerning accountable care organizations (ACO)?
    1. It is a legal entity.
    2. It is an organization of healthcare economists and accountants.
    3. It is responsible for promoting evidence-based medicine.
    4. To be eligible to participate in the ACO program, an ACO must have at least 50,000 Medicare beneficiaries assigned to it.
       A. 1, 3
       B. 2, 4
       C. 1, 2, 3
       D. All of the above

17) Which of the following statements about accountable care organizations is not true?
    1. They are shared risks programs, which only make money if they provide quality care at lower costs to Medicare beneficiaries.
    2. They must agree to participate in the program for not less than 10 years.
    3. They must provide a sufficient number of primary care physicians to care for all beneficiaries.
    4. The number of ACOs that are operating in the United States exceeds 2,000.
       A. 1, 3
       B. 2, 4
       C. 1, 2, 3
       D. None of the above

18) The Case Manager will find which of the following services difficult to arrange at home?
    A. Homemaker services
    B. Durable medical equipment
    C. Personal care
    D. All of the above
    E. None of the above

19) The Case Manager will find which of the following services difficult to arrange at home?
   1. Tocolytic therapy
   2. Respiratory therapy
   3. Infusion therapy
   4. Blood transfusions
   5. Dialysis
      A. 1, 2, 3
      B. 2, 3, 4
      C. 1, 4
      D. 4, 5
      E. None of the above

20) An example of a volunteer or charity organization is
   A. American Diabetes Association
   B. Veterans Administration
   C. Muscular Dystrophy Association
   D. A, B
   E. A, C

21) Case Managers should follow up on arrangements they have made for durable medical equipment to
   A. Determine if it is being used
   B. Determine if it was delivered
   C. Determine if the patient and caregiver are satisfied with the equipment
   D. Determine if it meets the current needs of the patient
   E. All of the above

22) _____ are facilities that provide lower-cost alternatives for complex cases that do not require the services of an acute care facility or specialized care center but require more care than can be provided at home.
   A. Subacute care centers
   B. Long-term care facilities
   C. Rehabilitation hospitals
   D. Convalescent hospitals

23) _____ are facilities for medically stable patients that offer services to patients requiring extended or respite care, such as wound management, pain management, dialysis, respiratory care, infusion therapy, physical therapy, occupational therapy, and speech therapy.
   A. Convalescent hospitals
   B. Subacute care centers
   C. Rehabilitation centers
   D. Acute care hospitals

24) The Case Manager is informed the rehabilitation facility she is presently negotiating with has CARF accreditation. CARF is
   A. A mandatory accreditation body
   B. A nonprofit organization established to adopt and apply standards
   C. A federally funded program
   D. A for-profit accreditation organization that produces rehabilitation guidelines

25) Which of the following statements is not true when negotiating for durable medical equipment?
    A. The deeper the discount agreed on, the later the vendor should be paid.
    B. Payer authorization and approval are required.
    C. Comparison of rental fees and purchase fees should be done.
    D. The needs of the patient are the first consideration.

26) A Case Manager has selected a durable medical equipment vendor for the equipment the patient needs. Which of the following should the Case Manager consider in determining whether a purchase or rental is more cost-effective?
    A. The costs of both the purchase and the rental
    B. The length of time the equipment will be required
    C. Availability and costs of maintenance and service
    D. All of the above
    E. None of the above

27) A Case Manager is planning rehabilitation for a spinal cord–injured patient. When choosing a facility, she or he should evaluate it in regard to which of the following?
    1. Peer support for the patient
    2. Specialization of the program and staff in spinal cord injury
    3. Credentials of the rehabilitation staff (are there physical and occupational therapists, rehabilitation nurses, social workers, etc.?)
    4. Speech therapy
        A. 1, 2, 3
        B. 2, 3, 4
        C. All of the above
        D. None of the above

28) Ancillary services can include which of the following?
    1. Laboratory medicine
    2. Diagnostic radiology
    3. Services that are adjuncts to the diagnosis and treatment of the patient's condition
    4. Therapeutic radiology
        A. 1, 2, 3
        B. 2, 3, 4
        C. 1, 2, 4
        D. All of the above
        E. None of the above

29) A Case Manager is frustrated by her inability to get her patient to agree to occupational therapy. The patient was involved in a high-speed motor vehicle accident and suffered severe head injuries. When encouraged to attend therapy sessions, the patient refuses, becomes verbally abusive, and hangs up the phone. Likely reason(s) for this patient's reaction is (are)
    A. Head injuries can result in emotional lability.
    B. Head injuries can result in cognitive impairments.
    C. Head injuries can result in prolonged head pain and mood depression.
    D. All of the above
    E. None of the above

30) _____ is the body's response to physical and psychological stress.
    1. Mutate
    2. Disease
    3. Eliminate toxins
    4. Adapt/cope
        A. 1, 3
        B. 2, 4
        C. All of the above
        D. None of the above

31) The definition of disease can include
    1. A disturbance of the homeostatic balance
    2. Imbalance in the internal environment of the body
    3. An attempt to restore balance in the body
    4. Mental illness
        A. 1, 2, 3
        B. 2, 3, 4
        C. All of the above
        D. None of the above

32) After a patient sustains a mild head injury, she continues to experience dizziness, headache, and inability to concentrate. These symptoms most likely are due to
    A. An aneurysm
    B. A subdural hematoma
    C. An arachnoid hemorrhage
    D. Postconcussion syndrome

33) A Case Manager expects a rehabilitation evaluation to be warranted for
    1. A brain-injured worker unable to perform his or her own activities of daily living
    2. A paraplegic with only manual labor work experience
    3. A back strain patient who is expected to return to work in 1 month
    4. An amputee who is expected to return to his regular job in 3 months
        A. 1, 2
        B. 2, 3, 4
        C. 2
        D. All of the above
        E. None of the above

34) The Case Manager knows that adaptive equipment, along with instruction and training in its use, results in
    A. Enhanced self-esteem
    B. Independence
    C. Decreased reliance on home health aides and others to perform activities of daily living
    D. All of the above
    E. None of the above

35) Which of the following statements is (are) true regarding the clinical consequences of head injuries?
    1. Patients may become depressed.
    2. A patient's cognitive ability may be impaired.
    3. Emotional lability is common.
    4. Chronic headaches may result.

A. 1, 3
B. 2, 4
C. 1, 2, 3
D. 1, 2, 4
E. None of the above

36) Which of the following statements is (are) not true regarding the clinical consequences of head injuries?
   1. Patients may become depressed.
   2. A patient's cognitive ability may improve as a result.
   3. Chronic headaches may result.
   4. Emotional lability is common.
      A. 1, 3
      B. 2, 4
      C. 1, 2, 3
      D. All of the above
      E. None of the above

37) When the Case Manager is planning for timely rehabilitation, she or he must do which of the following to provide for the coordination of the medical care the patient requires?
   A. Arrange for an objective second opinion.
   B. Request the diagnostic films for the medical director to read.
   C. Do an on-site evaluation.
   D. Develop and clarify the medical care plan of the attending physician.

38) A patient has just had a full diagnostic workup of his condition. The need for surgery has been ruled out, and the condition has been diagnosed as chronic. Which of the following is true of the patient's follow-up needs?
   A. The patient should be followed every 2 months by the surgeon, in case his or her condition changes and he or she requires surgery.
   B. Several other opinions should be sought to confirm the first diagnosis.
   C. Follow-up with the patient's primary care physician is indicated to obtain any needed treatment, monitoring, or medications required for the chronic condition.
   D. All of the above
   E. None of the above

39) Patients with chronic back pain require
   A. Supportive conservative treatment
   B. Whatever the patient and his or her various treating physicians determine is helpful
   C. Chiropractic care three times a week for life
   D. Continual testing to monitor the condition

40) Which of the following statements is not true about home infusion therapy?
   A. Infusion therapy can be safely administered in the home setting most of the time.
   B. It is always more cost-effective to arrange for infusion therapy to be given at home rather than at the hospital.
   C. Home-care patients must be stable to be set up for home infusion therapy.
   D. The primary caregiver must be capable of managing the infusion therapy at home.

41) _____ is the loss of the ability to express oneself and understand language.
   A. Dysphasia
   B. Aphasia
   C. Apraxia
   D. Amnesia

42) _____ is the impairment of speech resulting from a brain lesion.
   A. Dysphasia
   B. Aphasia
   C. Apraxia
   D. Amnesia

43) _____ is the inability to understand the meaning of things.
   A. Dysphasia
   B. Aphasia
   C. Apraxia
   D. Amnesia

44) _____ is the inability or difficulty in swallowing.
   A. Dysphasia
   B. Aphasia
   C. Apraxia
   D. Dysphagia

NOTES

Appendix 5-B

Healthcare Management and Delivery Answers

1) **ANSWER: E**
   This is part of assessing the resources available to meet the patient's needs. The Case Manager needs to use her or his professional and clinical judgment to choose cost-effective and quality providers.

2) **ANSWER: B**
   Personal Injury Protection (PIP) policy minimums are set by the state insurance department. These minimums may not be sufficient to cover the medical costs of more severe injuries.

3) **ANSWER: D**
   Group health, disability, and workers' compensation do not specifically provide for healthcare services that are required outside of an acute care facility for an extended period of time.

4) **ANSWER: A**
   Certifications should be time-limited, and progress reports should be evaluated before extending lengths of stay. Verifying the credentials of the facility and providers is important in choosing an appropriate facility for the patient.

5) **ANSWER: E**

6) **ANSWER: A**

7) **ANSWER: B**
   Discharge planning begins upon admission, especially in a spinal cord injury case.

8) **ANSWER: D**

9) **ANSWER: D**

10) **ANSWER: A**
    The complete communication of medical information from one provider to the next, including a complete medication list and comprehensive plans for follow-up, is associated with safe transfers of care. Each provider needs to understand the boundaries of his or her clinical responsibilities in a care transfer to ensure good clinical outcomes.

11) **ANSWER: C**

12) **ANSWER: D**
    It has been reported that 19% to 23% of patients suffer an adverse event, most frequently an adverse drug event.

13) **ANSWER: D**
Adverse clinical outcomes can include continuation or recurrence of a patient's symptoms, temporary or permanent disability, and death. An increase in healthcare costs is not a clinical outcome but a financial one.

14) **ANSWER: C**
The core principles of the ACO are provider-led organizations with a strong base of primary care that are collectively accountable for quality and total per capita costs across the full continuum of care for a population of patients; payments linked to quality improvements that also reduce overall costs; and reliable and progressively more sophisticated performance measurement, to support improvement and provide confidence that savings are achieved through improvements in care. ACOs do not charge additional copays or deductibles.

15) **ANSWER: C**
According to the Centers for Medicare & Medicaid Services, an ACO can be defined as "an organization of health care providers that agrees to be accountable for the quality, cost, and overall care of Medicare beneficiaries who are enrolled in the traditional fee-for-service program who are assigned to it."

16) **ANSWER: A**
An ACO is a legal entity recognized by the state. It is an organization of healthcare providers, who, in part, are responsible for promoting evidence-based medicine. To be eligible to participate in the ACO program, an ACO must have at least 5,000 Medicare beneficiaries assigned to it.

17) **ANSWER: B**
An ACO must agree to participate for a minimum of 3 years. Only a few ACOs are operating as pilot programs in the United States.

18) **ANSWER: E**

19) **ANSWER: D**
Blood transfusions are not usually done at home due to the risk of transfusion reaction. Although dialysis may be done at home, due to the associated risks, it is generally not done at home unless the patient is truly homebound.

20) **ANSWER: E**
The Veterans Administration is not a volunteer or charity organization.

21) **ANSWER: E**

22) **ANSWER: A**

23) **ANSWER: B**

24) **ANSWER: B**
CARF is a voluntary accreditation. The organization is not-for-profit and establishes national standards for rehabilitation facilities.

25) **ANSWER: A**
Generally, deeper discounts can be obtained with prompt payment agreements.

26) **ANSWER: D**

27) **ANSWER: A**
Patients with spinal cord injuries should not require the services of a speech therapist.

28) **ANSWER: D**
These are all charges outside the basic room and board that a hospital charges.

29) **ANSWER: D**

30) **ANSWER: B**
The body's attempt to adapt or cope with physical or psychological stress can result in disease if the adaptation is unsuccessful.

31) **ANSWER: C**

32) **ANSWER: D**

33) **ANSWER: C**

34) **ANSWER: D**

35) **ANSWER: D**

36) **ANSWER: B**

37) **ANSWER: D**
Second opinions and on-site evaluations are not required on every case. They may be necessary occasionally on a difficult case or a case in dispute. There is no medical necessity for the medical director to read the diagnostic films upon setting up a rehabilitation plan.

38) **ANSWER: C**
Chronic conditions not requiring surgery can be handled by the primary care physician, who can then make referrals when the patient's condition changes or he or she deems referrals medically necessary.

39) **ANSWER: A**
Supportive conservative care is the standard of care for chronic back pain.

40) **ANSWER: B**
If there are multiple infusions and frequent infusion administrations, it may be more cost-effective to administer the therapy in the hospital.

41) **ANSWER: B**

42) **ANSWER: A**

43) **ANSWER: B**

44) **ANSWER: D**

CHAPTER 6

Healthcare Reimbursement

PRIVATE BENEFIT PROGRAMS

The majority of a Case Manager's clients will have some type of health insurance. The health of the patient and his or her finances can depend on insurance benefits. A patient with a basic insurance package with high deductibles may have to pay high out-of-pocket fees. In contrast, a patient with a rich insurance package may have to pay little or nothing, despite high medical costs. Therefore, it is imperative that Case Managers understand the various types of insurance products their clients have purchased. This understanding allows Case Managers to advise their clients on how to get the most out of their current policy and counsel them on how to avoid incurring unnecessary out-of-pocket expenses. The most common types of insurance products are discussed below.

Indemnity Health Insurance Plans

An indemnity health insurance plan is a legal entity licensed by the state insurance department. The indemnity health insurance plan exists to provide health insurance to its enrollees. An indemnity health insurer "indemnifies," or reimburses, the enrollee for the costs of healthcare claims. Indemnity insurers historically did not spend money or time on utilization or quality management. Now, because of savings demonstrated by the managed care companies, indemnity companies have adopted many of managed care's cost-saving approaches. These enhanced indemnity companies are now referred to as "managed indemnity" companies.

Self-Insured Products

The high cost of health insurance premiums has encouraged employers to seek alternative ways to provide healthcare benefits to their employees. One option is to "self-insure." Self-insurance is one method of covering an employee's healthcare costs. A self-insured employer directly assumes the risk, in whole or in part, of providing health insurance for its employees rather than using an insurance company. In doing so the employer significantly decreases its cost of insurance.

In the self-insured scenario the employer is responsible for the cost of medical claims up to a "threshold" amount for the individual employee and the employed group. For costs incurred above this threshold amount, the employer purchases an insurance policy to limit any extraordinary liability. This insurance policy above the self-insured threshold is called reinsurance. Reinsurance policies are also referred to as "stop-loss" or "threshold" policies. These policies pay for healthcare claims above the threshold limit for both individual employees and for the self-insured group. For example, an employer may design a plan wherein it pays for all healthcare claims of each employee up to $100,000 annually. Additionally, the employer pays for all healthcare claims of its employees as a group, up to $1 million annually. In the situation in which an individual's healthcare costs exceed $100,000 or the group's healthcare costs exceed $1 million, the employer's reinsurance policy would pay the excess claims.

Benefits of a Self-Insured Program

A well-run self-insurance program can achieve the following benefits for an employer:

- Reduce the service costs usually incurred by conventional insurers; service costs include those expenses a traditional insurance company sustains with claims processing, underwriting, legal fees, actuarial expenses, and real estate
- Exempt the employer from providing benefits mandated by the Employee Retirement Income Security Act (ERISA)
- Eliminate the costs of premium taxes
- Improve cash flow
- Be flexible by offering extra-contractual benefits that are cheaper for the employer and more convenient for the patient, such as offering in-home rehabilitation rather than keeping the patient in the hospital to get the contractual benefit of in-hospital rehabilitation.

Because of these savings, large employers (more than 500 employees) tend to self-insure. Conversely, employers with fewer than 500 employees find it difficult to self-insure. Small employers lack the cash reserves necessary to handle large claims losses. An employer's decision to self-insure should be based on the size of the employee base, cash reserves, group claims experience, employee age and health status, and ability to find affordable reinsurance for catastrophic losses.

Third-Party Administrators

A third-party administrator (TPA) is an independent business that provides services to the self-insured employer. It is also referred to as an "administrative services only" company. A TPA's sole function is to perform "insurance-type" administrative services for self-insured employers. These services include, but are not limited to, performing claims adjudication and payment, maintaining all records, and providing utilization management, case management, and provider network management. Although it may act as an agent of the "insurer," the TPA is not party to the insurance contract between the employer and the employee. The TPA does not incur any financial risk for employer or employee losses.

Benefits of Using a TPA

Employers who self-insure often use a TPA for the following reasons:

- *Decrease start-up time:* The use of a TPA decreases the conversion time from external insurance coverage to self-insured coverage. It would be very time-consuming for the employer to develop the software systems for claims adjudication and payment alone.
- *Increased expertise:* The TPA "rents" the administrative talent that it would take years for the employer to develop in-house.
- *Decreased employee expense:* The employer does not incur the expense of hiring and finding space for full-time insurance administration personnel.
- *Decreased systems expense:* The TPA uses state-of-the-art hardware and software for claims administration. It would be prohibitively expensive for the employer to purchase the same equipment.
- *Privacy and objectivity:* The TPA ensures objectivity and discretion in claims adjudication, especially with the Health Insurance Portability and Accountability Act of 1996 (HIPAA) regulations that add additional layers of administrative complexity and federal compliance.

Automobile Insurance

Car owners are financially responsible for any accidents, damage to property, or injuries to people that they cause or someone else causes while driving their insured vehicle. Most states therefore require automobile insurance for those who own automobiles. Each state mandates the minimum allowable limits of policy coverage for medical expenses and lost wages. These policy limits vary from state to state. In some states, the policy limit is as low as $10,000.

The adjudication of car insurance claims is highly contentious and can be very costly. In an attempt to lower the costs, some states have enacted "no-fault" or personal injury protection (PIP) statutes to deter the incidence of tort claims. Under no-fault coverage the injured are paid, regardless of who is to blame for the accident. Under the PIP system, the individual can choose the payer—either the auto insurance company or the health insurance company that currently insures the person (unless Medicare or Medicaid is the health insurer; these federal programs do not allow PIP coverage of their insured). When a patient injured in an automobile collision makes a claim for benefits, a determination must be made as to whether the car in which he or she was riding had PIP coverage.

Patients injured in automobile accidents are characterized by many factors, including their youth, the severity of their injuries, the high incidence of head and spinal injuries, and the high rate of litigation in which they engage. Many patients are left permanently disabled as a result of automobile accidents. These patients can require long periods of rehabilitation, with extensive physical therapy, as well as speech, occupational, cognitive, and psychological therapy. Unlike workers' compensation, where there may be no limit to medically necessary care, automobile insurance has policy limits. Therefore, patients may not be able to afford all the care they require. Case Managers must plan for only necessary care and should be knowledgeable of community programs and resources that can supplement or replace purchased services.

Because of the frequency of litigation, many of these automobile accident cases will go to trial, and Case Managers' records can be subpoenaed. Case Managers must therefore keep clear, concise, and objective documentation of all patient and family interactions as well as all their decisions and recommendations.

When the source of payment for medical care is a tort claim and the funds available for treatment are extensive, the treating physicians have a tendency to treat the patient paternalistically. In other words, there is a tendency toward "over-treatment." The Case Manager must assess proposed care plans against the standard of what is reasonable and necessary.

Pharmacy Benefits

A pharmacy benefit is a contract between the insurance company and the employer that pays the costs of the pharmaceuticals and biological products prescribed for the insured. The pharmacy benefit is not a mandatory part of a commercial health insurance policy; rather it usually exists as a "rider" or amendment to the health insurance policy in exchange for additional premium dollars. Pharmacy benefits are not uniform, and their structures may vary dramatically between healthcare plans. What products the pharmacy benefit covers and how much it pays for each prescription are issues negotiated between the insurer and the employer.

The list of covered drugs in a pharmacy benefit is called the formulary. The formulary is created by the insurance company or other institution to ensure the quality and reduce the costs of pharmaceuticals. The formulary insures quality by excluding products that are known to be dangerous, have unsafe production methods, or are not approved by the U.S. Food and Drug Administration. Formularies reduce the cost of the pharmacy benefits by using the insurers' buying power to purchase drugs at lower prices. This buying power is increased when the number of products purchased is limited. Therefore, the more limited the formulary, the cheaper the cost of pharmacy benefit.

Pharmacy benefits are usually structured to increase the beneficiary's adherence to the formulary and by so doing to decrease the cost of the pharmacy benefit to the payer. Formulary adherence is encouraged by either categorically limiting the choice of drugs or increasing the out-of-pocket costs to the beneficiary. Mandatory use of generic drugs is a method of keeping the patient from purchasing the more expensive version of two or more equally effective drugs. Deductible fees, total dollar limits on the benefit, and copayments increase the out-of-pocket expense for the beneficiary when he or she chooses to purchase drugs not on the formulary.

A mandatory generic program is a stipulation in the insurance contract that states when a prescription is written for an insured and that drug is available in a generic version, only the generic version is covered by the benefit.

Deductible fees are an amount of money the insured must incur in drug purchases in 1 year before his or her insurance will begin to cover drug costs. The amount of the deductible is negotiated between the employer and the insurer. Higher deductible fees result in a less expensive pharmacy benefit but higher out-of-pocket costs for the insured with a lot of prescriptions.

Pharmacy benefit limits, also known as pharmacy caps, put a total dollar amount on the insured's drug benefit. For example, if an insured's drug benefit is $2,000, this is all the money the insurance company will pay for prescription drugs in that year. All prescription costs over this amount are paid out-of-pocket by the insured.

A copayment or copay is a payment made by the insured person each time a prescription is filled. The amount of this payment is described in the pharmacy benefit contract. Nearly all pharmacy benefit plans require some copayment to be charged to the patient for each prescription. This copayment system lowers the cost of the pharmacy benefit by sharing the costs of each prescription and discourages frivolous use. A tiered copay system is now a common method controlling pharmacy costs. With tiered copays each prescription drug on a formulary is assigned one of several levels, or "tiers." Each tier has a different copayment. The list of tiers and associated copayments are usually listed in the insured's plan document. For example,

- Tier-one prescription drugs are low-cost generics.
- Tier-two prescription drugs include higher-cost generics and lower-cost brand name drugs.
- Tier-three prescription drugs include higher-cost brand name drugs.
- Tier-four prescription drugs include much higher-cost medications (e.g., cancer drugs and biologicals).

Formulary directors can manage the utilization of drugs that are deemed to be the least cost-effective by assigning them to the higher tiers of copayment.

Deductible fees, pharmacy limits, and copayments were designed for two purposes: to lower pharmacy benefit costs through sharing and to encourage a dialogue between the insured and the treating physician that resulted in the physician ordering the most cost-effective drug, at the lowest effective dose and duration. Although these discussions do occur and unnecessary prescriptions are eliminated, unintended consequences have also been reported. For example, these financial incentives have been associated with reduced use of necessary and appropriate medications for chronic conditions such as asthma, chronic obstructive pulmonary disease, and breast cancer. RAND researchers concluded in their 2007 study that higher copayments were associated with lower rates of drug treatment, worse adherence among existing users, and more frequent discontinuation of therapy.[1]

Managed Care Reimbursement Concepts

Managed care is, at its base, a payer-driven system of cost containment. It is traditionally defined as any healthcare delivery system in which a third party (i.e., a party other than the physician or the patient) actively manages a defined, comprehensive set of healthcare benefits. The enrolled population is voluntary, and it pays premiums to the managed care organization for medical care.

Managed care medical insurance began in the 1930s when the first prepaid group practices were established as a way to improve access to quality health care and as a vehicle to provide preventive healthcare services. Included under the rubric of managed care organization are health maintenance organizations (HMOs), preferred provider organizations (PPOs), exclusive provider organizations (EPOs), and point of service (POS) plans.

Health Maintenance Organizations

The HMO is the most common form of managed care. It is a legal entity, licensed by the state or federal government as a healthcare insurer, and is regulated by state and federal HMO laws. It accepts premium payments in advance of disbursements and manages both the medical and the financial aspects of care. HMOs often use primary care physicians to act as coordinators (or gatekeepers) of the enrollee's health care. The coordinator's or gatekeeper's role in the HMO is to maximize the effectiveness of the care delivered and to do so at the least possible cost that is consistent with good medical care. There are four basic types of HMOs:

- *Staff model:* In this model the physicians are employed solely by the HMO. They see only the HMO's enrollees and are usually paid a salary. This is the oldest form of HMO and is rarely practiced today.
- *Group model:* The group model varies from the staff model in that the physicians are not employed by the HMO but are employed by the physician group. The physician group contracts with the HMO to provide a defined set of services for a fixed monthly rate per enrollee, which is known as a capitated rate. The physician group then distributes the proceeds of the capitated reimbursement to its physicians according to its own schedule.
- *Independent practice association (IPA) model:* In this model an IPA contracts with the HMO to provide medical services to its enrollees. An IPA is a legal entity sponsored by physicians that exists to contract with HMOs. An IPA is composed of physicians, or groups of physicians, who agree to be bound by the terms of a contract with an HMO. These physicians have their own practices, see their own patients (i.e., non-HMO patients), and care for the HMO's enrollees at the rate contracted by the IPA. The IPA negotiates payment for the physicians in the IPA as either a capitated fee or a discounted, fee-for-service rate.
- *Network model:* The HMO contracts individually with IPAs, medical groups, and independent physicians to form its provider network. Fees are negotiated as either a capitated rate or a discounted, fee-for-service rate. The physicians accept a discounted fee-for-service rate in exchange for an increased volume of patients.

The use of a gatekeeper is a method of physician case management practiced widely in HMOs, EPOs, and PPOs. The gatekeeper is a primary care physician who has a group of patients assigned to him or her by the HMO. The gatekeeper's responsibility to these patients is to provide primary medical and preventive care and to direct, authorize, and coordinate other medical care that is outside the scope of his or her practice. Before one of these assigned patients can receive health care that is reimbursable by the HMO, the gatekeeper must approve it.

Exclusions under the gatekeeper model include true medical or surgical emergencies and routine gynecological care. Benefits of the gatekeeper model are that it controls costs, controls utilization, and channels utilization of services to "in-network" providers.

This method of physician case management has proven effective in reducing unnecessary healthcare expenditures, especially when the gatekeeper is at financial risk for the cost of care. Although managed care companies have encouraged the gatekeeper concept, patients accustomed to referring themselves to specialists have chafed under this system.

Accusations that gatekeepers and HMOs deny medically appropriate care to save money have been leveled. The idea, however erroneous, that the gatekeeper model restricts patients' freedom and may not be in their best interest has gained currency with some consumers and the press. Further, physicians in the United States who are trained to provide the best care possible for each patient without regard to the patient's ability to pay may be uncomfortable in the role of gatekeeper, which sometimes puts them at odds with their patients and their training. Finally, primary care physicians may be pressured by HMOs to care for patients with diseases that, although not necessarily outside their training, may be outside their experience and comfort level. This could result in a patient receiving care that is below the level that a specialist, experienced in the care of that disease state, could offer.

Preferred Provider Organizations

As managed care became more popular, the perception grew that HMOs limited a patient's choice of provider. Consumers demanded more flexibility in choosing providers than that made available in the standard HMO. PPOs were formed to accommodate this desire for more freedom in provider selection. Typically, a PPO is formed when an insurer contracts with a large group of providers (i.e., a provider network) to provide medical services for its enrollees at a negotiated fee schedule. PPOs do not depend on gatekeepers to control specialty referrals, and they do not rely on capitation to control costs. Providers are usually paid on a discounted, fee-for-service schedule, and enrollees can seek specialty care as they see fit. Although enrollees are encouraged to seek care from the provider network, they can also receive care from nonaffiliated providers by paying a higher coinsurance fee. Aggressive utilization management and fee negotiations are used to control costs.

Exclusive Provider Organizations

An EPO uses the same model of organization as the PPO. It uses a network of contracted physicians who agree to care for the EPO's enrollees at a discounted rate. Gatekeepers and capitation are not employed. However, the enrollee is not free to choose a provider outside the network. Care from nonaffiliated providers is not reimbursed by the EPO.

Point of Service Plans

The POS plan is a hybrid between the PPO and the HMO. The POS plan uses a contracted network of providers. The primary care physician acts as a gatekeeper to control specialty referrals. Enrollees who seek care from network physicians pay little or no out-of-pocket expenses. Those who seek care from non-network physicians are reimbursed, but they are responsible for paying a higher deductible and coinsurance payment. Through this methodology insurers have managed to keep up to 85% of care provided within the HMO network.

Specialty Managed Care Arrangements (Carve-Outs)

As managed care became more prevalent, difficulties in managing medical specialty care arose. Typically, mental health and substance abuse, prescription drug services, dental care, and vision (prescription eyeglasses) care are "carved out" services. However, cancer care, HIV/AIDS care, cardiology, audiology, and radiology are also becoming common carve-outs. Escalating specialty costs and a lack of understanding of the intricacies of specialty care prompted managed care organizations to look for new options. New organizations with experience in handling specialty care began to negotiate with the managed care plans to provide services. These specialty organizations have their own contracted specialty provider panels and possess sophisticated management services that allowed them to offer the specialty care more efficiently and effectively.

Prospective Payment System: Capitation

Capitation is a payer-driven, prepayment methodology aimed at reducing costs. It accomplishes cost reduction by removing the provider's incentive to provide more services than are needed. This "perverse incentive" to over-prescribe and over-treat is seen commonly under the fee-for-service system. Physician motivations for over-prescribing services range from simply wanting to bill more, to intellectual laziness, to defensive medicine. Capitation permits the provider and the managed care organization to predict the expenses and revenues that will be generated by a defined population. The number of lives covered sets the capitated amount, rather than the number of services provided, and is usually expressed in units of dollars "per member per month," abbreviated and commonly referred to as PMPM.

This means the primary care physician is paid the same amount of money each month for a defined group of patients (the capitated population), regardless of how many times he or she sees those patients or what services he or she provides to those patients. This fixed payment amount provides no economic advantage for increasing utilization.

When catastrophic cases occur, requiring increased amounts of care, the primary care physician limits his or her degree of financial risk by purchasing reinsurance or stop-loss insurance. One of the advantages under capitation is the incentive for physicians to appreciate the need to manage the health of the entire population as a way of keeping costs under control. It brings into better focus the need to increase preventive services and to identify diseases early. For example, mammography screening becomes not just a public health issue, but it may save the physician the expense of caring for an end-stage breast cancer patient.

Critics of capitation have alleged that it encourages physicians to make choices that maximize practice revenue and minimize expense rather than ensuring the best care for their enrolled patients. That is, doctors will chose to deny necessary care to a patient to save him- or herself money. Although most physicians and their staffs are conscientious and ethical, a bias to minimize the utilization of capitated patients and to increase the utilization of fee-for-service patients does exist. This bias has done much to promote the impression that physicians are not working in the best interest of their patients, when their patients are capitated.

The following are advantages of capitation:

- Decreased utilization and costs associated with specialty services
- Decreased primary care physicians' tendency to over-treat
- Improved cash flow
- Increased tendency to offer preventive services
- Increased tendency to focus on the early detection of disease

There are disadvantages of capitation as well:

- Increased tendency to under-treat capitated patients
- Increased tendency of physicians to focus on fee-for-service patients to the detriment of the patients under capitated payment
- Increased suspicion of patients about motivations of physicians
- Regulatory and licensing issues when the physician acts as an insurer

Since the first edition of this book, capitated contracts have fallen out of vogue as a means of effectively controlling healthcare costs. The risks associated with capitation contracting have been responsible for the failure of many large, well-established physician practices. It was discovered that individual physicians and even large medical practices neither have the ability to accurately predict medical losses in their patient populations nor are able to maintain cash flow or purchase enough reinsurance to make the system work. Further, the practice of capitation contracting has been challenged in the courts in many states. It was argued that in the setting of capitation contracting, the physician acts as a health insurer and therefore should be subject to insurance regulation and licensing. There were also allegations of inappropriate denials of medical care based on costs. Excess medical costs could affect the economic viability of a physician's practice. It was believed that physicians managing capitated patients amounted to a serious conflict of interest. Capitated contracts are a rarity now.

HEALTHCARE INSURANCE PRINCIPLES

Coordination of Benefits

Coordination of benefits (COB) is a process used by insurers to fairly assign healthcare costs between payers when an individual is covered by more than one insurance policy. The COB process is structured so payments made to the insured do not exceed the expenses incurred. Without COB, an individual might be reimbursed more than 100% of the cost for medical care.

COB provisions were developed during the 1950s when it became common for people to have more than one source of insurance. Almost all group health insurers have COB provisions in their contracts with enrollees. COB rules are not federally mandated but are voluntarily adopted by states and individual insurance companies. Despite the voluntary nature of these rules, the compliance rate is very high. COB saves between 4% and 9% in claims costs.

The National Association of Insurance Commissioners has agreed to a set of common rules. The rules specify who pays for an individual's healthcare claims when the individual is a beneficiary of more than one insurance policy. Most states and insurance companies have adopted these rules. In fact, insurance plans without COB provisions are obligated to pay first. The rules of COB adopted by the National Association of Insurance Commissioners follow:

1. The insurance plan covering the individual as an employee pays first.
2. The plan covering the individual as a dependent pays second.
3. If both plans cover the individual as a dependent, the plan of the employee whose birthday occurs soonest in the year pays first. This rule (the "birthday rule") applies only if both plans have adopted the rule and if the parents are married.
4. If neither plan has adopted the birthday rule and if the parents are married, the plan of the male parent pays first.
5. If the parents are divorced, the plan awarded primary responsibility by the court pays first.

6. If the parents are divorced and there is no court-determined primary, then the following order is used:
   - The plan of the parent with custody of the child pays first.
   - The plan of the spouse of the parent with custody pays second (e.g., if a woman has custody of her child, then remarries, her new husband's insurance plan would pay second).
   - The plan of the parent without custody pays next (in the preceding scenario, the ex-husband's plan would pay next).
   - The plan of the spouse of the noncustodial parent pays last (in the preceding scenario, if the ex-husband remarried, his new wife's insurance plan would be responsible for her husband's child by his first marriage, as the last payer).
7. The plan covering an individual as an active employee pays first; the plan covering that individual as an inactive employee (such as a retiree or a laid-off employee) pays second.
8. The plan covering an individual due to Consolidated Omnibus Budget Reconciliation Act (COBRA) is secondary to a plan covering that individual as an employee, a member, or a dependent.
9. If none of the previous rules results in a determination, then the plan covering the individual for the longest period of time pays first.

Medical Necessity

Defining medical necessity is a problem that gets at the heart of health insurance. All health insurance policies state in some fashion that only "medically necessary" care will be reimbursed. However, the defining medical necessity is ambiguous at best and leads to a lack of consistency among insurance plans in the way they interpret medical necessity. In fact, a 1994 survey by the U.S. General Accounting Office revealed "substantial variation" in the denial rates for lack of medical necessity.

Problems with the Definition

Current corporate definitions of medical necessity are crafted in weak terms or in circular language. For example, a typical corporate definition describes medical necessity as "Those procedures, treatments or supplies that are recommended by a licensed physician, are appropriate, reasonable and accepted in the medical community for treating the disease in question, are not experimental or investigational, and are not custodial."

What is "appropriate, reasonable and acceptable"? What is experimental? What is custodial? It is not made clear to either the insured or the insurer's administrators.

Further complicating this issue is the fact that the insurer or the insurer's review organization typically reserves the right to determine what procedures are medically necessary. With the spectrum of meanings available in this definition, discrepancies over coverage issues naturally arise. When this issue is litigated, the courts have consistently construed the meaning of medical necessity in favor of the insured.

Reasonable Expectations

When cases of medical necessity are litigated, the courts place significant weight on the reasonable expectations of a layperson in the position of a patient. The court implies that if "reasonable laypersons" could expect a certain medical benefit under their contract, then they may be entitled to it. This expectation principle is used by the courts to justify granting a wide range of benefits to the subscriber that the insurer's policy language appears to exclude. In the case of *Ponder v. Blue Cross of Southern California*, for example, the insurer denied treatment for temporomandibular joint syndrome because it was excluded by the contract.[2] The fairness of the contract was questioned because the purchaser of the insurance did not understand the meaning of the exclusionary criteria in the contract. As the court stated, subscribers "could only discover what they had bought with their premiums as their diseases were diagnosed, and they found out to their sorrow, the true meaning of those mysterious words in their insurance contracts."[2]

Solutions

A procedural approach to defining medical necessity effectively bolsters an insurance company's contractual definition, especially when the definition is contested in court. The solution lies in the hands of the medical director. It is his or her responsibility to manage the "process" of claims adjudication for medical necessity. The medical director must ensure through this process that subscribers receive everything they paid for and are not subjected to ineffective or harmful treatment and that the process for making these decisions is fair, reproducible, and based on the best medical information available. This is called a "procedural definition" of medical necessity.

Therefore, the best solution lies not only in improving a contractual definition that contains exhaustive exclusionary criteria, but also in clearly defining the process for determining medical necessity. The goals of this process are to improve the health of subscribers and to protect them from harm through rigorous, scientifically sound, and manifestly fair methods. This process entails the following steps:

- *Firmly establish the intent of the medical necessity clause in all documentation:* The intent of medical necessity determinations is to protect the subscribers from irregular, dangerous, or unnecessary procedures. The intent of medical necessity should be clearly stated in the contract, the subscribers' handbook, and any other communications between the subscriber and the insurer.
- *Implement medical oversight:* The medical director, a physician licensed in the state in which the patient is treated, should review and approve all benefit denials.
- *Eliminate perverse incentives:* The compensation of the medical director and the utilization staff should not depend on the number of dollars saved through claims denials but rather on their adherence to the tenets and goals of the review process.
- *Be aware of high-profile cases:* The medical director, risk manager, and corporate counsel should be aware of all high-profile cases (i.e., those most likely to be legally contested or result in unfavorable media coverage—expensive, high-risk procedures, such as bone marrow transplants, neurosurgeries, or treatment of infants in pediatric intensive care units or oncology wards). These cases, which have a high potential for grievances and appeals, are more intensely scrutinized by subscribers, regulators, and the courts. They should therefore generate a commensurate amount of investigation and consideration by the medical director and the case management staff.
- *Consult objective specialists:* Cases that fall outside the medical director's area of expertise should be reviewed by independent, external, unbiased medical consultants.

- *Request and review the medical records:* The medical director must be alert to extenuating circumstances or clinical issues that may mitigate the claims denial. Medical directors should record the time, date, and findings from the chart review and any subsequent interviews or examination in their case notes.
- *Speak with the patient's attending physician:* To obtain the complete clinical picture, the medical director should speak with all physicians involved in the patient's care.
- *Document all decisions:* Documentation of decisions surrounding denials is essential. These documents should include both the cause of denial (e.g., not medically necessary) and the reasons for denial (e.g., does not meet inclusion criteria). Any literature or expert testimony relied on in making the decision should be included in the file.
- *Maintain denial database:* When denying claims, the medical director should review past decisions regarding the type of treatment under consideration. Lack of consistency in decision making opens the insurer to criticisms of arbitrary and capricious conduct. Insurers should maintain a database of prior decisions on medical necessity so these decisions can be reviewed and used to guide research and investigations into future claim issues. When a claim for a type of treatment is approved that has be denied in the past, the medical director should note in his or her record why this decision was made and how this case differs from the previous cases that were denied.
- *Address subscribers' expectations:* Insurers must address the reasonable expectations of their subscribers. Although a full explanation in the subscribers' manual is a good start, most subscribers do not read this document. Timely information about benefits and education about disease states is useful to subscribers and can be carried out by the case management staff.
- *Regularly review the medical adjudication procedures used in the utilization review process, including software edits in the claims system that define covered benefits:* Inaccuracies in the claims system may lead to unwarranted denials.

A comprehensive definition of medical necessity, although highly desirable, no longer satisfies subscribers or protects insurers against litigation. In determining medical necessity, insurers should strive to provide subscribers with the safest, most efficacious care needed. An insurer's attention to this process, rather than a slavish dependence on the definition alone, will improve subscriber satisfaction and decrease liability. Educating subscribers about the contract's benefits will temper their expectations when benefits are requested. The medical director should control the process of determining what is medically necessary, consult experts liberally, and document extensively.

An effective Case Manager should understand the definition of medical necessity as stated in the insured's contract, as well as the limitations of that definition. Counseling subscribers on what medical necessity means, how it is defined, and how discrepancies are adjudicated will help to manage their expectations and reduce needless anxiety.

Reinsurance or Stop-Loss Insurance

To reinsure is defined as the act of insuring again, especially by transferring in whole or in part a risk already covered under an existing contract. Reinsurance, then, is an insurance policy purchased by an insurer to reduce financial risk. Reinsurance policies protect the primary insurer against unexpected catastrophic losses.

Healthcare plans, insurance companies, and individual physicians (operating under risk contracts) purchase reinsurance policies to reduce their financial risk when paying the healthcare claims of an individual or a group. This reinsurance is sometimes called stop-loss or threshold insurance and may apply to the aggregate expense of multiple individuals (i.e., total claims for an insured population for 1 year) or to the expenses of a single enrollee. For example, health plan A receives $1 million of premium for providing health insurance to 1,000 enrollees. A single catastrophic case, such as a premature infant in the neonatal intensive care unit for 6 months, could eliminate all profits and perhaps bring the company to insolvency. Even a small group of severely ill patients could wipe out the health plan's earnings. For these types of occurrences the healthcare plan purchases stop-loss insurance or reinsurance. The first type of reinsurance sets a predefined dollar limit on any individual's loss, for example, $2,500 on any one enrollee. In this example the healthcare plan is at risk up to $2,500 on any one enrollee; after that, the reinsurance company pays the bills for that enrollee's care (up to a predefined dollar limit, e.g., $1 million). The second type of reinsurance sets a predefined dollar limit on the aggregate loss of the healthcare plan. To use healthcare plan A, as an example, it might buy a reinsurance policy that would set a limit of $500,000 in losses. After that limit is reached, the reinsurer would cover losses above $500,000.

Reinsurers of healthcare companies base their premiums (or cost of their insurance) on several variables:

- *Threshold:* At what dollar level does the reinsurer start paying? An insurer makes plans to cover healthcare claims up to a certain limit. This limit may be $5,000, $10,000, or $50,000. When claims are received for amounts above this limit, the reinsurer pays. The higher the threshold the insurer sets, the lower the premium rate or reinsurance will be.
- *Health risk of population:* Insurers and reinsurers base their premiums on the likelihood of the patients requiring medical services. The higher the risk of illness or injury, the higher the insurance premium will be. The risk of getting ill or injured is related to the age, occupation, and health experience of an individual or group. For example, those who work in heavy construction are more likely to get injured than those who perform office work; therefore, their health insurance premiums will be higher. Similarly, those groups or individuals who have a history of high medical resource utilization are expected to have a similar pattern of utilization in the future. They will, therefore, pay higher premiums for health insurance.
- *Benefits:* The liability or risk of exceeding the claims threshold is related to the benefits an insurer extends to a group. The more generous the benefit package, the easier it is for an individual or group to exceed its threshold. An insurer can reduce his or her risk of exceeding his or her reinsurance threshold by eliminating high cost or high utilization procedures or treatments from the benefits package. For example, cosmetic surgery or treatments for infertility are commonly excluded in health insurance policies.

CASE MANAGEMENT INTERVENTIONS

The Case Manager is given the ability to intervene in both the clinical and the financial aspects of patient care. That is, the Case Manager has positive interactions, not only between the medical provider and the patient but between the insurer and the patient.

In the following paragraphs the nature of these interactions is examined, along with their limitations and responsibilities.

Extra-Contractual Benefits

It should be noted that when a Case Manager (working for the insurer) extends extra-contractual benefits to an individual, this unfairly changes the assumptions upon which a reinsurer has based its premiums. To avoid a breach of the reinsurance contract, the insurer does not charge the costs of extra-contractual benefits against his or her reinsurance threshold.

Alternate Benefit Plans and Extra-Contractual Benefits

Alternate benefit plans and extra-contractual benefits are health insurance benefits given to a beneficiary that are not contained in the beneficiary's insurance policy. The insurer extends these benefits to the insured when two conditions can be met:

- The benefit will aid the patient (i.e., it is medically necessary for the patient).
- The utilization of the extra-contractual benefit will decrease the overall cost of care for the insurer (i.e., it will be financially advantageous to the insurer).

For example, an insured is an inpatient in the hospital receiving only wound care, a service that could be offered at home. The patient's insurance policy does not have a home care benefit; therefore, wound care must be offered at the hospital at considerable expense. It makes economic sense for the insurer to offer the patient a home care benefit, because doing so saves the insurer the cost of hospitalization.

The provision of extra-contractual benefits is not a discretionary right of the Case Manager. Case Managers, acting as agents for the insurer, are empowered to offer these extra-contractual benefits either through the Case Manager's job description or by provisions in the insurance contract between the insurance company and the insured. This is an instance in which the Case Manager's often competing obligations to act as an advocate for both the patient and the insurer are harmonious.

Case Managers' Responsibilities When Offering Alternate Benefit Plans and Extra-Contractual Benefits

To prevent confusion on the part of the patient and other insureds, the Case Manager should abide by the following rules when offering extra-contractual benefits:

- *Obtain approval from the referral source:* The referral source (i.e., the payer) must approve alternate benefit plans before the patient and provider are alerted. The request to the referral source is best done in person or over the telephone. In this way the Case Manager can present the entire case, including the rationale for "flexing" the benefit, the cost savings projected for the alternate benefit plan, and to answer any questions that may arise. It is prudent at this time for the Case Manager to obtain the approval in writing.
- *Inform the insured of the nature of the benefit:* The insured should be made aware that the benefit being offered is outside his or her benefit package and is being offered because it is financially advantageous for the insurer. It is helpful to

formalize this information in a letter to the insured. This will help to manage the patient's expectations before he or she requests other noncovered benefits.
- *Set time limits:* Extra-contractual benefits are financially advantageous to the insurer only when the extent of the benefit is known. For example, when offering home physical rehabilitation care to a patient recovering from an injury, a Case Manager assumes that the cost of home rehabilitation is cheaper than hospital-based rehabilitation. To correctly determine the cost of home rehabilitation versus the hospital-based rehabilitation, a Case Manager must know not just the per-diem cost but the total number of days of rehabilitation as well. Once begun, some benefits are difficult to stop, especially when the patient and family become accustomed to or dependent on the benefit. The costs of these "prolonged" benefits can far outstrip the costs of the more "expensive" care they were meant to replace. It is therefore imperative for the Case Manager to describe to the insured the reason for the benefit and to clearly articulate both the intensity (how many visits per day or per week) and the length of time it will be offered.
- *Document, document, and document:* As stated earlier, confusion can occur when extra-contractual benefits are offered. This confusion is not limited to the insured receiving the benefit. Other people insured by the same company might request benefits that they have seen other subscribers receive. These others may be family members, neighbors, coworkers, or healthcare providers. It becomes difficult to deny these requests when the insurer has no record of why the benefits contract was disregarded in the past. Accusations of arbitrary and capricious conduct or discrimination may be leveled at the insurer who appears to offer different levels of benefits to enrollees who have the same benefit plan. The need for adequate documentation is clear. The documentation should include but not be limited to:
  - A letter to the insurer notifying them what benefits are being offered, what they are replacing or trying to avoid, what the limits on the benefit will be, and what the cost and the savings will be
  - A letter to the employer (in the case of third-party administration) notifying them what benefits are being offered, what they are replacing or trying to avoid, what the limits on the benefit will be, and what the cost and the savings will be
  - A letter to the insured notifying him or her of the new benefit, the reason for the benefit, and the limits of the benefit
  - Letters to the providers of care in the case notifying them of the new benefit, the reason for the benefit, and the limits of the benefit
  - Letters to the claims administrator notifying them of the alternate benefit and what the limits on the benefit will be so that claims are adjudicated per the alternate benefit agreement
  - Case Manager's report documenting the narrative summary of individual case activity and cost savings
  - An extra-contractual benefits log should be created. It should contain the data for all extra-contractual benefits offered by the Case Manager or all Case Managers in a single office. These data should include the names of the insured, the benefit extended, the benefit replaced, and the savings accrued. Documenting who was notified of these benefits and when is also appropriate.

Extra-Contractual Benefits and Reinsurance

Reinsurance companies are institutions that indemnify insurance companies. The cost of extra-contractual benefits is the sole responsibility of the primary insurer, not the reinsurer. Therefore, the careful documentation of all costs associated with extra-contractual benefits must be reported to the insurer so the reinsurer is not billed.

Prior Approval

It is important for Case Managers to understand the insurance policy and benefits the patient has when planning his or her care. One of the most important aspects of the policy is whether there is a precertification requirement and, if so, which benefits require prior approval. The Case Manager needs to coordinate the needed referrals for precertification with the primary physician. The limitations of certain benefits can be seen in the setting of a patient who requires extensive rehabilitation, for example:

- Does the patient have a maximum of 40 visits per calendar year for physical therapy?
- Is the patient's inpatient rehabilitation benefit unlimited?
- Does the patient only have access to a durable medical equipment benefit if arranged through a specific network vendor?
- Does the case management benefit allow for free rein in choosing providers and arranging alternate benefit plans?

Most payers want to be involved in approving alternate benefit plans or extra-contractual benefits. It is important to document the payer source's approval and to communicate that approval to the claims processor. The Case Manager should speak to the person delegated to approve or deny such benefit plan recommendations before putting the request in writing. That way, any questions about benefit limitations, plan exclusions, and the cost-effectiveness of the outlined plan can be answered immediately and the patient's expectations for future care can be appropriately managed. It is important to communicate estimated time frames, negotiated rates, and comparisons with other treatments that are contemplated. For instance, if the patient's plan has no "home care benefit" without a prior hospitalization and a patient requires a course of intravenous antibiotics for 6 weeks, it is very effective to compare the cost of the hospitalization versus the cost of home intravenous therapy. That difference in these costs are often called "hard savings." The total daily rate for the hospitalization that was avoided is referred to as "soft savings" or "potential savings."

Another way of looking at the hard savings is as the difference between the costs that would have been incurred had there been no case management intervention and the actual cost due to case management intervention. Soft savings are usually "in lieu" of some other therapy or treatment plan. The savings realized from subtracting the cost of a subacute facility from an acute care facility is considered soft savings, whereas the savings from negotiating off the usual fee at the subacute facility is considered hard savings. After the payer or referral source has agreed to the alternate benefit plan or extra-contractual benefit, a specific letter detailing the agreement should be faxed or mailed to the payer or referral source for signature and be returned for the Case Manager's records. If the bills are sent to the Case Manager for approval before sending them for claims adjudication, it is advantageous to attach a copy of the extra-contractual agreement to ensure proper payment.

Negotiations

Case Managers need to maintain a file of basic costs for the items they negotiate routinely. Most insurance companies have predetermined fee schedules for these common items based on what is termed reasonable and customary fees (also called usual and customary fees). Although there are many methods to determine usual and customary fees, they are generally created by averaging fees derived from bills submitted in a geographical region. Alternatively, some large databases, such as Health Insurance Association of America, can be used to create the usual and customary fee. A third method is to base usual and customary fees on the Medicare fee schedule. It is common to negotiate durable medical equipment, intravenous medications, nursing visits, and so forth at some percentage of the Medicare fee schedule. The *Red Book*[3] is an invaluable tool when negotiating prescription medications. Among other important information, the *Red Book* lists the average wholesale price for all medications sold in the United States. The Case Manager can be more effective when using national resources such as the *Red Book* as a basis for negotiating discounts.

Utilization Management and Utilization Review

Utilization review is a management process used by health insurance companies to control the cost and quality of healthcare services. This process ensures that requested services are covered under the insurance contract and that the appropriate service is being performed at the appropriate level of care, by the appropriate provider, and at an appropriate cost. Utilization review can be prospective (e.g., precertification of an elective hospital admission), concurrent (e.g., an immediate adjudication of an unexpected or emergent admission), or retrospective (e.g., when claims are received and reviewed after services have been rendered).

Although the terms "utilization management" and "utilization review" are often used interchangeably, they are two distinct processes. They both involve the review of medical care based on necessity and appropriateness; however, utilization management usually refers to requests for approval of future medical needs (prospective review), such as the precertification of admissions or surgical procedures, whereas utilization review refers to reviews of past medical treatment (retrospective review). The process of utilization review involves the collection of clinical data from the treating physician, including the results of the medical history, physical examination, lab results, and imaging procedures. These data are compared against an explicit criteria set to determine if the treatment is medically necessary and appropriate. This determination is made by a licensed physician (the medical director) in the employ of the utilization review organization. If claim for the treatment is denied and the patient or the treating physician disagrees with that decision, they are invited to make an appeal. The appeals process, also a part of the utilization review process, involves another review of the case. The medical director collects more clinical data, discusses the case with the treating physician, and may ask for a review by an independent third-party physician with expertise in the clinical discipline in question before making another determination on the case.

Utilization review is especially effective in identifying patients who would benefit by case management services. Utilization review can positively affect the length of stay and patient outcome. An example of this improved length of stay and outcome occurs when a patient scheduled for a hip replacement is taught physical therapy exercises and obtains a raised toilet seat and a walker before the surgery. This reduces discharge planning delays associated with getting equipment and teaching the patient ambulation with a walker. The patient can also get more out of the teaching before the surgery, when he or she is not distracted because of pain or less alert from taking pain medications.

One of the most noted consequences of utilization review is the improved outcomes associated with its sentinel effect. The sentinel effect is akin to the "Hawthorne effect" described in industrial psychology research. The premise of both is that a group of people will perform their jobs better if they know they are being observed. In the case of the sentinel effect, it has been observed that a case will be better managed, and therefore less costly, simply because a neutral, third party was observing.[4] In other words, for the purposes of utilization review, the knowledge that someone is doing utilization review positively affects the process. Those being "observed" are aware and want to do well; thus, more timely interventions and discharges occur.

FEDERAL LEGISLATION IMPORTANT TO THE CASE MANAGER

Tax Equity and Fiscal Responsibility Act of 1982

Among various federal legislation that are pertinent to the Case Manager is the Tax Equity and Fiscal Responsibility Act of 1982. This legislation was designed to provide providers incentives for cost containment and provided the following:

- Established a case-based reimbursement system, known as diagnosis-related groups. This prospective payment system determined the cost of care for selected diagnoses, while also placing limits on rate increases in hospital revenues.
- Exempted medical rehabilitation from diagnosis-related groups. Rehabilitation would continue as a cost-based reimbursement system, subject to certain limits.
- Amended the Social Security Act and made Medicare secondary to employer group health plans for active employees 65 to 69 years old and their spouses in the same age group.
- Revised the Age Discrimination in Employment Act of 1967 by requiring employers to offer active employees age 65 to 69 and their spouses the same health benefits as those made available to younger employees.
- Established peer review organizations. A peer review organization is an entity selected by the Centers for Medicare & Medicaid Services (CMS) to reduce costs associated with the hospital stays of Medicare and Medicaid patients. Further, peer review organizations are charged with conducting reviews of hospital-based care on these patients to ensure quality of care and appropriateness of admissions, readmissions, and discharges. Through this review procedure, peer review organizations can maintain or lower admission rates and reduce lengths of stay while ensuring against inadequate treatment.

Mental Health Parity Act of 1996

The Mental Health Parity Act (MHPA) of 1996 is a federal law that protects individuals with mental health problems against discrimination by prohibiting lifetime or annual dollar limits on mental health care, unless comparable limits apply to medical or surgical treatment. Enforcement began during plan years beginning on or after January 1, 1998.

The scope of the MHPA is limited, as is its likely impact on mental health services. Some important issues in this law are as follows:

- The MHPA's definition of mental health excludes treatments associated with substance abuse. Therefore, plans have separate limits for the treatment of substance abuse.
- Under the MHPA, health insurance plans are not required to cover mental health treatment. However, if a plan does have mental health coverage, it cannot set a separate dollar limit from medical care.
- Although annual or lifetime dollar limits cannot be set under the provisions of the MHPA, other limits are allowed, for example:
  - Limited number of annual outpatient visits
  - Limited number of annual inpatient days
  - A per-visit fee limit
  - Higher deductibles and copayments, without parity in medical and surgical benefits.

Some employers are exempt from this law. These include employers with 50 or fewer employees and any group plan that can demonstrate that the MHPA's requirements will result in a significant financial hardship. Specifically, if parity would require an increase of 1% or more in its healthcare costs, the plan is exempt.

Pregnancy Discrimination Act

The Pregnancy Discrimination Act is a federal law that extends to the disabilities associated with pregnancies and childbirth the same rights and benefits offered to employees with other medical disabilities. This federal law was created as an amendment to Title VII of the Civil Rights Act of 1964.

The Pregnancy Discrimination Act expects employers to treat individuals with disabilities attendant to medical and surgical conditions the same as they do disabilities associated with pregnancy and childbirth. This "same treatment" includes

- Health insurance benefits
- Short-term sick leave
- Disability benefits
- Employment policies (such as seniority, leave extensions, and reinstatement)

The "same treatment" means that in regard to choice, access, cost, and quality, maternity benefits will equal medical benefits. An individual cannot be discriminated against in any of the following ways:

- Limiting the number of physicians or hospitals that provide maternity care, when medical and surgical care providers are not limited
- Limiting the number of plans that offer maternity care, without corresponding limits on medical and surgical care
- Limiting the reimbursement for maternity care, when there are no corresponding limits on medical and surgical care
- Exacting higher deductibles, copayments, or out-of-pocket maximums for maternity care than for medical and surgical care

Who Is Covered by the Pregnancy Discrimination Act?

The courts have interpreted coverage standards for employees broadly, and all of the following are considered eligible under the Pregnancy Discrimination Act:

- Full-time employees
- Part-time employees
- Independent contractors
- Employees of successor corporations
- Employees of parent-subsidiary groups

The Pregnancy Discrimination Act is enforced, independent of the marital status of the employee. Benefits not covered under the Pregnancy Discrimination Act include abortions and mandatory maternity leave.

As with most laws, some employers are exempt from the Pregnancy Discrimination Act's restrictions. These include private employers with fewer than 15 employees.

Newborns' and Mothers' Health Protection Act of 1996

Among the phrases brought into common parlance by the managed care industry, the term "drive-through delivery" engendered more controversy than most. This term refers to insurers who would cover only 24 hours of hospitalization for mother and child after a normal vaginal delivery or 3 days for a cesarean section. Although little clinical evidence linked this policy with increased risk to mother or child, a few tragic cases of out-of-hospital morbidity and mortality began a call for reform. On September 26, 1996, the Newborns' and Mothers' Health Protection Act (NMHPA) was enacted to provide protection for mothers and newborns with regard to hospital lengths of stay after childbirth.

Compliance with the Act

This law applies to private and public employer plans and health insurance issuers. Nonfederal governmental, self-insured plans may elect to opt out of this Act's requirements, in the same manner as they may opt out of the requirements of HIPAA, the MHPA, and the Women's Health and Cancer Rights Act.

Under NMHPA, group health plans and health insurance issuers may not do the following:

- Restrict benefits for any hospital length of stay in connection with childbirth for mother or newborn child to less than 48 hours after a normal vaginal delivery or less than 96 hours after a delivery by cesarean section
- Require a provider to obtain authorization for prescribing a length of stay up to 48 hours for a normal vaginal delivery or 96 hours for a delivery by cesarean section
- Increase an individual's coinsurance for any later portion of a 48-hour (or, if applicable, 96-hour) hospital stay
- Deny a mother or her newborn child eligibility or continued eligibility to enroll, or to renew coverage, under the terms of the plan solely to avoid the NMHPA requirements
- Provide monetary payments, payments in kind, or rebates to a mother to encourage her to accept less than the minimum protections available under the NMHPA

- Penalize, or otherwise reduce or limit, the reimbursement of an attending provider because the provider furnished care to a mother or newborn in accordance with the NMHPA
- Provide monetary or other incentives to an attending provider to induce the provider to furnish care to a mother or newborn in a manner inconsistent with the NMHPA

An attending physician may discharge the mother and/or child before the 48- and 96-hour limits when both the mother and the physician agree that it is safe and appropriate to do so.

How Does the NMHPA Law Define the Hospital Length of Stay?

The hospital stay begins at the time of the newborn's delivery, when that delivery occurs in the hospital. In the event of multiple births, the time and date of the last delivery begins the hospital stay. When the delivery occurs outside the hospital, the hospital length of stay begins at the time the mother or newborn is admitted to the hospital in connection with the childbirth. The physician alone will determine if the hospital admission is "in connection with childbirth."

Health Insurance Portability and Accountability Act of 1996

> The case manager should adhere to applicable local, state, and federal laws, as well as employer policies, governing the client, client privacy, and confidentiality rights and act in a manner consistent with the client's best interest.
>
> —CMSA Standards of Practice for Case Management, Revised 2010

HIPAA was signed into law on August 21, 1996,[5] in an effort by the Clinton Administration to reform health care. It includes important new protections for millions of working Americans and their families who have preexisting medical conditions or might suffer discrimination in health coverage based on an individual's health status. HIPAA's provisions amend Title I of ERISA of 1974, as well as the Internal Revenue Code and the Public Health Service Act. HIPAA has significantly changed the way healthcare providers and payers do business. In fact, the HIPAA legislation has been described as the most important legislation to affect health care since the Medicare program of 1965. Its wide-ranging scope places new requirements on healthcare providers, hospitals, clinics, employer-sponsored group health plans, insurance companies, and HMOs.

The HIPAA legislation has four primary objectives:

- *Portability:* Ensures health insurance portability by eliminating "job lock" due to preexisting medical conditions; further, it prohibits discrimination against employees and dependents based on their health status, protects many workers who lose health coverage by providing better access to individual health insurance coverage, and guarantees renewability and availability of health coverage to certain employers and individuals.
- *Integrity:* Reduces healthcare fraud and abuse.

- *Efficiency:* Encourages administrative simplification by establishing and enforcing standards for health information to streamline industry inefficiencies and to reduce paperwork.
- *Privacy:* Guarantees security and privacy of health information.

These four goals are built into the legislation. This legislation is organized into five sections, or titles:

- Title I: This title guarantees health insurance access, portability, and renewal through laws guaranteeing coverage and renewal of health insurance, eliminates some preexisting condition exclusions from insurance contracts, and prohibits discrimination based on health status.
- Title II: This title creates fraud and abuse controls, demands adherence to standards to ensure administrative simplification, and establishes medical liability reform. It also establishes security standards that protect the confidentiality and integrity of "individually identifiable health information."
- Title III: Medical savings accounts are established in Title III. Additionally, tax deductions are created for health insurance premiums paid by the self-employed.
- Title IV: This title empowers the Office of Civil Rights to enforce these health plan provisions.
- Title V: This title establishes revenue offset provisions.

HIPAA Review

The focus of this section is Title II, which establishes the majority of rules and requirements the healthcare industry has to follow, and its provisions mainly have to do with administrative simplification. These provisions are intended to reduce the costs and administrative burdens of health care by making possible the standardized, electronic transmission of administrative and financial transactions that are currently executed manually and on paper.

Put simply, this rule requires providers, insurers, payers, and, to a small extent, employers to submit enrollments, eligibility, and claims processing via standardized electronic data interchange transactions. Electronic data interchange is essentially a set of very specific rules governing how information will be packaged electronically to send orders, invoices, statements, and payments from one trading partner to another.

The government has adopted this standard as a way of ensuring that providers, payers, insurers, and employers have a uniform way of communicating and sending information to each other. Properly done, electronic data interchange transactions do not require human intervention; therefore, transactions such as electronic eligibility, benefit inquiries, and claims can be processed very quickly.

Specifically, Title II of HIPAA calls for the following:

- Standardization of electronic patient health, administrative, and financial data
- Unique health identifiers for individuals, employers, health plans, and healthcare providers
- Security standards protecting the confidentiality and integrity of "individually identifiable health information," past, present, or future

The Standards for Privacy of Individually Identifiable Health Information[6] are designed to help guarantee privacy and confidentiality of patient medical records. These new

Standards for Privacy are quite extensive, and a full discussion of their content is beyond the scope of this book. Case Managers should review this rule and its requirements in great detail with the intent to update and replace any current internal guidelines and ensure HIPAA compliance.

Achieving HIPAA compliance for Case Managers is not easy. Case Managers, unlike insurers, also have to deal with payers, providers, patients, and family members in the course of performing their duties. Dealing with these numerous clients—along with other problems posed by ensuring the secure transfer of information between these clients via phone, fax, and Internet—makes the protection of individually identifiable patient information a major challenge.

The following sections include explanations or amplifications of HIPAA terms or policies.

What Is a Preexisting Condition?

A preexisting condition is a medical condition that a subscriber has and that is diagnosed and treated by a medical professional before the enrollment date in any new health plan. Under HIPAA the only preexisting conditions that may be excluded under preexisting condition exclusions are those for which medical advice, diagnosis, care, or treatment was recommended or received within the 6-month period before the enrollment date. If a subscriber had a medical condition in the past but had not received any medical advice, diagnosis, care, or treatment within the 6 months before his or her enrollment date in the plan, the old condition is not a preexisting condition for which exclusion can be applied.

Does HIPAA Prohibit All Preexisting Condition Exclusions?

No, under HIPAA, employers and states may impose preexisting condition exclusions and still be compliant. A group health plan or a health insurance issuer offering group health insurance coverage may impose a preexisting condition exclusion. However, to do so the following requirements must be satisfied:

- A preexisting condition exclusion must relate to a condition for which medical advice, diagnosis, care, or treatment was recommended or received during the 6-month period before an individual's enrollment date.
- A preexisting condition exclusion may not last for more than 12 months (18 months for late enrollees) after an individual's enrollment date.
- This 12- or 18-month period must be reduced by the number of days of the individual's prior creditable coverage, excluding coverage before any break in coverage of 63 days or more.

What Is Job Lock?

Job lock refers to the situation that occurs when an employee refuses to seek other employment for fear that a new employer's insurance benefits will exclude his or her current medical conditions or those of his or her dependents under a preexisting condition exclusion. Because of this fear, the employee feels "locked into" his or her current job.

How Does HIPAA Prevent Job Lock?

Under HIPAA, the time period of these restrictions is limited so that most plans must cover an individual's preexisting condition after 12 months. Under HIPAA, a new employer's plan is required to give credit for the length of time that the employee had continuous health insurance coverage. The amount of time previously insured (continuously) will reduce the 12-month exclusion period.

If, for example, at the time an employee changes jobs he or she already has had 12 months of continuous health coverage (without a break in coverage of 63 days or more), he or she will not have to start over with a new 12-month exclusion for any preexisting conditions. In this case, coverage for preexisting conditions under the new health plan will begin immediately.

What Preexisting Conditions Cannot Be Excluded From Coverage?

Preexisting condition exclusions cannot be applied to pregnancy, regardless of whether the woman had previous coverage. In addition, a preexisting condition exclusion cannot be applied to a newborn, an adopted child under age 18, or a child under 18 placed for adoption as long as the child became covered under the health plan within 30 days of birth, adoption, or placement for adoption and provided the child does not incur a subsequent 63-day or longer break in coverage.

How Is It Determined That a Person Is Subject to a Preexisting Condition Exclusion?

Many health insurance plans do not exclude coverage for preexisting conditions. However, if a plan does, it must tell the subscriber that it has a preexisting condition exclusion period (and can only exclude coverage for a preexisting condition after the subscriber has been notified). The plan must also notify the subscriber of his or her right to show proof of prior creditable coverage to reduce the preexisting condition exclusion period.

If the plan does apply a preexisting condition exclusion period, the plan must make a determination regarding the creditable coverage and the length of any preexisting condition exclusion period that applies to a subscriber. Generally, this determination must occur within a "reasonable time" after a subscriber has provided the plan with a certificate or other information relating to creditable coverage.

The plan is required to notify the subscriber of its determination to impose a preexisting condition period. The notice must also inform the subscriber of the basis of the determination, including the source and substance of any information on which the plan relied and any appeals procedures that are available to the subscriber.

If, at a later date, the plan determines the claimed creditable coverage was in error or was insufficient, it may modify its initial determination. In this circumstance the plan must notify the subscriber of its reconsideration, and until a final determination is made, the plan must act in accordance with its initial determination for purposes of approving medical services.

Can States Modify HIPAA's Portability Requirements?

Yes, HIPAA requirements do not supersede state requirements. If the state has laws that are stricter in protecting medical records privacy, the state law prevails. States may impose stricter obligations on health insurance providers in the following seven areas:

1. Shorten the 6-month "look-back" period before the enrollment date to determine what is a preexisting condition
2. Shorten the 12- and 18-month maximum preexisting condition exclusion periods

3. Increase the 63-day significant break in coverage period
4. Increase the 30-day period for newborns, adopted children, and children placed for adoption to enroll in the plan so that no preexisting condition exclusion period may be applied thereafter
5. Expand the prohibitions on conditions and people to whom a preexisting condition exclusion period may be applied beyond the "exceptions" described in federal law (the exceptions under federal law are for certain newborns, adopted children, children placed for adoption, and pregnant women)
6. Require additional special enrollment periods
7. Reduce the maximum HMO affiliation period to less than 2 months (3 months for late enrollees)

Therefore, if a person's health coverage is offered through an HMO or an insurance policy issued by an insurance company, he or she should check with the State Insurance Commissioner's Office to find out the rules or their modifications in his or her state.

What Constitutes a Significant Break in Coverage?

According to HIPAA legislation, a significant break in coverage is a time period of 63 days or longer that a subscriber has been without health insurance coverage (not including waiting periods).

What Is a Waiting Period?

A waiting period is a period of time, specified by the health insurance contract, that occurs between signing up for insurance and the beginning of health insurance coverage. The time in a waiting period cannot be counted as creditable coverage time. Health insurance coverage can be obtained during this waiting period through the COBRA benefits from prior employment.

- *Establishing waiting periods:* HIPAA does not prohibit a plan or issuer from establishing a waiting period. However, if a plan has a waiting period and a preexisting condition exclusion period, the preexisting condition exclusion period begins when the waiting period begins; that is, the periods must run concurrently.
- *Creditable coverage:* Creditable coverage refers to a period of time during which a person was covered under a health insurance policy. Most health coverage is creditable coverage, such as coverage under a group health plan (including COBRA continuation coverage), HMO, individual health insurance policy, military-sponsored health plan, Medicaid, or Medicare. Creditable coverage does not include coverage consisting solely of "excepted benefits," such as coverage solely for dental or vision benefits. Days in a waiting period during which a person does not have any coverage are not considered creditable coverage under the plan, nor are these days taken into account when determining a significant break in coverage (a break of 63 days or more). In the standard method for calculating creditable coverage, a subscriber will receive credit for previous coverage that occurred without a break in coverage of 63 days or more. Any coverage occurring before a break in coverage of 63 days or more will not be credited against a preexisting condition exclusion period. To illustrate, suppose an individual had health insurance coverage for 2 years, followed by a break in coverage of 70 days, and then resumed coverage for 8 months. That individual would only

receive credit for 8 months of coverage; no credit would be given for the 2 years of coverage before the break in coverage of 70 days.

It is also important to remember that during any preexisting condition exclusion period under a new plan, a subscriber may be entitled to COBRA continuation coverage under his or her previous health insurance benefits plan. COBRA is the name for a federal law that provides workers and their families the opportunity to purchase group health coverage through their employer's health plan for a limited period of time (generally 18, 29, or 36 months) if they lose coverage due to specified events, including termination of employment, divorce, or death. Workers in companies with 20 or more employees generally qualify for COBRA. Some states have laws similar to COBRA that may apply to smaller companies.

Certification of Creditable Coverage

Group health plans and health insurance issuers are required to furnish a certificate of coverage to provide documentation of the individual's prior creditable coverage. A certificate of creditable coverage

- Must be provided automatically by the plan or issuer when an individual either loses coverage under the plan or becomes entitled to elect COBRA continuation coverage and when an individual's COBRA continuation coverage ceases
- Must also be provided, if requested, before the individual loses coverage or within 24 months of losing coverage
- May be provided through use of the model certificate

Nondiscrimination Requirements

Individuals may not be excluded from coverage under the terms of the plan, or charged more for benefits offered by a plan or issuer, based on specified factors related to health status. Group health plans and issuers may not establish rules for eligibility (including continued eligibility) of any individual to enroll under the terms of the plan based on "health status–related factors." These factors are a subscriber's health status, medical condition (physical or mental), claims experience, receipt of health care, medical history, genetic information, evidence of insurability, or disability. For example, a subscriber cannot be excluded or dropped from coverage under his or her health plan just because the health plan knows that the subscriber will require a liver transplant in the next year. Plans may, however, establish limits or restrictions on benefits or coverage for similarly situated individuals. In addition, plans may change covered services or benefits if they give participants notice of such "material reductions" within 60 days after the change is adopted. Also, plans may not require an individual to pay a premium or contribution greater than that for a similarly situated individual based on a health status–related factor. This includes plans that require a preemployment physical examination. The results of preemployment examinations may not be used to discriminate in employment opportunity or insurance eligibility.

Unique Identifiers for Providers, Employers, Health Plans, and Patients

HIPAA guidelines propose standard identifiers for providers, employers, health plans, and patients. The current insurance system allows entities to have multiple identification numbers when dealing with each other. HIPAA sees this as confusing, conducive to error, and costly. It is expected that these unique identifiers will reduce these problems.

Security of Health Information and Electronic Signature Standards

The final security rule was published on February 20, 2003, and provides a uniform level of protection of all health information that

- Is housed or transmitted electronically
- Pertains to an individual

The security standard mandates safeguards for physical storage and maintenance, transmission, and access to individual health information. It applies not only to the transactions adopted under HIPAA but also to all individual health information that is maintained or transmitted. However, the electronic signature standard applies only to the transactions adopted under HIPAA.

The security standard does not require specific technologies to be used; solutions will vary from business to business, depending on the needs and technologies in place. Also, no transactions adopted under HIPAA currently require an electronic signature.

Women's Health and Cancer Rights Act of 1998

This law was enacted as part of the Omnibus Appropriations Bill and became effective for plan years beginning on or after October 21, 1998. This Act amended ERISA to require group health plans, including self-insured plans, which provide coverage for mastectomies to provide certain reconstructive and related services after mastectomies.

What Is Covered?

These services mandated by the Act are as follows:

- Reconstruction of the breast upon which the mastectomy has been performed
- Surgery and reconstruction of the other breast to produce a symmetrical appearance
- Breast prosthesis
- Treatment for physical complications attendant to the mastectomy, for example, lymphedema

It should be noted the law specifically states that these services may be subject to annual deductibles and coinsurance under the plan's normal terms.

Prohibitions

This Act imposes prohibitions on the insurers that include the following:

- A group health plan is prohibited from denying a patient eligibility to enroll or renew coverage solely for the purpose of avoiding the requirements of the Act.
- A group health plan is prohibited from inducing an attending physician to limit the care that is required under the Act, whether that takes the form of penalizing, reducing, or limiting the reimbursement to such physician. This prohibition should not be thought of as an impediment to effective price negotiation. The Act specifically states that its provisions shall not be construed to prevent a group health plan from negotiating the level and type of reimbursement with a provider for care provided in accordance with the Act.

This law applies to private and public employer plans and health insurance issuers. Nonfederal governmental, self-insured plans may elect to opt out of this Act's requirements, in the same manner as they may opt out of the requirements of HIPAA, the MHPA, and the NMHPA.

PUBLIC BENEFIT PROGRAMS

Centers for Medicare & Medicaid Services

The CMS (formerly known as the Health Care Financing Administration) is a federal agency within the U.S. Department of Health and Human Services. CMS runs (among others) the Medicare and Medicaid programs—two national healthcare programs that benefit about 75 million Americans. Working with the Health Resources and Services Administration, CMS runs the State Children's Health Insurance Program (SCHIP), which is expected to cover many of the approximately 10 million uninsured children in the United States. (A detailed description of this program is found later in this chapter.)

CMS also regulates all laboratory testing (except research) performed on humans in the United States. Approximately 158,000 laboratory entities fall within CMS's regulatory responsibility. CMS, with the U.S. Departments of Labor and Treasury, helps millions of Americans and small companies get and keep health insurance coverage and helps eliminate discrimination based on health status for people buying health insurance (see the section on HIPAA, above).

CMS spends more than $503 billion a year buying healthcare services for beneficiaries of Medicare, Medicaid, and SCHIP. In this context, CMS

- Ensures that Medicaid, Medicare, and SCHIP are properly run by the contractors and state agencies
- Establishes policies for paying healthcare providers
- Conducts research on the effectiveness of various methods of healthcare management, treatment, and financing
- Assesses the quality of healthcare facilities and services
- Takes enforcement actions as appropriate

CMS protects the fiscal integrity of Medicare, Medicaid, and SCHIP. Working with other federal departments and state and local governments, CMS has a comprehensive program to combat fraud and abuse. Strong enforcement action against those who commit fraud and abuse protects taxpayer dollars and guarantees security for these programs.

CMS is improving the quality of health care provided to Medicare, Medicaid, and SCHIP beneficiaries. Quality improvement is based on

- Developing and enforcing standards through surveillance
- Measuring and improving outcomes of care
- Educating healthcare providers about quality improvement opportunities
- Educating beneficiaries to make good healthcare choices

Medicare

The Medicare program was created by Title XVIII of the Social Security Act. The Social Security Administration first administered the program, which went into effect in 1966. In 1977 the Medicare program was transferred to the newly created Health Care Financing Administration, now known as CMS.

Medicare is divided into two parts, Part A and Part B. Part A is the Hospital Insurance Program, which is funded by Social Security taxes and is provided to eligible individuals at no personal expense. As one might suspect, Part A is a basic hospital insurance plan covering hospital care, extended care, home health services, and hospice care for terminally ill patients. Part B helps pay for doctor services, outpatient hospital services, medical equipment and supplies, and other health services and supplies. Both parts are described in more detail later in this chapter.

Who Is Eligible for Medicare Benefits?

As previously stated, CMS administers Medicare, the nation's largest health insurance program, which covers 40 million Americans. Medicare provides insurance to the following individuals:

- *Persons aged 65 years:* Generally, people over the age of 65 are eligible for Medicare benefits on their own or through their spouse's employment. Any one of the following must be true:
  - The patient receives benefits under Social Security or the Railroad Retirement System.
  - The patient is eligible for benefits under Social Security or the Railroad Retirement System but has not filed for them.
  - The patient's spouse has Medicare-covered government employment.
- *Those who are disabled:* A person becomes entitled to Medicare on the basis of disability after he or she has been entitled to Social Security disability benefits for 24 months. An individual has a 5-month waiting period before receiving Social Security disability payments, which means, in most instances, there will be a 29-month period before the individual becomes entitled to Medicare.
- *Those diagnosed with permanent kidney failure:* A person is considered to have end-stage renal disease (ESRD) if he or she has irreparable kidney damage that requires a transplant or dialysis to maintain life. A person becomes eligible for Medicare if he or she requires dialysis, has a kidney transplant, and meets the following requirements:
  - The patient has worked the required amount of time under Social Security, the Railroad Retirement Board, or as a government employee.
  - The patient is receiving or is eligible for Social Security or Railroad Retirement benefits.
  - The patient is a spouse or dependent child of a person who has worked the required amount of time or who is receiving Social Security or Railroad Retirement benefits.
  - If a person becomes entitled to Medicare solely because of ESRD, he or she has a 3-month wait until coverage begins (or the 3rd month after the month in which a regular course of dialysis starts).
  - For those beneficiaries entitled to Medicare solely because of ESRD, Medicare protection ends 12 months after the month the patient no longer requires maintenance dialysis treatments or 36 months after a successful kidney transplant.
  - It should also be noted that if a person less than 65 years old becomes eligible for Medicare due to ESRD, the benefits extended to the patient by Medicare will cover only those medical expenses that are attendant to the treatment of the disease. For example, if a person under 65 who was eligible for Medicare because of ESRD were to also suffer from rheumatoid arthritis, the cost of the medical care for the treatment of arthritis would not be covered by Medicare, but the cost for renal dialysis would be.
  - If a patient has permanent kidney failure, he or she cannot join a Medicare managed care plan/HMO. However, if the patient is already enrolled in the Medicare HMO, the plan will provide, pay for, or arrange for the patient's care.

What Are the Benefits from Medicare?

Medicare benefits come in two parts: hospital insurance (Part A) and medical insurance (Part B). Medicare Part A benefits provide coverage for inpatient hospital services, skilled nursing facilities, home health services, and hospice care. Medicare Part A helps pay for up to 90 days of medically necessary inpatient hospital care in each benefit period. From the 1st through the 60th day of in-hospital treatment, Medicare pays for all covered services (except the Part A deductible) during each benefit period. During the 61st to the 90th day of in-hospital treatment, Medicare pays for all medically necessary services, except for an amount called Part A coinsurance (Table 6-1). Medicare Part A helps pay for up to 100 days in a skilled nursing facility after a hospital stay (under certain conditions; Table 6-2). Medicare Part A helps pay for up to 210 days of hospice care. When necessary, an extended period of coverage may be allowed. Patients pay no deductible but may pay a coinsurance amount for outpatient drugs and respite care (Table 6-3).

Medicare Part B helps pay for the cost of physician services, outpatient hospital services, medical equipment and supplies, and other health services and supplies.

TABLE 6-1 Medicare Payments for Hospital Treatment

In-Hospital Days	Medicare Pays	Patient Pays
1st–60th	100% of allowable charges – Deductible	Part A deductible = $764.00
61st–90th	100% of allowable charges – Part A coinsurance	Part A coinsurance = $191.00*
91st–151st	100% of allowable charges – Part A coinsurance	Part A coinsurance = $382.00*

*Amount charged per day.

TABLE 6-2 Medicare Payments for Skilled Nursing Facility

Skilled Nursing Facility Days	Medicare Pays	Patient Pays
1st–20th	100% of allowable charges	0
21st–100th	100% of allowable charges	Part A coinsurance = $95.00*

*Amount charged per day.

TABLE 6-3 Medicare Payments for Hospice Care

Hospice Care	Medicare Pays	Patient Pays
1st–210th	100% of allowable charges	0
Outpatient drugs	100% of allowable charges – coinsurance	Coinsurance
Respite care	100% of allowable charges – coinsurance	Coinsurance

What Is a Benefit Period?

Medicare defines a benefit period as that period of time that begins the first day of a patient's admission to a hospital, skilled nursing facility, or hospice and ends after he or she has been discharged for 60 contiguous days. There is no limit to the number of benefit periods a beneficiary may have for hospital and skilled nursing care, but there is a limit to the number of days of care for which a beneficiary may claim payment.

What Is a Reserve Day?

A reserve day is one of 60 "extra days" of hospital care that Medicare will pay for during the lifetime of a beneficiary. Medicare Part A includes an extra 60 hospital days that can be used if the patient has a prolonged illness necessitating a hospital stay of longer than 90 days. A Medicare beneficiary has only 60 nonrenewable, reserve days in a lifetime. The beneficiary has the right to choose when to use these reserve days.

Medicare Prescription Drug Coverage

Medicare Part D

Americans spend more on pharmaceuticals and pay the highest prices for pharmaceuticals than any country. In 2004 Americans spent $188.5 billion on prescription drugs. From 1994 to 2005, the number of prescriptions purchased increased 71% (from 2.1 billion to 3.6 billion), compared to a U.S. population growth of 9%. The elderly use more prescription drugs than any other age group and thus bear a disproportionate amount of this financial burden. This spending occurs at a time in their lives when their incomes are often fixed and their assets dwindling.

To help defer the costs of prescription drugs in this population, Medicare created a plan, called Medicare Part D, and began enrolling participants on January 1, 2006. Medicare prescription drug coverage is a type of insurance. It is designed to help patients pay for their current prescription drugs and also to protect them against future higher drug costs. To get the drug coverage, Medicare recipients must enroll in a Medicare-approved private drug plan. There are many plans to choose from, so patients can choose the one that best suits their unique needs.

Who Is Eligible to Participate in This Plan?

All Medicare recipients are eligible to participate in this plan, regardless of income, health status, or how they currently pay for prescription drugs.

How Does This Plan Work?

Medicare provides coverage to help pay for both brand-name and generic drugs that patients need. To get Medicare prescription drug coverage, patients must choose and join a Medicare drug plan. Medicare drug plans are offered by insurance companies and other private companies approved by Medicare.

Is There Only One Type of Medicare Prescription Coverage Plan?

There are two types of Medicare prescription coverage plans:

- Supplemental plan: This Medicare prescription drug plan adds coverage to another Medicare plan, such as the original Medicare plan, Medicare private fee-for-service plans that don't offer Medicare prescription drug coverage, and Medicare cost plans.

- Prescription drug coverage is also a part of Medicare advantage plans (like an HMO, a PPO, or a private fee-for-service plan) and other Medicare health plans. A patient can get all of her or his health care, including prescription drug coverage, through these plans.

What Are the Costs to the Patient for This Plan?

The costs of a plan vary depending on which plan is chosen. In general, patients may pay a monthly premium and a yearly deductible (up to the first $320). Keep in mind, this premium is an addition to a patient's monthly premium for Medicare Part B or other insurance plans she or he may have. Each person must pay a premium as an individual. There are no discounts for married couples.

Unlike a typical indemnity plan, the Medicare prescription coverage plan is a bit complex. In this plan the patient and Medicare share the costs of coverage according to a fixed schedule that varies slightly, depending on which insurance company the patient chooses.

For a patient that joins the plan in 2012, she or he would pay the following for covered drugs:

- A monthly premium (varies depending on the plan chosen): Average premium in 2006 is estimated to be $54 per month. This adds (on average) an additional $648 to a patient's yearly drug costs.
- The first $320 per year for prescriptions: This is called the deductible.

The following are the changes in the "Standard Benefit Plan" that can be expected in 2012 according to CMS. The initial deductible will be increased by $10 to $320 and the initial coverage limit will increase from $2,840 in 2011 to $2,930. A Medicare recipient can expect that the out-of-pocket threshold will increase from $4,550 to $4,700. The coverage gap, or donut hole, begins once the patient reaches the Medicare Part D plan's initial coverage limit ($2,930) and ends when he or she spends a total of $4,700. While in the donut hole Part D enrollees will continue to receive a 50% discount on the total cost of their brand-name drugs. The government's intention is to incrementally close the coverage gap (eliminate the donut hole) in Medicare Part D. Case Managers can expect significant changes in this coverage in the years to come.

After the patient pays the $320 deductible, here's how the costs work:

- The patient pays 25% of her or his yearly drug costs from $320 to $2,930 and her or his plan pays the other 75% of these costs, then
- She or he pays 100% of the next $3,727.50 in drug costs (this coverage gap, or "donut hole," is where the patient pays 100% of drug cost, with a 50% discount on brand-name drugs), then
- The patient pays 5% of the drug costs (or a small copayment) for the rest of the calendar year after she or he has spent $$4,835.13 out-of-pocket (not including premiums). The plan pays the rest. This is called "catastrophic benefit" or "catastrophic coverage," and it protects the patient from high drug costs associated with catastrophic illnesses.

How Can Patients Maximize Coverage?

Patients can maximize coverage by reducing the cost of drugs they use. Costs can be reduced by requesting the doctor use the least expensive drug that is safe and effective for their condition. Further, patients can reduce costs by requesting generic rather than brand-name drugs.

What If the Patient Can't Afford to Participate in the Medicare Prescription Plan?

If the patient has a limited income and resources, he or she may get assistance in paying the Medicare drug plan costs. Medicare and Social Security have a program for people with limited income and resources that helps them pay for their monthly premiums, annual deductibles, and prescription copayments related to a Medicare prescription drug plan; this program is called "Extra Help." People with the lowest incomes and resources will get the most help. People who qualify for the most help will pay no premiums or deductibles, and their copayments for each prescription will be $2.60 for generics and $6.50 for brand-name drugs. People in nursing homes with both Medicare and Medicaid will pay nothing for their prescriptions.

Those with somewhat higher incomes will pay reduced monthly premiums and a reduced annual deductible of $50 a year. Their copayments will be 15% of the cost of each prescription. Everyone who qualifies for Extra Help will get continuous drug coverage throughout the year. Some people automatically qualify for Extra Help and will not need to apply for it (Medicare has already notified them about this).

Who Is Eligible for Extra Help in Paying for Prescription Drugs?

To be eligible for the Extra Help program, a Medicare beneficiary must qualify as follows:

- He or she must reside in 1 of the 50 states or the District of Columbia.
- His or her resources must be limited to $12,640 for an individual or $25,260 for a married couple living together. Resources counted toward eligibility include such things as bank accounts, stocks, and bonds. Medicare does not count the home, car, and any life insurance policy as resources.
- His or her annual income must be limited to $16,335 for an individual or $22,065 for a married couple living together. If the Medicare recipient's annual income is higher, he or she still may be able to get some help. Some examples where a Medicare recipient's income may be higher and still be eligible include
  - If he or she and spouse support other family members who live with them or
  - If he or she lives in Alaska or Hawaii.

Medigap Insurance

Although Medicare covers many healthcare costs, patients will still have to pay Medicare's coinsurance and deductible fees. There are also many medical services that Medicare does not cover (e.g., dental care); because of this, Medicare recipients sometimes buy a Medicare supplemental insurance (Medigap) policy. Medigap is private insurance designed to help pay the patient's Medicare cost-sharing amounts. There are 10 standard Medigap policies, and each offers a different combination of benefits. The best time to buy a policy is during the Medigap open enrollment period. For a period of 6 months from the date a patient is first enrolled in Medicare Part B and is age 65 or older, he or she has a right to buy the Medigap policy of his or her choice; that period is the person's open enrollment period. Patients cannot be turned down or charged higher premiums because of poor health if they buy a policy during this period. After the Medigap open enrollment period ends, the patient may not be able to buy the policy of his or her choice. The patient may have to accept whatever Medigap policy an insurance company is willing to sell him.

If the patient has Medicare Part B but is not yet 65, his or her 6-month Medigap open enrollment period begins when he or she turns 65. However, several states (Connecticut, Maine, Massachusetts, Minnesota, New Jersey, New York, Oklahoma, Oregon, Pennsylvania, Virginia, Washington, and Wisconsin) require at least a limited Medigap open enrollment period for Medicare beneficiaries under 65. The state health insurance assistance program can answer questions about Medicare and other health insurance for patients. The services are free.

Medicare Select

Medicare Select is another type of Medicare supplemental health insurance. Insurance companies and HMOs throughout the United States sell it. Medicare Select is the same as standard Medigap insurance in nearly all respects. The only difference between Medicare Select and standard Medigap insurance is that Medicare Select operates like a managed care plan. That is, each insurer has specific hospitals and, in some cases, specific doctors that the patient must use, except in an emergency, to be eligible for full benefits. Medicare Select policies generally have lower premiums than other Medigap policies because of this requirement.

When Do Other Insurance Policies Pay Before Medicare?

Other health insurance policies may have to pay before Medicare pays its share of a patient's bill. For those patients who have other health insurance policies and are eligible for Medicare (not including Medigap policies), the other insurance will pay first if

- The patient is 65 or older.
- The patient (or spouse) is currently working for an employer with 20 or more employees and has group health insurance based on that employment.
- The patient is under age 65 and is disabled.
- The patient or any member of his or her family is currently working for an employer with 100 or more employees, and he or she has group health insurance based on that employment.
- The patient has Medicare because of permanent kidney failure (discussed in more detail below).
- The patient has an illness or injury that is covered under workers' compensation, the federal black lung program, no-fault insurance, or any liability insurance.

Before enactment of the Balanced Budget Act of 1997, Medicare benefits were secondary to benefits payable under a group health plan in the case of patients entitled to benefits on the basis of ESRD during a 30-month coordination period. This coordination period begins with the first month the patient is eligible for Medicare, whether or not the patient is actually entitled or enrolled. Medicare is secondary during this period even though the employer policy or plan contains a provision stating that its benefits are secondary to Medicare, or otherwise excludes or limits payments to Medicare beneficiaries. Under this provision, the group health plan must be billed first for services provided to the Medicare ESRD beneficiary. If the group health plan does not pay for covered services in full, Medicare may pay secondary benefits in accordance with current billing instructions. This provision applies to all Medicare-covered items and services (not just those pertaining to ESRD) furnished to beneficiaries who are in the coordination period.

Assistance for Low-Income Beneficiaries

For patients who have a low income and limited resources, the state may pay for their Medicare costs, including premiums, deductibles, and coinsurance. To qualify, the patient must be entitled to Medicare hospital insurance (Part A), his or her annual income level must be at or below the national poverty guidelines, and he or she cannot have resources such as bank accounts or stocks and bonds worth more than $6,680 for one person or $10,020 for a couple (his or her home and first car do not count).

Medicaid

Medicaid is a national insurance program aimed at serving the poor and the "needy." All 50 states, the District of Columbia, Guam, Puerto Rico, and the Virgin Islands operate Medicaid plans. It was created by Title XIX of the Social Security Act and is part of the federal and state welfare system. State welfare or health departments usually operate the Medicaid program, within the guidelines issued by the CMS, and are funded by the general tax revenues of the federal and state governments. Persons covered by the Medicaid program have no out-of-pocket expense for coverage.

Although Medicaid benefits can vary from state to state, the program must furnish the federally mandated services that include

- Inpatient hospital care and outpatient services
- Physicians' services
- Skilled nursing home services for adults
- Laboratory and x-ray services
- Family planning services
- Early and periodic screening, diagnosis, and treatment for children under age 21

Eligibility requirements for Medicaid benefits are set by each state, although the CMS has set some minimum standards. The people who are eligible under these standards include the categorically needy and the medically needy.

The categorically needy are a group that includes families and certain children who qualify for public assistance. Therefore, they are eligible for Aid to Families with Dependent Children (AFDC) or Supplemental Security Income (SSI). Common examples are the aged, blind, and physically disabled adults and children.

The medically needy comprise a group who earn enough to meet their basic needs but have inadequate resources to pay healthcare bills. For example, persons infected with tuberculosis (TB) are financially eligible for Medicaid at the SSI level (but only for TB-related ambulatory services and TB drugs).

Mandatory Coverage for the Categorically Needy

States have some discretion in determining which groups their Medicaid programs cover and the financial criteria for Medicaid eligibility. To be eligible for federal funds, states are required to provide Medicaid coverage for most individuals who receive federally assisted income maintenance payments, as well as for related groups not receiving cash payments. The following are examples of the mandatory Medicaid eligibility groups:

- AFDC recipients.
- SSI recipients (or, in states using more restrictive criteria, aged, blind, and disabled individuals who meet criteria that are more restrictive than those of the SSI program and that were in place in the state's approved Medicaid plan as of January 1, 1972).
- Infants born to Medicaid-eligible pregnant women. (Medicaid eligibility must continue throughout the first year of life so long as the infant remains in the mother's household and she remains eligible or would be eligible if she were still pregnant.)
- Children under age 6 and pregnant women who meet the state's AFDC financial requirements or whose family income is at or below 133% of the federal poverty level (FPL). (The minimum mandatory income level for pregnant women and infants in certain states may be higher than 133% if the state had established a higher percentage for covering those groups. States are required to extend Medicaid eligibility until age 19 to all children born after September 30, 1983 in families with incomes at or below the FPL. This coverage was phased in to cover all poor children under age 19 by the year 2002. Once eligibility is established, pregnant women remain eligible for Medicaid through the end of the calendar month ending 60 days after the end of the pregnancy, regardless of any change in family income. States are not required to have a resource test for these poverty-level related groups. However, any resource test imposed can be no more restrictive than that of the AFDC program for infants and children and the SSI program for pregnant women.)
- Recipients of adoption assistance and foster care under Title IV-E of the Social Security Act, certain Medicare beneficiaries (described below), and special protected groups who lose cash assistance because of the cash programs' rules, but who may keep Medicaid for a period of time. (Examples are persons who lose AFDC or SSI payments due to earnings from work or increased Social Security benefits and two-parent, unemployed families whose AFDC cash assistance time is limited by the state and who are provided a full 12 months of Medicaid coverage after termination of cash assistance.)

Optional Coverage for the Categorically Needy

States also have the option to provide Medicaid coverage for other categorically needy groups. These optional groups share characteristics of the mandatory groups, but the eligibility criteria are somewhat more liberally defined. Examples of the optional groups that states may cover as categorically needy (and for which they will receive federal matching funds) under the Medicaid program are as follows:

- Infants up to age 1 and pregnant women not covered under the mandatory rules whose family income is below 185% of the FPL (the percentage to be set by each state)
- Certain aged, blind, or disabled adults who have incomes above those requiring mandatory coverage but below the FPL
- Children under age 21 who meet income and resources requirements for AFDC but who otherwise are not eligible for AFDC

- Institutionalized individuals with income and resources below specified limits
- Persons who would be eligible if institutionalized but who are receiving care under home and community-based services waivers
- Recipients of state supplementary payments
- TB-infected persons who would be financially eligible for Medicaid at the SSI level (only for TB-related ambulatory services and TB drugs)

Medically Needy Eligibility Groups

The option to have a medically needy program allows states to extend Medicaid eligibility to additional qualified persons who may have too much income to qualify under the mandatory or optional categorically needy groups. This option allows them to "spend down" to Medicaid eligibility by incurring medical or remedial care expenses to offset their excess income, thereby reducing it to a level below the maximum allowed by that state's Medicaid plan. States may also allow families to establish eligibility as medically needy by paying monthly premiums to the state in an amount equal to the difference between family income (reduced by unpaid expenses, if any, incurred for medical care in previous months) and the income eligibility standard.

Eligibility for the medically needy program does not have to be as extensive as the categorically needy program. However, states that elect to include the medically needy under their plans are required to include certain children under age 18 and pregnant women who, except for income and resources, would be eligible as categorically needy. These states may choose to provide coverage to other medically needy persons: aged, blind, and/or disabled persons; certain relatives of children deprived of parental support and care; and certain other financially eligible children up to age 21. In 1995, 40 medically needy programs provided at least some services to recipients.

Amplification on Medicaid Eligibility

Medicaid coverage may be applied retroactively for up to 3 months before application if the individual would have been eligible during that period. Coverage generally stops at the end of the month in which a person's circumstances change. Most states have additional "state-only" programs to provide medical assistance for specified poor persons who do not qualify for the Medicaid program. No federal funds are provided for state-only programs.

Medicaid does not provide medical assistance for all poor persons. Even under the broadest provisions of the federal statute (except for emergency services for certain persons), the Medicaid program does not provide healthcare services, even for very poor persons, unless they are in one of the groups designated previously. Low income is only one test for Medicaid eligibility; assets and resources are also tested against established thresholds. As noted earlier, categorically needy persons who are eligible for Medicaid may or may not also receive cash assistance from the AFDC program or from the SSI program. Medically needy persons who would be categorically eligible except for income or assets may become eligible for Medicaid solely because of excessive medical expenses.

States may use more liberal income and resources methodologies to determine Medicaid eligibility for certain AFDC-related and aged, blind, and disabled individuals under Section 1902(r)(2) of the Social Security Act. The more liberal income methodologies cannot result in the individual's income exceeding the limits prescribed for federal matching (for those groups that are subject to these limits).

Significant changes were made in the Medicare Catastrophic Coverage Act of 1988 that affected Medicaid. Although much of the Medicare Catastrophic Coverage Act was repealed, the portions affecting Medicaid remain in effect. The law also accelerated Medicaid eligibility for some nursing home patients by protecting assets for the institutionalized person's spouse at home at the time of the initial eligibility determination after institutionalization. Before an institutionalized person's monthly income is used to pay for the cost of institutional care, a minimum monthly maintenance needs allowance is deducted from the institutionalized spouse's income to bring the income of the community spouse up to a moderate level.

Medicaid–Medicare Relationship

The Medicare program (Title XVIII of the Social Security Act) provides hospital insurance, also known as Part A coverage, and supplementary medical insurance, which is known as Part B coverage. For people aged 65 and older (and for certain disabled persons) who have insured status under Social Security or Railroad Retirement, coverage for hospital insurance is automatic. Coverage for supplementary medical insurance, however, requires payment of a monthly premium. Some aged and/or disabled persons are covered under both the Medicaid and Medicare programs.

For Medicare beneficiaries who are also fully eligible for Medicaid, Medicare coverage is supplemented by healthcare services that are available under the state's Medicaid program. If a person is a Medicare beneficiary, payments for any services covered by Medicare are made by the Medicare program before the Medicaid program makes any payments. Medicaid is always the "payer of last resort." As each state elects, the Medicaid program may provide services such as eyeglasses, hearing aids, and nursing facility care not covered by Medicare.

Limited Medicaid benefits are available for certain qualified disabled working individuals who have earnings sufficiently high to preclude entitlement to Medicare coverage, except if the individual purchases coverage, and whose earnings are less than 200% of the FPL. State Medicaid programs must pay the hospital insurance premium for qualified disabled working individuals with income less than 150% of the FPL and may pay some or the entire hospital insurance premium for qualified disabled working individuals with earnings between 150% and 200% of the FPL. Medicaid does not pay supplementary medical insurance premiums for these individuals.

For certain poor Medicare recipients known as qualified Medicare beneficiaries—those beneficiaries with incomes below the FPL and with resources at or below twice the standard allowed under the SSI program—the Medicaid program pays the Medicare premiums and cost-sharing expenses for Medicare hospital and supplement insurances. For specified low-income Medicare beneficiaries—those like qualified Medicare beneficiaries but with slightly higher incomes—the Medicaid program pays only the supplemental medical insurance premiums.

Spousal Impoverishment

Placing a spouse in a nursing home can be a very expensive proposition. With monthly expenses running $2,000 to $3,000 it does not take very long for these bills to wipe out a lifetime of savings and leave the community-based spouse destitute. This situation has come to be called spousal impoverishment.

In an attempt to prevent such spousal impoverishment, Congress enacted provisions in 1988 that allow a couple to have Medicaid benefits without spending down their resources. These provisions help ensure that spousal impoverishment will not occur and that community spouses are able to live out their lives with independence and dignity.

To be eligible for Medicaid under this provision, the member of the couple who is in a nursing facility or medical institution must be expected to remain there for at least 30 days. The state then evaluates the couple's resources. After the state's evaluation, it determines the spousal resource amount (SRA). The SRA is the number the state measures against its minimum resource standard for an institutionalized patient to receive Medicaid. An institutionalized spouse who has less than this amount is eligible for Medicaid. The SRA is equal to the following: the combined spousal assets, minus the house, car, household goods, and burial costs, divided by 2. It is described in the following formula:

$$SRA = \frac{1}{2} \times ([\text{couple's combined assets}] - [\text{house, car, etc.}])$$

To determine whether the spouse residing in a medical facility is eligible for Medicaid, the SRA must be less than the state's minimum resource standard. As an example, this number was $109,560 in New York State in 2011 (http://www.nyc.gov/html/hra/downloads/pdf/income_level.pdf viewed 12/3/11). If the SRA is greater than the state's minimum resource standard, the remainder becomes attributable to the spouse who is residing in a medical institution as countable or depletable resource.

The community spouse is entitled to protection of a certain amount of the couple's combined assets under this provision. These assets are known as the spouse's protected resource amount. Said another way, the protected resource amount is that amount of the couple's combined assets that the community spouse keeps for his or her own benefit and that is not available to the institutionalized spouse. This protected resource amount is the greatest of

- The spousal resource amount
- The state spousal resource standard, which is the amount the state has determined is protected for the community spouse
- An amount transferred to the community spouse for her or his support as directed by a court order
- An amount designated by a state hearing officer to raise the community spouse's protected resources up to the minimum monthly maintenance needs standard

If the amount of resources for the institutionalized spouse is below the state's resource standard, the individual is eligible for Medicaid. After resource eligibility is determined, resources of the community spouse are not attributed to the spouse in the medical facility.

The community spouse's income is not considered available to the spouse who is in the medical facility, and the two individuals are not considered a couple for these purposes. The state is to use the income eligibility standards for one person rather than two. Therefore, the standard income eligibility process for Medicaid is used.

Although the income of the community spouse is not considered available to the institutionalized spouse, this is not the case for the institutionalized spouse's income. How much of that spouse's income is to be contributed to the cost of his or her own care is determined through the posteligibility process. This process is followed after an individual in a nursing facility or other medical institution is determined to be eligible for Medicaid. This process also determines how much of the income of the spouse who is in the medical facility is actually protected for use by the community spouse. Deductions are made from the total income of the spouse who is residing in the medical facility in the following order:

- A personal needs allowance is the reasonable amount of money for clothing and other personal needs of the individual while in the institution. This protected personal needs allowance is approximately $60 a month for an individual and $120 a month for an institutionalized couple. The amount of this allowance can vary by state.
- Maintenance needs of the community-based spouse. For an institutionalized individual with a spouse at home, an additional amount of money is allocated for the maintenance needs of that community-based spouse. This amount must be based on a reasonable assessment of need.
- A family monthly income allowance: For an institutionalized individual with a family at home, an additional amount of money is allocated for the maintenance needs of the family. This amount must be based on a reasonable assessment of their financial need and be adjusted for the number of family members living in the home.
- An amount of money for medical expenses that are incurred by the institutionalized spouse when these expenses are not covered by Medicaid. These expenses may include Medicare and other health insurance premiums, deductibles, or coinsurance charges as well as any necessary medical or remedial care recognized under state law but not covered under the state's Medicaid plan.

The sum of these deductions subtracted from the income of the individual who is in the medical facility will result in the amount the individual must contribute to his or her cost of care.

Home Equity

The Deficit Reduction Act of 2005 states that applicants who have home equity in excess of $500,000 are ineligible for Medicaid. In some states this threshold is increased to $750,000. Therefore, people contemplating an application to Medicaid would need to sell their house or take out a reverse mortgage.

Transfers of Assets Before Institutionalization or Medicaid Application

When a patient is transferred to any of the following facilities (long-term care, receiving home, or community-based waiver services) and state/federal funding is requested, the state will examine the financial records of the individual for assets transferred for less than their fair market value. In common parlance, this financial examination undertaken by the state is called a "look back." (For the state's purposes, assets are defined both as real financial assets and as income.)

States "look back" into an individual's financial records during the evaluation of eligibility for Medicaid. The state looks to find transfers of assets for 60 months before the date the individual is institutionalized or, if later, the date he or she applies for Medicaid. For certain trusts this look-back period extends to 60 months. If a transfer of assets for less than fair market value is found, the state imposes a period of ineligibility, or a penalty period. A penalty period is that amount of time that a state will withhold payment for a nursing facility and certain other long-term care services. There is no statutory limit to the length of the penalty period.

The penalty period is calculated by determining the fair market value of the transferred asset and dividing the value of the asset by the average monthly private pay rate of a nursing facility in that state. For example, if an asset worth $120,000 has been transferred, and the average cost of a nursing facility in that state is $2,000 per month, then the penalty period would be calculated as $120,000/$2,000 per month = 60 months penalty period.

For certain types of transfers, these penalties are not applied. The principal exceptions are as follows:

- Reducing existing debt, such as mortgage or credit card debt.
- Making certain types of purchases, such as for home modifications. When such purchases and payments convert a countable resource, such as money in the bank, to noncountable resources, such as household goods, they effectively reduce the assets that are counted when determining Medicaid eligibility.
- To a spouse or to a third party for the sole benefit of the community spouse.
- By an institutionalized spouse to a third party for the sole benefit of the community spouse.
- Transfers of money to certain disabled individuals (a child) or to trusts established for those individuals.
- Transfer of property ownership. Medicaid allows individuals to transfer ownership of their home, without penalty, to certain relatives, including a spouse or a child under age 21.
- Financial instruments: Some financial instruments, namely annuities and trusts, have been used to reduce countable assets to enable individuals to qualify for Medicaid.
- Personal services contract or care agreement: Personal services contracts or care agreements are arrangements in which an elderly or disabled individual pays another person, often an adult child, to provide certain services. Based on CMS guidance, relatives can be legitimately paid for care they provide, but there is a presumption that services provided without charge at the time they were rendered were intended to be provided without compensation. Under this presumption, payments provided for services in the past would result in a penalty period.
- For a purpose other than to qualify for Medicaid.
- Where imposing a penalty would cause undue hardship.

Treatment of Annuities

An annuity contract is an insurance product. It is created when an insured party, usually an individual, pays a life insurance company a single premium that will later be distributed back to the insured party over time. Annuity contracts traditionally provide a guaranteed distribution of income over time, until the death of the person or persons named in the contract or until a final date, whichever comes first.

Annuities have become a common method for individuals to reduce countable resources for the purpose of becoming eligible for Medicaid because they are used to convert countable resources, such as money in the bank, to a resource that is not counted (an insurance policy) and a stream of income. However, this was changed under the Deficit Reduction Act of 2005. Now, if a person applying for Medicaid buys an annuity, the annuity may be seen as an uncompensated transfer. If the annuitant (the person who receives the income from the annuity) is the community spouse or a disabled child, then the annuity is not deemed an uncompensated transfer. If the annuity income goes to the Medicaid applicant, then the purchase will be subject to a penalty period unless the state is named as the remainder beneficiary in the first position for at least the total amount of medical assistance paid for on behalf of the Medicaid applicant, or the state is named as the remainder beneficiary in the second position after the community spouse or minor or disabled child.

Treatment of Trusts

A trust is a legal title to property, held by one party for the benefit of another. There are usually three parties involved in a trust. The first is the grantor. The grantor is the person or entity who establishes the trust and donates the assets. A trustee is a person or qualified trust company who holds and manages the assets for the benefit of another. The beneficiary is the recipient of some or all of the trust's assets. The assets held by a trust can exist in many forms, for example, money, real estate, art, businesses, stocks, bonds, or other tangible assets. Trusts usually come in two varieties: revocable trusts (those trusts whose terms or beneficiaries can be changed) and irrevocable trusts (those trusts whose terms and beneficiaries are unchangeable).

Putting an asset in a trust transfers that asset from the individual's ownership to that of the trustee, who holds the property for the beneficiary(ies). For most purposes the law looks at these assets as if the trustee now owned them. However, the CMS does not. The CMS wants to prevent asset transfers made only to ensure the individual appears eligible for Medicaid benefits. It therefore has a process to evaluate the financial history of individuals applying for benefits and for imposing penalties for what it terms inappropriate transfers of assets.

Trusts and Medicaid Eligibility

How a trust is treated by CMS depends to some extent on the type of trust it is (e.g., whether it is revocable or irrevocable) and what specific requirements and conditions the trust contains. In general, however, payments actually made to or for the benefit of the individual are treated as income to the individual. CMS considers amounts that could be paid to or for the benefit of the individual but are not as available resources. Further, amounts that could be paid to or for the benefit of the individual but are paid to someone else are treated as transfers of assets for less than fair market value. Amounts that cannot, in any way, be paid to or for the benefit of the individual are also treated as transfers of assets for less than fair market value.

Certain trusts are not counted as being available to the individual:

- Established by a parent, grandparent, guardian, or court for the benefit of an individual who is disabled and under the age of 65, using the individual's own funds
- Established by a disabled individual, parent, grandparent, guardian, or court for the disabled individual, using the individual's own funds, where the trust is made up of pooled funds and managed by a nonprofit organization for the sole benefit of each individual included in the trust
- Composed only of pension, Social Security, and other income of the individual, in states that make individuals eligible for institutional care under a special income level, but do not cover institutional care for the medically needy
- In which the state determines that counting the trust would cause an undue hardship

In all these instances the trust must provide that the state receives any funds, up to the amount of Medicaid benefits paid on behalf of the individual, remaining in the trust when the individual dies.

When an individual, his or her spouse, or anyone acting on the individual's behalf establishes a trust using at least some of the individual's funds, that trust can be considered available to the individual for purposes of determining eligibility for Medicaid.

Social Security

Social Security is a group of federally funded public programs designed to provide income and services to individuals in the event of retirement, sickness, disability, death, or unemployment. Social Security is the largest expenditure in the federal budget, exceeding the costs of both national defense and Medicare/Medicaid. In 2011 there will be 56 million beneficiaries and 158 million workers paying into the fund.

The Social Security Act that established these programs was enacted in 1935. The six original program titles of the Social Security Act were Old-Age Assistance, Old-Age (retirement) Benefits, Unemployment Compensation, Aid to Dependent Children, Maternal and Child Welfare, and Aid to the Blind. Title II, Old-Age Benefits for retired adults, was the keystone measure of the Act and is the portion most often referred to as Social Security. Monthly cash benefit payments are made to the following:

- Retired workers who have reached at least the age of 62
- Spouses and dependents of retired workers
- Divorced spouses of retired or disabled workers
- Workers who become disabled
- Spouses and dependents of disabled workers
- Survivors of deceased workers
- Divorced spouses of deceased workers

To be eligible to collect Social Security benefits, an individual must meet two criteria. First, the individual must have worked 40 quarters (or 10 years) in a job that paid Social Security premiums to be fully insured. (Individuals who have less than 10 years may not be excluded, as there are many exceptions to this rule.) Second, the individual must meet the requirements to collect the benefits (i.e., be the right age, be able to prove disability or dependence on an insured worker, or be the survivor of an insured deceased worker).

Since its inception in 1935 the Social Security Act has been modified more than 20 times by major amendments. A 1950 amendment to Social Security added Cost of Living Adjustments to increase benefit payments in keeping with inflation. Another major amendment to the Act in 1956 added benefits for disabled workers. All amendments up to this time created what is now known as the centerpiece of Social Security: Old-Age, Survivors' and Disability Insurance (OASDI). A 1965 amendment created a program that provides hospital insurance to the elderly, along with supplementary medical insurance for other medical costs. In 1972 the original Old-Age Assistance and Aid to the Blind titles were combined with new provisions for assistance to disabled people to create the SSI program.

In 1983 concern for the financial integrity of Social Security prompted the passage of major legislative changes, including the ending and, in some cases, taxation of certain benefits. At this time Congress also legislated a gradual increase in the standard retirement age, raising it from 65 to 67 for individuals born in 1960 or later. In 1996 welfare reform bills were submitted by Congress that created Temporary Aid for Needy Families as a replacement for the AFDC program, which was a revision of the original Aid to Dependent Children title. These bills also made changes to the provision of SSI, in particular, denying benefits for most noncitizens.

Temporary Aid for Needy Families is administered by state governments and is supported by the Administration for Children and Families within the U.S. Department of Health and Human Services, which took over the health and social welfare components of the Department of Health, Education, and Welfare in 1979. The Social Security Administration and the CMS jointly administer Medicare, as mentioned previously, whereas the U.S. Employment and Training Administration of the Department of Labor administers unemployment compensation.

Programs

OASDI, Medicare hospital insurance, and Medicare supplementary medical insurance are separately financed segments of the Social Security program. The OASDI program provides benefits for the aged, for the disabled, and for survivors of deceased workers. The cash benefits for OASDI are financed by earmarked payroll taxes levied on employees, their employers, and the self-employed. The rate of these contributions is based on the employee's taxable earnings, up to a maximum taxable amount, with the employer contributing an equal amount. Self-employed people contribute twice the amount levied on payrolled employees.

The hospital insurance portion of Medicare is, for the most part, similarly financed through payroll taxes. The amount of a person's cash benefits is determined by the combined wages, salaries, and self-employment income of the primary earner or earners in a family; dependent children and a noncontributing spouse receive additional amounts. The law specifies certain minimum and maximum monthly benefits. To keep the cash benefits in line with inflation, they are annually indexed to the increase in the cost of living as it is gauged in the consumer price index.

The 1986 amendments to the Age Discrimination in Employment Act state that, with some exceptions (such as firefighters, police officers, and tenured university faculty), an individual cannot be compelled to retire because of age. Since 2000 individuals aged 65 and older are entitled to receive full Social Security benefits even if they continue working. For other eligible workers, the amount of benefits is based on age and earnings. For example, working persons at full retirement age with earnings of $14,160 in 2011 and $14,640 in 2012 or less would not lose any Social Security benefits. For those at full retirement $1 is deducted from the social security benefit for every $3 made over that limit. For those under their age for full retirement $1 is deducted from their social security benefit for every $2 made over the limit. In accordance with the automatic adjustment provisions of the law, these limits are raised yearly in proportion to the increase in average annual wages.

Social Security benefits replace a stated portion of a person's former earned income, expressed as a percentage of earnings in the year before retirement. Low earners receive a larger percentage of their former income as benefits than recipients from higher income brackets. An earner's noncontributing spouse, first claiming benefits at age 65 or older, receives 50% of the amount paid to the earner. Similar percentages are payable to disabled individuals and their spouses. Surviving spouses and children receive a percentage of the retirement benefit computed from the earnings of the deceased earner.

Under the SSI, the federal government provides payments to needy aged, blind, and disabled individuals. Although the SSI program is run by the Social Security Administration, an individual does not have to be eligible for Social Security to receive benefits (i.e., a work history is not needed). Eligibility criteria for SSI include an individual with very limited personal property and at least one of the following characteristics: 65 years or older, blind, or disabled.

SSI criteria for disability include the following three items:

1. An individual is unable to engage in substantial gainful employment.
2. An individual cannot engage in work due to a medically determinable physical or mental impairment.
3. The medically determinable impairment can be expected to result in death, or in a disability lasting at least 12 months.

Children as well as adults can get benefits because of a disability.

In determining the amount of aid given, programs take into consideration the income and resources of individuals and families. However, once an individual qualifies for disability benefits, payments continue for as long as he or she remains medically disabled and unable to work. Periodic medical reviews are made to determine his or her health status. Those who receive SSI can receive Social Security benefits at the same time. Individuals who receive SSI are eligible in most states to receive medical care through the Medicaid program and food stamps. The basic monthly SSI check is the same in all states. As of January 2009 the SSI payment for an eligible individual is $674 per month and $1,011 per month for an eligible couple. Beneficiaries may be able to receive SSI in addition to monthly Social Security benefits, if the Social Security benefit is low enough to qualify.

Not all who are eligible get this exact amount, however. Individuals may get more if they live in a state that supplements the SSI check. Less may be given if the individual or his or her family has another source of monthly income.

CMS defines income as money the individual has coming in, such as earnings, Social Security checks, and pensions. Noncash items received, such as food, clothing, or shelter, also count as income. Federal eligibility rules define limited income and personal property as less than $2,000 in assets for an individual or $3,000 for a couple. However, the amount an individual can have each month and still get SSI depends on where he or she lives. In some states an individual can have more income than other states. Generally, the more income an applicant has, the less his or her SSI benefit will be. If an applicant's countable income is over the allowable limit, he or she cannot receive SSI benefits. Not all income is countable in an eligibility determination. For example, earnings up to $1,640 per month to a maximum of $6,600 per year (effective January 2011) for a student under age 22 are not counted when applying for SSI.

As with so many of these laws, some assets are protected or exempt from this calculation:

- An individual's home
- Household goods up to $2,000
- Wedding rings
- Car (especially if it is needed for employment or getting to medical appointments)
- Trade or business property needed for self-support
- Value of burial plot

- Up to $1,500 burial expense
- Cash value of life insurance, if the face value is less than $1,500 (if the face value is higher, it is considered an asset)

Unemployment Compensation

The U.S. Unemployment Compensation program (established by the Social Security Act of 1935) and employment service programs (established in 1933) form a federal–state cooperative system. The federal Unemployment Tax Act levied taxes on employers' payrolls to finance unemployment payments. Most of this federal tax can be offset by employer contributions to state funds under an approved state unemployment compensation law. The federal government, to pay for the administrative costs of the unemployment compensation and employment service programs and for loans to states whose funds run low, retains a small portion of the tax.

State financing and benefit laws vary widely. In general, unemployment compensation benefits under state laws are intended to replace about 50% of an average worker's previous wages. Maximum weekly benefits provisions, however, result in benefits of less than 50% for most higher-earning workers. All states pay benefits to some unemployed persons for 26 weeks. In some states the duration of benefits depends on the amount earned and the number of weeks worked in a previous year. In others, all recipients are entitled to benefits for the same length of time. During periods of heavy unemployment federal law authorizes extended benefits, in some cases up to 39 weeks; in 1975 extended benefits were payable for up to 65 weeks. Extended benefits are financed in part by federal employer taxes.

State Children's Health Insurance Program

At least 5 million children in the United States have no health insurance coverage. Responsive to this need, the federal government designed SCHIP to increase coverage for uninsured children. Run by CMS, together with the Health Resources and Services Administration, it provides $24 billion in federal matching funds to the states, beginning in 1997.

Like Medicaid, states set eligibility and coverage but must follow federal guidelines. Basic eligibility requirements mandate that recipients must have low incomes, be otherwise ineligible for Medicaid, and be uninsured. State programs differ, but all states must cover at least these services:

- Inpatient and outpatient hospital services
- Doctors' surgical and medical services
- Laboratory and x-ray services
- Well-baby/child care, including immunizations

Some states may provide additional benefits.

COBRA

In 1986, Congress passed the landmark law, called the Consolidated Omnibus Budget Reconciliation Act, or COBRA. The law amended ERISA, the Internal Revenue Code, and the Public Health Service Act. It provides workers and their families who lose their health benefits the opportunity to continue group health benefits provided by their group health plan. These benefits are made available to the ex-employee for limited periods of time under certain circumstances, such as voluntary or involuntary job loss, reduction in the hours worked, transition between jobs, death, divorce, and other life events.

Those who elect to purchase group health coverage under COBRA often find their premiums are more expensive for the same health coverage they had when they were active employees. This is because the employer often paid a part of the premium for active workers. Individuals who qualified for COBRA coverage may be required to pay up to 102% of the cost to the plan. The additional 2% is the cost of administrative charges. As a result, only 9% of Americans who were eligible for COBRA insurance in 2006 used it, many because they were unable to afford to pay the full premium after their job loss.[8] As an example, a survey of unemployed Americans in 41 states performed by the nonprofit organization Families USA found that although unemployment insurance benefits vary by state, the national average unemployment insurance benefit is $1,278. However, the average COBRA premium for family coverage is $1,069, or about 84% of those funds (http://www.familiesusa.org/resources/newsroom/press-releases/2009-press-releases/cobra-premiums-for-family.html viewed on 12/15/11), Despite this, the cost of group health coverage under COBRA is ordinarily significantly less expensive than purchasing health coverage as an individual.

The duration of COBRA coverage varies depending on the circumstances of the beneficiary. In most cases COBRA allows for coverage for up to 18 months. If the Social Security Administration determines that the individual is disabled, coverage may continue for up to 29 months. In the case of divorce from the former employee, the former spouse's coverage may continue for up to 36 months. In the case of death of the former employee, the widow's coverage may continue for up to 36 months.

At the time of job termination, an employer is obliged to notify the employee in writing of his or her rights under COBRA. The employee then has 60 days from the date of the notice or from the date his or her health insurance ended to enroll or sign up for coverage under COBRA. If the employee does not enroll during this 60-day period, his or her health insurance benefits under COBRA are no longer available. In addition, if the employee's company canceled their health insurance plan for all employees, went out of business, or went bankrupt, COBRA is not available.

REFERENCES

1. Goldman, D. P., Joyce, G. F., & Zheng, Y. (2007). Prescription drug cost sharing: Associations with medication and medical utilization and spending and health. *Journal of the American Medical Association, 298,* 61–69.
2. *Ponder v. Blue Cross of Southern California*, 193: Rptr. 632, Cal. App. 1983. The health insurance policy had an exclusion denying payment for dental care including "treatment for or prevention of temporomandibular joint syndrome." The Appellate Court held that this was not an effective exclusion.
3. *Red book: Pharmacy's fundamental reference.* (2010). Montvale, NJ: Medical Economics.
4. Thorne, K. (1990). *The birth of third generation of case management.* Canoga Park, CA: Thorne Associates.
5. The Health Insurance Portability and Accountability Act. (1996). Public Law, 104–191.
6. Standards for Privacy of Individually Identifiable Health Information. Title 45 Code of Federal Regulations: Parts 160 and 164.
7. Retrieved from http://www.medicaid.gov/Medicaid-CHIP-Program-Information/By-Topics/Eligibility/Spousal-Impoverishment-Page.html
8. Doty, M. M., Rustgi, S. D., Schoen, C., & Collins, S. R. (2009). *Maintaining health insurance during a recession: Likely COBRA eligibility.* The Commonwealth Fund.

Appendix 6-A

Healthcare Reimbursement Questions

1) The hypothesis that states a case would be better managed, and therefore less costly, simply because a neutral party is observing is known as
   A. The sentinel effect
   B. Utilization review
   C. The Hawthorne effect
   D. None of the above

2) When the Case Manager is arranging for durable medical equipment ordered by the physician, she or he should
   1. Order the equipment as quickly as possible without contacting the payer for approval to avoid delays in delivery
   2. Determine if renting or purchasing is more cost effective
   3. Monitor progress, patient recovery, and use of equipment to avoid charges for unused equipment
   4. Contact the insurer to request information on benefits, preferred providers, and any other pertinent information required
      A. 1, 3
      B. 2, 3
      C. 2, 3, 4
      D. All of the above
      E. None of the above

3) When the Case Manager arranges for medical supplies to be delivered to the patient's home, she or he should keep the following in mind:
   A. The best selection is the vendor recommended by the attending physician, regardless of price and other factors.
   B. The goal is to meet the patient's needs in a safe and cost-effective manner to maintain quality.
   C. The goal is to pick the most expensive vendor because this ensures quality service.
   D. The goal is to maximize the patient's benefit dollars; therefore, the least expensive vendor should always be chosen.

4) When the Case Manager is arranging for supplies and services, it is important for him or her to know the following:
   1. The patient's diagnosis and support system
   2. The physician's orders and treatment plan
   3. The benefit coverage and any guidelines to be used in obtaining supplies and services
   4. Any barriers to delivery or use of the supplies or services in the home

A. 1, 2, 3
B. 2, 3, 4
C. All of the above
D. None of the above

5) Which of the following is not one of the primary objectives of the Health Insurance Portability and Accountability Act (HIPAA) of 1996 legislation?
   A. Ensure health insurance portability by eliminating job lock due to preexisting medical conditions
   B. Reduce healthcare fraud and abuse
   C. Increase documentation and paperwork
   D. Guarantee security and privacy of health information

6) Which of the following entities is (are) covered by the HIPAA requirements?
   A. Insurance companies
   B. Hospitals
   C. Individual physician's offices
   D. All of the above

7) Which of the following statements is true regarding HIPAA?
   A. States can modify the "portability requirements."
   B. States can refuse insurance portability based on preexisting conditions.
   C. States can refuse portability if the patient was covered by a managed care plan.
   D. States can refuse electronic data interchange (EDI) if it is too expensive.

8) Under HIPAA provisions, a group health plan may charge a higher insurance premium to one subscriber compared with another similarly situated subscriber based on which of the following?
   A. Family history of mental illness
   B. Previous history of hypertension
   C. Preexisting renal failure
   D. None of the above

9) Under HIPAA provisions, which of the following statements is true?
   A. Employers are mandated to offer standard health insurance benefits.
   B. Employers are mandated to offer health insurance benefits that are the same or better than an employee's previous health benefit package.
   C. Employers are mandated to offer affordable health insurance benefits.
   D. None of the above

10) Under HIPAA, the term "preexisting condition" is best described by which of the following statements?
    A. A medical condition that a person has had before enrollment in his or her current insurance plan
    B. A medical condition that a subscriber has, which is diagnosed and treated by a medical professional, within the 6 months before the enrollment date in any new health plan
    C. A medical condition that a person develops during the 6-month waiting period for insurance coverage
    D. A medical condition that a person may develop during the first 6 months of the insurance coverage period

11) Under HIPAA, which of the following preexisting conditions cannot be excluded under a preexisting condition exclusion?
   A. Pregnancy
   B. Conditions affecting newborns
   C. Conditions affecting adopted children under 18 years of age
   D. All of the above

12) Under HIPAA, which of the following insurance types constitutes creditable coverage?
   A. Group health insurance
   B. Medicare, Medicaid
   C. COBRA health insurance
   D. All of the above

13) Under HIPAA, which of the following types of insurance is considered creditable coverage?
   A. Vision and eyeglass benefits
   B. Dental care coverage
   C. Group health plan coverage
   D. Long-term disability insurance

14) Utilization review can be done in the following manner:
   1. Retrospectively
   2. Prospectively
   3. Concurrently
   4. Ambulatory
      A. 1, 2, 3
      B. 2, 3, 4
      C. None of the above
      D. All of the above

15) Which of the following is a type of utilization review?
   A. Preadmission/precertification
   B. Concurrent
   C. Retrospective
   D. All of the above

16) Utilization review evaluates the following in regard to medical services:
   1. The medical appropriateness
   2. The medical necessity
   3. The efficiency
   4. The level of care
   5. The provider of care
      A. 1, 2, 3, 4
      B. 2, 3, 4, 5
      C. All of the above
      D. None of the above

17) Which of the following statements about indemnity health insurance plans is (are) true?
   1. It is a legal entity.
   2. It is licensed by the U.S. Department of the Interior.
   3. It exists to provide health insurance to enrollees.
   4. It reimburses enrollees for the cost of any health care they desire.

A. 1, 3
B. 2, 4
C. 1, 2, 3
D. All of the above
E. None of the above

18) Which of the following statements about indemnity health insurance plans is (are) not true?
    1. It is a legal entity.
    2. It is licensed by the U.S. Department of the Interior.
    3. It exists to provide health insurance to enrollees.
    4. It reimburses enrollees for the cost of any health care they desire.
        A. 1, 3
        B. 2, 4
        C. 1, 2, 3
        D. All of the above
        E. None of the above

19) Which of the following benefits accrue to employers who choose to self-insure their employees' healthcare costs?
    1. Increased service costs above those usually incurred by conventional insurers
    2. Exemption from providing benefits mandated by ERISA
    3. Increased costs of premium taxes
    4. Improved cash flow
        A. 1, 3
        B. 2, 4
        C. 1, 2, 3
        D. All of the above
        E. None of the above

20) Which of the following benefits do not accrue to employers who choose to self-insure their employees' healthcare costs?
    1. Increased service costs above those usually incurred by conventional insurers
    2. Exemption from providing benefits mandated by ERISA
    3. Increased costs of premium taxes
    4. Improved cash flow
        A. 1, 3
        B. 2, 4
        C. 1, 2, 3
        D. All of the above
        E. None of the above

21) Which of the following reason(s) is (are) important when considering whether an employer should self-insure for employee healthcare costs?
    1. Size of the president's yearly production bonus
    2. Size of employees' cash reserves
    3. Claims processing speed of the production workers
    4. Employer health status
        A. 1, 3
        B. 2, 4
        C. 1, 2, 3
        D. All of the above
        E. None of the above

CHAPTER SIX

22) Which of the following statements is (are) not true regarding third-party administrators (TPAs)?
   1. The TPA usually operates in the environment of the self-insured employer.
   2. The TPA is an agent of the insurer.
   3. The TPA is not party to the insurance contract and is not liable for losses incurred by employees.
   4. The TPA's sole function is to provide "insurance-type" administrative services to the employer.
      A. 1, 3
      B. 2, 4
      C. 1, 2, 3
      D. All of the above
      E. None of the above

23) Which of the following function(s) is (are) normally provided by TPAs for employers?
   1. Medical claims adjudication and payment
   2. Maintaining all records
   3. Providing case management, utilization management, and quality management
   4. Collecting and investing premium dollars
      A. 1, 3
      B. 2, 4
      C. 1, 2, 3
      D. All of the above
      E. None of the above

24) All the following are functions normally provided by TPAs for employers, except
   1. Medical claims adjudication and payment
   2. Providing medical care for the employees
   3. Providing case management, utilization management, and quality management
   4. Collecting and investing premium dollars
      A. 1, 3
      B. 2, 4
      C. 1, 2, 3
      D. All of the above
      E. None of the above

25) Which of the following benefit(s) is (are) associated with employers using a TPA?
   1. Access to state-of-the-art hardware and software claims processing systems
   2. Collection of premiums and investment of premium dollars for the employer
   3. Objectivity and privacy in claims processing
   4. Risk sharing with the TPA
      A. 1, 3
      B. 2, 4
      C. 1, 2, 3
      D. All of the above
      E. None of the above

26) Which of the following benefit(s) is (are) not associated with employers using a TPA?
   1. Access to state-of-the-art hardware and software claims processing systems
   2. Collection of premiums and investment of premium dollars for the employer
   3. Objectivity and privacy in claims processing
   4. Risk sharing with the TPA

A. 1, 3
B. 2, 4
C. 1, 2, 3
D. All of the above
E. None of the above

27) Which of the following is (are) not financially responsible for any personal injury or damaged property caused by car accidents?
   1. The state insurance fund
   2. The car owner
   3. The highway department
   4. The car owner's insurer
      A. 1, 3
      B. 2, 4
      C. 1, 2, 3
      D. All of the above
      E. None of the above

28) Which of the following determines minimum policy limits of personal injury protection (PIP) automobile insurance?
   1. State insurance department
   2. Accident rate in local community
   3. State insurance commissioner
   4. Driver's record of accidents
      A. 1, 3
      B. 2, 4
      C. 1, 2, 3
      D. All of the above
      E. None of the above

29) Which of the following does not determine minimum policy limits of PIP automobile insurance?
   1. State insurance department
   2. Accident rate in local community
   3. State insurance commissioner
   4. Driver's record of accidents
      A. 1, 3
      B. 2, 4
      C. 1, 2, 3
      D. All of the above
      E. None of the above

30) Which of the following characteristic(s) is (are) common to victims of automobile accidents?
   1. Senescence
   2. Seriousness of injuries
   3. Low incidence of head injuries
   4. High incidence of spinal injuries
      A. 1, 3
      B. 2, 4
      C. 1, 2, 3
      D. All of the above
      E. None of the above

31) Which of the following characteristic(s) is (are) not common to victims of automobile accidents?
   1. Senescence
   2. Seriousness of injuries
   3. Low incidence of head injuries
   4. High incidence of spinal injuries
      A. 1, 3
      B. 2, 4
      C. 1, 2, 3
      D. All of the above
      E. None of the above

32) PIP is designed to provide insurance coverage for which of the following people?
   1. Passengers involved in an auto accident
   2. Drivers involved in an auto accident
   3. Pedestrians involved in an auto accident
   4. A window washer who falls off a ladder while at work
      A. 1, 3
      B. 2, 4
      C. 1, 2, 3
      D. All of the above
      E. None of the above

33) PIP is designed to provide insurance coverage for which of the following people?
   1. Passengers involved in an auto accident
   2. Pedestrians involved in a drive-by shooting
   3. Pedestrians involved in an auto accident
   4. A window washer who falls off a ladder while at work
      A. 1, 3
      B. 2, 4
      C. 1, 2, 3
      D. All of the above
      E. None of the above

34) Which of the following people are protected by a PIP policy?
   1. Passengers involved in an auto accident
   2. Pedestrians involved in a slip-and-fall accident
   3. Pedestrians involved in an auto accident
   4. A driver who is the victim of domestic violence
      A. 1, 3
      B. 2, 4
      C. 1, 2, 3
      D. All of the above
      E. None of the above

35) Which of the following people are not protected by a PIP policy?
   1. Passengers involved in an auto accident
   2. Pedestrians involved in a slip-and-fall accident
   3. Pedestrians involved in an auto accident
   4. A driver who is the victim of domestic violence

A. 1, 3
B. 2, 4
C. 1, 2, 3
D. All of the above
E. None of the above

36) Many victims of automobile accidents have which of the following needs?
A. Speech therapy
B. Cognitive therapy
C. Occupational therapy
D. All of the above
E. None of the above

37) PIP insurance is the portion of an automobile policy that covers
A. Damage to the owner's automobile
B. Damage to another's automobile
C. Bodily injury to the drivers, passengers, or pedestrians
D. Damage to engine, drive train, and transmission only
E. All of the above

38) A driver has a no-fault policy. An uninsured driver strikes him while driving his vehicle. The uninsured driver of the second vehicle is noted to have alcohol on his breath, and subsequent testing reveals a blood alcohol level of 203 mg/dl. Both drivers are seriously injured. The first driver's insurance company can successfully deny medical coverage to the uninsured driver because
A. He was driving while intoxicated.
B. He was driving while uninsured.
C. He has demonstrated negligence and disregard for safety.
D. All of the above
E. None of the above

39) A hybrid insurance plan that provides the employee with provider choice and a contracted network with a gatekeeper is known as
A. PPO
B. HMO
C. Point of service
D. Indemnity

40) _____ is an organization that collects a predetermined fee per member per month, provides health care for a geographical area, and accepts responsibility to deliver a specified health benefit package to a voluntary enrolled group of employees.
A. A PPO
B. An HMO
C. A point of service plan
D. An indemnity program

41) Which of the following types of insurance is subject to the guidelines of the state in which the policy is written?
A. Short-term disability
B. Long-term disability
C. Group medical insurance
D. Workers' compensation insurance

42) _____ is a system of cost containment programs.
   A. Case management
   B. Managed care
   C. Workers' compensation
   D. All of the above

43) _____ is a system of healthcare delivery focused on managing the cost and quality of access to health care. It is used by HMOs, PPOs, and certain indemnity plans to improve the delivery of healthcare services and contain costs.
   A. Capitation
   B. Workers' compensation
   C. Managed care
   D. All of the above

44) In complex or disputed cases, _____ may be done to determine an individual's diagnosis, present status, need for continued treatment, type of appropriate treatment, degree of disability, or ability to return to work.
   A. A second surgical opinion
   B. An agreed-on medical exam
   C. A qualified medical exam
   D. An independent medical exam

45) A(n) _____ is an employee who has the necessary skills to examine claims and make decisions on whether to approve, investigate, or deny the claims.
   A. Medical examiner
   B. Claims examiner
   C. Insurance investigator
   D. Case Manager

46) HMOs designate that all primary care physicians are the _____ in the patient's care regarding specialty referrals and needs.
   A. Internal medicine doctors
   B. Chiropractors
   C. Gatekeepers
   D. Medical directors

47) The amount payable by the insurer to the insured under his or her group health coverage is called
   A. Coinsurance
   B. Copayment
   C. Deductible
   D. Benefits

48) Which of the following statements are true regarding current definitions of medical necessity in insurance contracts?
   1. They are clear.
   2. They are concise.
   3. They are unambiguous.
   4. They are uniform throughout the industry.
      A. 1, 3
      B. 2, 4
      C. 1, 2, 3
      D. All of the above
      E. None of the above

49) In standard health insurance contracts, which of the following terms is (are) made clear in the definition of medical necessity?
   1. Appropriate medical care
   2. Reasonable medical are
   3. Custodial medical care
   4. Experimental medical care
      A. 1, 3
      B. 2, 4
      C. 1, 2, 3
      D. All of the above
      E. None of the above

50) Which of the following statements is (are) true regarding the definition of medical necessity in insurance contracts?
   1. It is largely a "nonissue" discussed only by academics.
   2. It is an important issue that affects the adjudication of all health insurance claims.
   3. It is a problem solved easily by crafting the "right words" into the definition.
   4. The definition of what is medically necessary is best approached through a "procedural methodology."
      A. 1, 3
      B. 2, 4
      C. 1, 2, 3
      D. All of the above
      E. None of the above

51) When determining what is medically necessary in a particular case, which of the following should be evaluated?
   1. The reasonable expectations of the patient
   2. The opinion of objective specialists in the field of medicine in question
   3. The patient's medical record
   4. The opinion of the treating physician
      A. 1, 3
      B. 2, 4
      C. 1, 2, 3
      D. All of the above
      E. None of the above

52) Which of the following is (are) not important in the determination of what is medically necessary in a particular case?
   1. The reasonable expectations of the patient
   2. The opinion of objective specialists in the field of medicine in question
   3. The patient's medical record
   4. The opinion of the treating physician
      A. 1, 3
      B. 2, 4
      C. 1, 2, 3
      D. All of the above
      E. None of the above

53) Which of the following describes the intent of the insurance company when making a determination of what is medically necessary?
   1. Protect the subscriber from irregular medical practices
   2. Protect the subscriber from dangerous medical treatments
   3. Protect the subscriber from ineffective medical treatments
   4. Assure the policy holders that the insurer is paying only for care that is necessary and appropriate
      A. 1, 3
      B. 2, 4
      C. 1, 2, 3
      D. All of the above
      E. None of the above

54) When making a determination of what care is medically necessary, the medical director's intent should include all except which of the following?
   1. Protect the subscriber from dangerous medical treatments
   2. Decrease the utilization of medical resources at all costs
   3. Protect the subscriber from ineffective medical treatments
   4. Decease medical costs to raise the medical director's year-end bonus
      A. 1, 3
      B. 2, 4
      C. 1, 2, 3
      D. All of the above
      E. None of the above

55) Which of the following statements should characterize the decision-making process that determines what is medically necessary?
   1. The process is fair.
   2. The process uses the best available information.
   3. The process is reproducible.
   4. The process is managed by the insurance carrier's medical director.
      A. 1, 3
      B. 2, 4
      C. 1, 2, 3
      D. All of the above
      E. None of the above

56) The decision to deny a claim payment because it is determined the proposed treatment was not medically necessary should be made by whom?
   A. Senior vice president of claims operations
   B. Claims manager
   C. Case Manager
   D. Medical director
   E. Manager of network services

57) Aside from the medical director, who should be authorized to make claim denials for lack of medical necessity?
   1. Claims supervisor
   2. Manager of the provider network
   3. Chief operating officer
   4. Vice president of medical informatics

A. 1, 3
B. 2, 4
C. 1, 2, 3
D. All of the above
E. None of the above

58) Which of the following is (are) true about an indemnity health insurance plan?
1. It is a legal entity.
2. It is licensed by the state insurance department.
3. It exists to provide health insurance to enrollees.
4. It reimburses enrollees for the cost of healthcare goods and services covered in the insurance contract.
    A. 1, 3
    B. 2, 4
    C. 1, 2, 3
    D. All of the above
    E. None of the above

59) Which of the following is (are) true about indemnity health insurance companies?
1. They historically have had very active utilization review departments.
2. They historically have invested heavily in healthcare quality managed programs.
3. They exert tight control on network physicians.
4. They negotiate prices with capitated contracts.
    A. 1, 3
    B. 2, 4
    C. 1, 2, 3
    D. All of the above
    E. None of the above

60) Which of the following benefits accrue to employers who choose to self-insure?
1. Reduced service costs that are usually incurred by conventional insurers
2. Exemption from providing benefits mandated by ERISA
3. Elimination of the costs of premium taxes
4. Improved cash flow
    A. 1, 3
    B. 2, 4
    C. 1, 2, 3
    D. All of the above
    E. None of the above

61) Which of the following is (are) important when considering whether an employer should self-insure for employee healthcare costs?
1. Size of the employee base
2. Size of cash reserves
3. Group claims experience
4. Employee health status
    A. 1, 3
    B. 2, 4
    C. 1, 2, 3
    D. All of the above
    E. None of the above

62) Which of the following is (are) financially responsible for any personal injury or damaged property caused by car accidents?
   1. The state insurance fund
   2. The car owner
   3. The highway department
   4. The car owner's insurer
   5. The U.S. Department of the Interior
      A. 1, 3
      B. 2, 4
      C. 1, 2, 3
      D. All of the above
      E. None of the above

63) A type of automobile insurance in which each person's own insurance company pays for injury or damage up to a certain limit, regardless of whether its insured was actually at fault, is referred to as
   A. Malpractice insurance
   B. Excess and omission insurance
   C. No-fault insurance
   D. Personal injury protection
   E. Reinsurance

64) Of the following, who determines the minimum allowable limits of car insurance coverage for medical expenses and lost wages?
   A. Car manufacturers
   B. Federal government
   C. State government
   D. Car owner
   E. Insurance companies

65) Which of the following statements is (are) true concerning coordination of benefits (COB) as a process used by insurance companies?
   1. Coordinates claims payments between two or more insurance companies
   2. Helps human resources departments determine which of their employees requires which type of insurance
   3. Ensures that the claimant does not receive more than 100% of the cost of medical care
   4. Helps charitable organizations coordinate the financial gifts of donors
      A. 1, 3
      B. 2, 4
      C. 1, 2, 3
      D. All of the above
      E. None of the above

66) Of the following statements, which is (are) not true concerning COB rules?
   1. Almost all group health insurers have COB provisions in their contracts.
   2. COB provisions are federally mandated.
   3. Compliance with COB rules is voluntary.
   4. Compliance rates among insurers are low.
      A. 1, 3
      B. 2, 4
      C. 1, 2, 3
      D. All of the above
      E. None of the above

67) A man is hospitalized for treatment of his chronic gallbladder disease. He is covered by his employer-sponsored health plan, and he is covered as a dependent on his wife's employee-sponsored health plan. According to COB rules, which of the following policies pays first for his health care?
   A. His wife's health insurance policy
   B. His employee health insurance policy
   C. His workers' compensation policy
   D. His wife's no-fault insurance policy
   E. His excess and omissions policy

68) A man is hospitalized for treatment of his chronic gallbladder disease. He is covered by his employer-sponsored health plan, and he is covered as a dependent on his wife's employee-sponsored health plan. According to COB rules, which of the following policies will pay second for his health care?
   A. His wife's health insurance policy
   B. His employee health insurance policy
   C. His workers' compensation policy
   D. His wife's no-fault insurance policy
   E. His excess and omissions policy

69) A nurse is hospitalized for treatment of a ruptured ovarian cyst. She has health insurance coverage by her employee-sponsored health plan and is covered as a dependent on her husband's health plan. According to COB rules, which of the following policies pays first for her health care?
   A. Her husband's health insurance policy
   B. Her employee health insurance policy
   C. Her workers' compensation policy
   D. Her husband's no-fault insurance policy
   E. Her excess and omissions policy

70) A nurse is hospitalized for treatment of an arthritic ankle. She has health insurance coverage by her employee-sponsored health plan and is covered as a dependent on her husband's health plan. According to COB rules, which of the following policies pays second for her health care?
   A. Her husband's health insurance policy
   B. Her employee health insurance policy
   C. Her workers' compensation policy
   D. Her husband's no-fault insurance policy
   E. Her excess and omissions policy

71) When determining the order of insurance payment for a dependent child, when is the "birthday rule" invoked?
   1. When the parents are divorced
   2. When both the insurance companies involved have adopted the birthday rule in their contracts
   3. When the parents agree to coordinate benefits
   4. When each of the married parents has named the child as a dependent in their health insurance policies
      A. 1, 3
      B. 2, 4
      C. 1, 2, 3
      D. All of the above
      E. None of the above

72) Which of the following statements concerning the "birthday rule" in the coordination of the benefits process is (are) true?
   1. It is invoked when two or more plans cover an individual as a dependent.
   2. It bases the order of payment on the order of birthdays of the parents of the dependent.
   3. It can be used only when both insurance companies have adopted the birthday rule.
   4. It bases the order of payment on the birthday of the claimant.
      A. 1, 3
      B. 2, 4
      C. 1, 2, 3
      D. All of the above
      E. None of the above

73) When a child is covered as a dependent on both of his parents' policies, if the mother's insurance company does not ascribe to the "birthday rule," which insurance company pays first?
   A. The father's insurance company will sue the mother's insurer to invoke the birthday rule.
   B. The father's insurance company will pay in accordance with the male/female rule.
   C. The mother's insurance company will pay first in accordance with the male/female rule.
   D. The mother's insurance company will pay first because they have not adopted the birthday rule.
   E. Neither insurance company pays, and the claim is sent to the national insurance fund for payment.

74) A child of divorced parents becomes ill. Which of the following statements is (are) true regarding the coordination of benefits for the case?
   1. The insurance plan that is awarded primary responsibility by the courts pays first.
   2. The insurance plan of the parent with the earliest birthday pays first, if the courts have not determined a primary carrier.
   3. The insurance plan of the parent with custody pays first, if the courts have not determined a primary carrier.
   4. The insurance plan of the parent without custody pays first, if the courts have not determined a primary carrier.
      A. 1, 3
      B. 2, 4
      C. 1, 2, 3
      D. All of the above
      E. None of the above

75) A couple is divorced; they have four children from that union. The father has custody of the children. The mother of the children remarries, whereas the father of the children remains single. When one of the children becomes ill, whose insurance company pays first?
   A. The mother's insurance carrier
   B. The father's insurance carrier
   C. The mother's spouse's insurance carrier
   D. The father's girlfriend's insurance carrier
   E. The National Allied Insurance Fund (NAIF)

76) A couple is divorced; they have four children from that union. The father has custody of the children. The mother of the children remarries, whereas the father of the children remains single. When one of the children becomes ill, whose insurance company pays second?
   A. The mother's insurance carrier ✓
   B. The father's insurance carrier
   C. The mother's spouse's insurance carrier
   D. The father's girlfriend's insurance carrier
   E. The National Allied Insurance Fund (NAIF)

77) A couple with a single child is divorced; the mother has custody of the child. Each of the parents subsequently remarries. When the child gets ill, which of the following insurance companies pays first?
   A. The mother's insurance carrier ✓
   B. The father's insurance carrier
   C. The mother's spouse's insurance carrier
   D. The father's spouse's insurance carrier
   E. The National Adoption Insurance Fund

78) A couple with a single child is divorced; the mother has custody of the child. Each of the parents subsequently remarries. When the child gets ill, which of the following insurance companies pays second?
   A. The mother's insurance carrier
   B. The father's insurance carrier
   C. The mother's spouse's insurance carrier ✓
   D. The father's spouse's insurance carrier
   E. The National Adoption Insurance Fund

79) A couple with a single child is divorced; the mother has custody of the child. Each of the parents subsequently remarries. When the child gets ill, which of the following insurance companies pays last?
   A. The mother's insurance carrier
   B. The father's insurance carrier
   C. The mother's spouse's insurance carrier
   D. The father's spouse's insurance carrier
   E. The National Adoption Insurance Fund

80) A nurse, after working in a hospital for 25 years, retires with retiree health insurance benefits. She subsequently takes a job as an executive in an insurance company. When she becomes ill, which insurance company pays health insurance costs first?
   A. Her retiree health insurance benefit from the hospital, because that is where she was insured first
   B. The current employer's insurance carrier, because that is where she is insured now
   C. Her spouse's insurance company
   D. Her malpractice insurance company
   E. Her workers' compensation insurance

81) A police officer retires after 30 years on the force. Her retirement package includes healthcare benefits. She takes a full-time job as a security guard; this job has health insurance as a benefit to full-time employees. When she gets ill, which insurance entity pays first?
   A. Her retiree health insurance benefit from the police force, because that is where she was insured first
   B. The current employer's insurance carrier, because that is where she is insured now as an active employee
   C. Her spouse's health insurance company
   D. Her professional malpractice insurance company
   E. Her husband's workers' compensation insurance policy

82) A man usually employed as a bricklayer is laid off. He is able to maintain his health benefits as a laid-off employee. He also has healthcare benefits as a dependent on his wife's health insurance policy. When he becomes ill, which carrier pays first?
   A. His health insurance benefit from his job as a bricklayer
   B. Workers' compensation insurance
   C. His spouse's health insurance company, where he is covered as a dependent
   D. His unemployment insurance benefit
   E. His wife's workers' compensation insurance policy

83) A man usually employed as a bricklayer is laid off. He is able to maintain his health benefits as a laid-off employee. He also has healthcare benefits as a dependent on his wife's health insurance policy. When he becomes ill, which carrier pays second?
   A. His health insurance benefit from his job as a bricklayer
   B. Workers' compensation insurance
   C. His spouse's health insurance company, where he is covered as a dependent
   D. His unemployment insurance benefit
   E. His wife's workers' compensation insurance policy

84) A nurse, after working in a hospital for 25 years, retires with retiree health insurance benefits. She subsequently takes a job as an executive in an insurance company. When she becomes ill, which insurance entity pays health insurance costs second?
   A. Her retiree health insurance benefit from the hospital, because she is covered under an active employee plan
   B. The current employer's insurance carrier, because that is where she is insured now
   C. Her spouse's insurance company
   D. Her malpractice insurance company
   E. Her workers' compensation insurance

85) A hospital employee is fired from his job. He continues his health insurance benefits under COBRA, although he is also a dependent on his wife's employer-sponsored health insurance policy. He subsequently is employed as a day laborer without benefits. If he becomes ill, who pays his medical bills first?
   A. His current employer's excess and omissions insurance plan
   B. His health insurance plan maintained by his COBRA coverage
   C. His wife's insurance plan, where he is listed as a dependent
   D. Unemployment benefits insurance plan
   E. National Laborer's Relief Organization (NLRO)

86) A hospital employee is fired from his job. He continues his health insurance benefits under COBRA, although he is also a dependent on his wife's employer-sponsored health insurance policy. He subsequently is employed as a day laborer without benefits. If he becomes ill, who pays his medical bills second?
   A. His current employer's excess and omissions insurance plan
   B. His health insurance plan maintained by his COBRA coverage
   C. His wife's insurance plan, where he is listed as a dependent
   D. Unemployment benefits insurance plan
   E. National Laborer's Relief Organization (NLRO)

87) Victims of automobile accidents are characterized by which of the following?
   1. Youth
   2. Seriousness of injuries
   3. High incidence of head injuries
   4. High incidence of spinal injuries
   5. High incidence of permanent disability
      A. 1, 3
      B. 2, 4
      C. 1, 2, 3
      D. All of the above
      E. None of the above

88) When managing a patient who was injured in a car accident, the Case Manager needs to be knowledgeable regarding charitable and not-for-profit programs and services available in the community because
   A. They are qualitatively superior to those that can be purchased privately.
   B. PIP policy limits may restrict the range of options available to the client.
   C. A higher quality-of-life index is associated with these programs.
   D. All of the above
   E. None of the above

89) Utilization review is a process that
   1. Reviews medical bills to identify overcharging, billing errors, and overutilization
   2. Screens hospital admissions for appropriateness of service and service site
   3. Compares medical services to national standards of care to determine appropriateness of care for specific diagnoses
   4. Reviews ambulatory procedures for reasonable and customary charges
      A. 1, 2
      B. 1, 3
      C. 2, 3
      D. 2, 4

90) Which of the following is (are) true regarding a "claims edit"?
   1. It is software logic within an electronic claims processing system.
   2. It selects certain claims for evaluation.
   3. It compares certain claims against normative data.
   4. It can "decide" to pay the claim in full or in part.
      A. 1, 3
      B. 2, 4
      C. 1, 2, 3
      D. All of the above
      E. None of the above

91) Which of the following is (are) true regarding a "claims edit"?
1. It is software logic within an electronic claims processing system.
2. It randomly selects claims for evaluation.
3. It compares certain claims against normative data.
4. It can only "suspend" claims for manual review.
   A. 1, 3
   B. 2, 4
   C. 1, 2, 3
   D. All of the above
   E. None of the above

92) Which of the following is (are) not true regarding a "claims edit"?
1. It is software logic within an electronic claims processing system.
2. It randomly selects claims for evaluation.
3. It compares certain claims against normative data.
4. It can only "suspend" claims for manual review.
   A. 1, 3
   B. 2, 4
   C. 1, 2, 3
   D. All of the above
   E. None of the above

93) Which of the following is (are) true regarding "authoritative evidence"?
1. It is written medical or scientific conclusions.
2. It demonstrates the effectiveness of a treatment or procedure.
3. It is produced by controlled clinical trials.
4. It is produced by assessments initiated by CMS.
   A. 1, 3
   B. 2, 4
   C. 1, 2, 3
   D. All of the above
   E. None of the above

94) Which of the following statements is (are) correct?
1. COB coordinates workers' compensation with group health coverage.
2. With COB, patients can obtain benefits exceeding 100% of the fee charged.
3. COB rules are national.
4. COB determines the manner in which medical and dental benefits will be paid when a patient has coverage from multiple healthcare insurers.
   A. 1, 2
   B. 3, 4
   C. All of the above
   D. None of the above

95) Which of the following statements is (are) incorrect?
1. COB coordinates workers' compensation with group health coverage.
2. With COB, patients can obtain benefits exceeding 100% of the fee charged.
3. COB rules are national.
4. COB determines the manner in which medical and dental benefits will be paid when a patient has coverage from multiple healthcare insurers.

A. 1, 2
B. 2, 3, 4
C. All of the above
D. None of the above

96) Which of the following statements is (are) true regarding current definitions of medical necessity in insurance contracts?
1. They are inconsistent.
2. They are concise.
3. They are ambiguous.
4. They are uniform throughout the industry.
    A. 1, 3
    B. 2, 4
    C. 1, 2, 3
    D. All of the above
    E. None of the above

97) Which of the following statements is (are) not true regarding current definitions of medical necessity in insurance contracts?
1. They are inconsistent.
2. They are concise.
3. They are ambiguous.
4. They are uniform throughout the industry.
    A. 1, 3
    B. 2, 4
    C. 1, 2, 3
    D. All of the above
    E. None of the above

98) In standard health insurance contracts, which of the following terms is (are) not made clear in the definition of medical necessity?
1. Appropriate medical care
2. Reasonable medical care
3. Custodial medical care
4. Experimental medical care
    A. 1, 3
    B. 2, 4
    C. 1, 2, 3
    D. All of the above
    E. None of the above

99) Which of the following statements is (are) not true regarding the definition of medical necessity in insurance contracts?
1. It is largely a "nonissue" discussed only by academics.
2. It is an important issue that affects the adjudication of all health insurance claims.
3. It is a problem solved by easily crafting the "right words" into the definition.
4. The definition of what is medically necessary is best approached through a "procedural methodology."
    A. 1, 3
    B. 2, 4
    C. 1, 2, 3
    D. All of the above
    E. None of the above

100) When determining what is medically necessary in a particular case, which of the following should be evaluated?
1. The reasonable expectations of the hospital's nursing staff
2. The opinion of objective specialists in the field of medicine in question
3. The patient's financial record
4. The opinion of the treating physician
   A. 1, 3
   B. 2, 4
   C. 1, 2, 3
   D. All of the above
   E. None of the above

101) When determining what is medically necessary in a particular case, which of the following should not be evaluated?
1. The reasonable expectations of the hospital's billing staff
2. The opinion of objective specialists in the field of medicine in question
3. The patient's financial record
4. The opinion of the treating physician
   A. 1, 3
   B. 2, 4
   C. 1, 2, 3
   D. All of the above
   E. None of the above

102) When determining the medical necessity of a claim, which of the following is (are) true regarding the "reasonable expectations" of the claimant?
1. The reasonable expectations of the claimant are unimportant in the adjudication of the claim.
2. If a certain medical benefit can be reasonably expected, then the claimant should be entitled to it.
3. The ability for the insured to understand the complex terminology in the contract is irrelevant.
4. The fairness of any insurance contract is suspect when the claimant does not or cannot understand its benefits or the meaning of its exclusions.
   A. 1, 3
   B. 2, 4
   C. 1, 2, 3
   D. All of the above
   E. None of the above

103) When determining the medical necessity of a claim, which of the following is (are) not true regarding the "reasonable expectations" of the claimant?
1. The reasonable expectations of the claimant are unimportant in adjudication of the claim.
2. If a certain medical benefit can be reasonably expected, then the claimant should be entitled to it.
3. The ability for the insured to understand the complex terminology in the contract is irrelevant.
4. The fairness of any insurance contract is suspect when the claimant does not or cannot understand its benefits or the meaning of its exclusions.

A. 1, 3
B. 2, 4
C. 1, 2, 3
D. All of the above
E. None of the above

104) When determining the medical necessity of a claim, which of the following is (are) not true regarding the "reasonable expectations" of the claimant?
1. The reasonable expectations of the claimant are unimportant in adjudication of the claim.
2. Just because a certain medical benefit can be reasonably expected by the average layperson does not mean the claimant should be entitled to it.
3. The ability for the insured to understand the complex terminology in the contract is irrelevant.
4. The fairness of any insurance contract is suspect when the claimant does not or cannot understand its benefits or the meaning of its exclusions.
    A. 1, 3
    B. 2, 4
    C. 1, 2, 3
    D. All of the above
    E. None of the above

105) Which of the following is (are) true of utilization review?
1. Utilization review reviews services for medical appropriateness.
2. Utilization review reviews services for medical necessity.
3. Utilization review is only done retrospectively.
4. Utilization review compares services rendered to nationally acceptable standards and protocols.
5. Utilization review denies care over certain preestablished dollar amounts.
    A. 1, 2, 3
    B. 1, 2, 4
    C. 1, 3, 5
    D. All of the above
    E. None of the above

106) When managing a patient who was injured in a car accident, the Case Manager needs to be knowledgeable regarding charitable and not-for-profit programs and services available in the community. Which of the following statements is (are) not true in regard to these programs?
1. They are qualitatively superior to those that can be purchased privately.
2. PIP policy limits may restrict the range of options available to the client.
3. A higher quality-of-life index is associated with these programs.
4. The costs of health care may exceed the finances of the patient and insurer.
    A. 1, 3
    B. 2, 4
    C. 1, 2, 3
    D. All of the above
    E. None of the above

107) While driving and dialing his cell phone, the driver hits another car. The driver of the first car suffers bilateral femur fractures. The driver of the second car has facial fractures. Witnesses report the first driver was driving erratically and was seen using his cell phone. Both drivers have no-fault automobile insurance. The second driver's insurance company can successfully deny medical coverage because
   A. The first driver was clearly at fault.
   B. The first driver was breaking the "hands-free use" law for cell phones.
   C. The first driver's insurance coverage has a higher limit.
   D. All of the above
   E. None of the above

108) Which of the following statements is (are) true regarding unemployment insurance?
   1. Financing of unemployment benefits is uniform from state to state.
   2. Unemployment compensation benefits guarantee a replacement of 50% of salary.
   3. Benefits are never extended past the usual maximum length of benefit.
   4. All states pay a minimum of 46 weeks of unemployment benefits.
      A. 1, 3
      B. 2, 4
      C. 1, 2, 3
      D. All of the above
      E. None of the above

109) Which of the following statements is (are) true regarding unemployment insurance?
   1. Financing of unemployment benefits varies from state to state.
   2. Unemployment compensation benefits guarantee a replacement of 50% of salary.
   3. Benefits may be extended past the usual maximum length of benefit, during periods of heavy unemployment.
   4. All states pay a minimum of 46 weeks of unemployment benefits.
      A. 1, 3
      B. 2, 4
      C. 1, 2, 3
      D. All of the above
      E. None of the above

110) Which of the following statements is (are) true regarding unemployment insurance?
   1. Financing of unemployment benefits is uniform from state to state.
   2. Unemployment compensation benefits are intended to replace 50% of an average worker's salary.
   3. Benefits are never extended past the usual maximum length of benefit.
   4. All states pay a minimum of 26 weeks of unemployment benefits.
      A. 1, 3
      B. 2, 4
      C. 1, 2, 3
      D. All of the above
      E. None of the above

111) Which of the following statements is (are) not true regarding unemployment insurance?
   1. Financing of unemployment benefits varies from state to state.
   2. Unemployment compensation benefits guarantee a replacement of 50% of salary.
   3. Benefits may be extended past the usual maximum length of benefit, during periods of heavy unemployment.
   4. All states pay a minimum of 46 weeks of unemployment benefits.

A. 1, 3
B. 2, 4
C. 1, 2, 3
D. All of the above
E. None of the above

112) Which of the following statements is (are) not true regarding unemployment insurance?
1. Financing of unemployment benefits is uniform from state to state.
2. Unemployment compensation benefits are guaranteed to replace 50% of an average worker's salary.
3. Benefits are never extended past the usual maximum length of benefit.
4. All states pay a minimum of 26 weeks of unemployment benefits.
A. 1, 3
B. 2, 4
C. 1, 2, 3
D. All of the above
E. None of the above

113) All except which of the following asset transfers are exempted from state-imposed penalties during a "look back" for inappropriately transferred assets?
A. Transfers to a spouse or to a third party for the sole benefit of the spouse
B. Transfers by a spouse to a third party for the sole benefit of the spouse
C. Transfers to a sibling for the sole benefit of the sibling
D. Transfers for a purpose other than to qualify for Medicaid
E. Transfers in which imposing a penalty would cause undue hardship

114) An individual transfers his house to his sister for consideration of $1, one year before his entrance into a nursing home. The house's fair market value is $100,000. During the state's look back, they find this asset transfer and apply a penalty period. If the average cost of the individual's medical care is $500 per month, the average pharmacy cost is $50 per month, and the average nursing home cost in that state is $2,000 per month, how long is the penalty period?
A. 50 months
B. 100 months
C. 200 months
D. 2,000 months
E. None of the above

115) The time limit for a state-imposed "penalty period" for the inappropriate transfer of assets is
A. 100 months
B. 60 months
C. 36 months
D. No limits
E. None of the above

266 CHAPTER SIX

116) The "look-back" period for asset transfer, performed by the state for a Medicaid applicant, is
   A. 60 months before the date the individual is institutionalized or, if later, the date he or she applies for Medicaid
   B. 360 months for certain types of trusts
   C. 90 months before the date the individual is institutionalized or, if later, the date he or she applies for Medicaid
   D. A only
   E. A, C

117) Which of the following results in a "penalty period" imposed by the state when the state reviews financial records during a "look back" for a Medicaid applicant?
   A. When an individual's financial asset is transferred at a cost higher than fair market value
   B. When an individual's financial asset is transferred at a cost of the fair market value
   C. When an individual's financial asset is transferred for a cost less than the fair market value
   D. All of the above
   E. None of the above

118) A healthy individual creates an irrevocable trust and makes his grandson the beneficiary of his trust. He transfers the majority of his real estate holdings into this trust. Six months elapse, and the individual suffers a massive stroke and requires nursing home care. Which of the following is (are) true regarding how Medicaid will view the assets in trust?
   A. The assets will be considered not available to the individual because they are placed in an irrevocable trust.
   B. The assets will be considered not available to the individual because the title to the assets is held by the trust.
   C. The assets will be considered available to the individual because the trust was established within the look-back period.
   D. None of the above
   E. All of the above

119) A father establishes a trust for his 12-year-old mentally retarded son. The trust is funded by the son's Social Security benefits. Which of the following statements describes how CMS will view these assets upon the son's application for Medicaid benefits?
   A. The assets will be considered not available to the individual because they are placed in an irrevocable trust.
   B. The assets will be considered not available to the individual because the title to the assets is held by the trust.
   C. The assets will be considered available to the individual because the trust was established within the look-back period.
   D. None of the above
   E. All of the above

120) _____ made the employer's health plan the primary payer for all active Medicare-eligible employees and their spouses, regardless of age; mandated the extension of medical benefits after termination from employment and after a person becomes ineligible under a medical plan; and required that employers with healthcare plans provide healthcare coverage to former employees, divorced or widowed spouses of employees, and former dependent children of employees at group rates for a specific time frame.
   A. Medicare
   B. COBRA
   C. SSI
   D. Federal Employee Liability Act (FELA)

121) Which of the following statements about unemployment compensation is (are) true?
   1. It is a program established by the Social Security Act of 1935.
   2. It is designed to replace 100% of an employee's previous wages.
   3. It is financed by unemployment taxes or by employer contributions to an approved state unemployment fund.
   4. The minimum duration of benefits is 26 weeks.
      A. 1, 3, 4
      B. 2, 4
      C. 1, 2, 3
      D. All of the above
      E. None of the above

122) Which of the following statements about unemployment compensation is (are) true?
   1. It is a program established by the Unemployment Act of 1952.
   2. It is designed to replace 50% of an employee's previous wages.
   3. It is financed by state sales tax.
   4. The minimum duration of benefits is 26 months. WEEKS
      A. 1, 3, 4
      B. 2, 4
      C. 1, 2, 3
      D. All of the above
      E. None of the above

123) Eligibility criteria for the State Children's Health Insurance Program include all except which of the following?
   1. Recipients must have been insured in the previous 12 months.
   2. Recipients must be from families with low incomes.
   3. Recipients must be between the ages of 10 and 19 years.
   4. Recipients must be uninsured.
   5. Recipients must be otherwise ineligible for Medicaid.
      A. 1, 3
      B. 2, 4
      C. 1, 2, 3
      D. All of the above
      E. None of the above

124) Which of the following benefits is (are) federally mandated for the State Children's Health Insurance Program?
1. Inpatient and outpatient hospital services
2. Doctor's surgical and medical services
3. Laboratory and x-ray services
4. Well baby/child care, including immunizations
    A. 1, 3
    B. 2, 4
    C. 1, 2, 3
    D. All of the above
    E. None of the above

125) "Utilization of services that are in excess of a beneficiary's medical needs or receiving a capitated Medicare payment and failing to provide services to meet a beneficiary's medical needs" defines which of the following terms, according to CMS?
    A. Inappropriate utilization
    B. Abuse
    C. Fraud
    D. Theft
    E. Collusion

126) Which of the following is (are) true regarding the Medicare program?
1. It was created by Title XVIII of the Social Security Act.
2. It went into effect in 1966.
3. It is currently managed by the Centers for Medicare & Medicaid Services (CMS).
4. It was started as a "make work" program for underutilized physicians.
    A. 1, 3
    B. 2, 4
    C. 1, 2, 3
    D. All of the above
    E. None of the above

127) Which of the following statements is (are) true concerning the Medicare program?
1. It is divided into two parts, Part A and Part B.
2. Part A is the Hospital Insurance program.
3. Part B is the out-of-hospital care and physicians' services insurance program.
4. Part A is funded by Social Security taxes.
    A. 1, 3
    B. 2, 4
    C. 1, 2, 3
    D. All of the above
    E. None of the above

128) Medicare provides health insurance benefits to whom?
1. Persons 65 years old who receive Social Security benefits
2. Persons 65 years old who receive Railroad Retirement benefits
3. Persons 65 years old who have a spouse who has Medicare-covered government employment
4. Persons 65 years old who have never worked or been married to a worker who has paid Social Security taxes

A. 1, 3
B. 2, 4
C. 1, 2, 3
D. All of the above
E. None of the above

129) Which of the following statements is (are) not true concerning the Medicare program?
1. Part B is the Hospital Insurance program.
2. It was enacted under Title XIV of the Social Security Act.
3. Part A is the out-of-hospital care and physicians' services insurance program.
4. Part A is funded by Social Security taxes.
    A. 1, 3
    B. 2, 4
    C. 1, 2, 3
    D. All of the above
    E. None of the above

130) Medicare provides health insurance benefits to whom of the following?
1. Persons 55 years old who receive Social Security benefits
2. Persons 55 years old who receive Railroad Retirement benefits
3. Persons 55 years old who have a spouse who has Medicare-covered government employment
4. Persons 55 years old who have never worked or been married to a worker who has paid Social Security taxes
    A. 1, 3
    B. 2, 4
    C. 1, 2, 3
    D. All of the above
    E. None of the above

131) Which of the following is (are) not true regarding the Medicare program?
1. It was created by Title XVIII of the Social Security Act.
2. It went into effect in 1956.
3. It is currently managed by the Centers for Medicare & Medicaid Services (CMS).
4. It was started as a "make work" program for underutilized physicians.
    A. 1, 3
    B. 2, 4
    C. 1, 2, 3
    D. All of the above
    E. None of the above

132) Medicare provides health insurance benefits to whom of the following?
1. Persons who have been entitled to Social Security benefits for 24 months
2. Persons who have been in active duty in the armed forces
3. Persons who are disabled and who are entitled to Social Security benefits
4. Persons who have been treated in a Veterans Administration hospital
    A. 1, 3
    B. 2, 4
    C. 1, 2, 3
    D. All of the above
    E. None of the above

133) A patient is entitled to Medicare benefits if he or she has permanent kidney failure and if which of the following is (are) also true?
   1. He or she has worked the required amount of time under Social Security or the Railroad Board or is a government employee.
   2. He or she is receiving or is eligible to receive Social Security or Railroad Retirement case benefits.
   3. He or she is the spouse or a dependent child of a person who has worked the required amount of time or who is receiving Social Security or Railroad case benefits.
   4. He or she is a foreign national who has never worked in this country, or he or she is not a dependent of an eligible worker.
      A. 1, 3
      B. 2, 4
      C. 1, 2, 3
      D. All of the above
      E. None of the above

134) A patient is not entitled to Medicare benefits if he or she has permanent kidney failure and if which of the following is (are) also true?
   1. He or she has not worked the required amount of time under Social Security or the Railroad Board and is not is a government employee.
   2. He or she is receiving or is eligible to receive Social Security or Railroad Retirement case benefits.
   3. He or she is not the spouse or a dependent child of a person who has worked the required amount of time or who is receiving Social Security or Railroad case benefits.
   4. He or she is a foreign national who has never worked in this country, or he or she is not a dependent of an eligible worker.
      A. 1, 3, 4
      B. 2, 4
      C. 1, 2, 3
      D. All of the above
      E. None of the above

135) Medicare will not provide health insurance benefits to whom of the following?
   1. Patients who are not entitled to Social Security benefits
   2. Patients who have been in active duty in the armed forces but are not entitled to Social Security benefits
   3. Patients who have been treated in a Veterans Administration hospital
   4. Patients who are disabled and who are entitled to Social Security benefits
      A. 1, 3
      B. 2, 4
      C. 1, 2, 3
      D. All of the above
      E. None of the above

136) When a patient becomes entitled to Medicare solely because of end-stage renal disease, he or she must wait how long until he or she is covered by Medicare?
   A. 1 month
   B. 2 months
   C. 3 months
   D. 4 months
   E. 5 months

137) Which of the following is (are) true regarding Medicare coverage for a patient with end-stage renal disease?
1. He or she is considered to have end-stage renal disease if he or she has irreparable damage that requires a transplant or dialysis to maintain life.
2. If he or she becomes entitled to Medicare benefits solely because of end-stage renal disease, he or she must wait 3 months before he or she is covered by Medicare benefits.
3. If he or she becomes entitled to Medicare benefits solely because of end-stage renal disease, his or her protection ends 12 months after the month he or she no longer needs maintenance dialysis treatments.
4. If he or she becomes entitled to Medicare benefits solely because of end-stage renal disease, his or her protection ends 36 months after a successful kidney transplant.
   A. 1, 3
   B. 2, 4
   C. 1, 2, 3
   D. All of the above
   E. None of the above

138) If a patient is entitled to Medicare benefits solely because of end-stage renal disease, when do his or her benefits expire?
1. His or her protection ends 3 years after maintenance dialysis begins.
2. His or her protection ends 12 months after the month he or she no longer needs maintenance dialysis treatments.
3. His or her protection ends 24 months after his or her diagnosis of end-stage renal disease is made.
4. His or her protection ends 36 months after a successful kidney transplant.
   A. 1, 3
   B. 2, 4
   C. 1, 2, 3
   D. All of the above
   E. None of the above

139) Which of the following is (are) not true regarding Medicare coverage for a patient with end-stage renal disease?
1. He or she is considered to have end-stage renal disease if he or she has irreparable damage that requires a transplant or dialysis to maintain life.
2. If he or she becomes entitled to Medicare benefits solely because of end-stage renal disease, he or she must wait 6 months before he or she is covered by Medicare benefits.
3. If he or she becomes entitled to Medicare benefits solely because of end-stage renal disease, his or her protection ends 12 months after the month he or she no longer needs maintenance dialysis treatments.
4. If he or she becomes entitled to Medicare benefits solely because of end-stage renal disease, his or her protection ends 12 months after a successful kidney transplant.
   A. 1, 3
   B. 2, 4
   C. 1, 2, 3
   D. All of the above
   E. None of the above

140) Medicare benefits under the Part A program include which of the following?
1. Inpatient hospital services
2. Skilled nursing facilities
3. Home health services
4. Hospice care
   A. 1, 3
   B. 2, 4
   C. 1, 2, 3
   D. All of the above
   E. None of the above

141) Medicare benefits under the Part A program include all except which of the following?
1. Physician fees
2. Skilled nursing facilities
3. Outpatient hospital services
4. Hospice care
   A. 1, 3
   B. 2, 4
   C. 1, 2, 3
   D. All of the above
   E. None of the above

142) Medicare benefits under the Part A program include which of the following?
1. Inpatient hospital services
2. Hemodialysis (outpatient)
3. Home health services
4. Ambulatory surgery
   A. 1, 3
   B. 2, 4
   C. 1, 2, 3
   D. All of the above
   E. None of the above

143) Which of the following statements is (are) true regarding Medicare Select?
1. It is more expensive than Medigap insurance.
2. It offers benefits similar to Medigap.
3. The federal government sells it.
4. It limits treatment to specific hospitals and physicians except in emergencies.
   A. 1, 3
   B. 2, 4
   C. 1, 2, 3
   D. All of the above
   E. None of the above

144) Medicare Part A pays for how many days of inpatient hospital care for each benefit period?
   A. Medicare pays for 90 days of medically necessary inpatient hospital care.
   B. Medicare pays for 60 days of medically necessary inpatient hospital care.
   C. Medicare pays for 50 days of medically necessary inpatient hospital care.
   D. Medicare pays for 120 days of medically necessary inpatient hospital care.
   E. Medicare pays for 90 days of medically unnecessary inpatient hospital care.

145) **Medicare Part A helps pay for how many days of care in a skilled nursing facility for each benefit period?**
   A. Medicare pays for 160 days of medically necessary care in a skilled nursing facility after a hospital stay.
   B. Medicare pays for 50 days of medically necessary care in a skilled nursing facility after a hospital stay.
   C. Medicare pays for 100 days of medically necessary care in a skilled nursing facility after a hospital stay.
   D. Medicare pays for 90 days of medically necessary care in a skilled nursing facility after a hospital stay.
   E. Medicare pays for 100 days of medically necessary care in a skilled nursing facility without a hospital stay.

146) **Medicare Part A helps pay for how many days of hospice care?**
   A. Medicare helps pay for 220 days of hospice care.
   B. Medicare helps pay for 310 days of hospice care.
   C. Medicare helps pay for 90 days of hospice care.
   D. Medicare helps pay for 210 days of hospice care.
   E. Medicare helps pay for 50 days of hospice care.

147) **Which of the following statements is (are) true regarding the Medicare Part A program?**
   1. Medicare Part A helps pay for 210 days of hospice care.
   2. Medicare pays for 100 days of medically necessary care in a skilled nursing facility after a hospital stay.
   3. Medicare pays for 90 days of medically necessary inpatient hospital care.
   4. Medicare pays for 50 days of medically unnecessary inpatient hospital care.
      A. 1, 3
      B. 2, 4
      C. 1, 2, 3
      D. All of the above
      E. None of the above

148) **Which of the following statements is (are) not true regarding the Medicare Part A program?**
   1. Medicare Part A helps pay for 210 days of hospice care.
   2. Medicare pays for 200 days of medically necessary care in a skilled nursing facility after a hospital stay.
   3. Medicare pays for 90 days of medically necessary inpatient hospital care.
   4. Medicare pays for 50 days of medically unnecessary inpatient hospital care.
      A. 1, 3
      B. 2, 4
      C. 1, 2, 3
      D. All of the above
      E. None of the above

149) Medicare Part B helps pay for the cost of which of the following services?
1. Physician services
2. Outpatient hospital services
3. Medical equipment and supplies
4. Inpatient hospital stays
    A. 1, 3
    B. 2, 4
    C. 1, 2, 3
    D. All of the above
    E. None of the above

150) Medicare Part B helps pay for the cost of all except which of the following services?
1. Physician services
2. Hospice care services
3. Medical equipment and supplies
4. Inpatient hospital stays
    A. 1, 3
    B. 2, 4
    C. 1, 2, 3
    D. All of the above
    E. None of the above

151) A 45-year-old patient becomes eligible for Medicare benefits solely because of end-stage renal disease. Which of the following services is (are) covered by Medicare?
1. Hemodialysis
2. Arthroscopic surgery to treat osteoarthritis of the knee
3. Surgical placement of an arteriovenous fistula for hemodialysis access
4. Retinal surgery
    A. 1, 3
    B. 2, 4
    C. 1, 2, 3
    D. All of the above
    E. None of the above

152) A 33-year-old patient becomes eligible for Medicare benefits solely because of end-stage renal disease. Which of the following services is (are) not covered by Medicare?
1. Hemodialysis
2. Speech therapy
3. Surgical placement of an arteriovenous fistula for hemodialysis access
4. Clipping of a cerebral aneurysm surgery
    A. 1, 3
    B. 2, 4
    C. 1, 2, 3
    D. All of the above
    E. None of the above

153) Which of the following statements is (are) true regarding Medicare "reserve days"?
1. The beneficiary has the right to choose when to use a reserve day.
2. It is one of 60 extra days of hospital care for which Medicare pays.
3. There are only 60 reserve days in a beneficiary's lifetime.
4. They can be used if the patient has a prolonged illness necessitating a hospital stay longer than 90 days.

A. 1, 3
B. 2, 4
C. 1, 2, 3
D. All of the above
E. None of the above

154) **Which of the following statements is (are) not true regarding Medicare "reserve days"?**
 1. Only the provider has the right to choose when to use a reserve day.
 2. It is one of 60 extra days of hospital care for which Medicare pays.
 3. There are only 90 reserve days in a beneficiary's lifetime.
 4. They can be used if the patient has a prolonged illness necessitating a hospital stay longer than 90 days.
    A. 1, 3
    B. 2, 4
    C. 1, 2, 3
    D. All of the above
    E. None of the above

155) **Which of the following statements is (are) true regarding a Medicare "benefit period"?**
 1. A benefit period begins the first day of a patient's admission to a hospital, skilled nursing facility, or hospice.
 2. A benefit period ends after the patient has been discharged for 60 contiguous days.
 3. There is no limit to the number of benefit periods a patient may have for hospital and skilled nursing facilities.
 4. There is no limit to the number of days a beneficiary may claim payment for during a benefit period.
    A. 1, 3
    B. 2, 4
    C. 1, 2, 3
    D. All of the above
    E. None of the above

156) **Which of the following statements is (are) not true regarding a Medicare "benefit period"?**
 1. A benefit period begins the first day of a patient's admission to a hospital, skilled nursing facility, or hospice.
 2. A benefit period ends after the patient has been discharged for 90 contiguous days.
 3. There is no limit to the number of benefit periods a patient may have for hospital and skilled nursing facilities.
 4. There is no limit to the number of days a beneficiary may claim payment for during a benefit period.
    A. 1, 3
    B. 2, 4
    C. 1, 2, 3
    D. All of the above
    E. None of the above

157) Which of the following statements is (are) true regarding a Medicare "benefit period"?
1. A benefit period begins the first day of a patient's admission to a hospital, skilled nursing facility, or hospice.
2. A benefit period ends after the patient has been discharged for 90 contiguous days.
3. There is no limit to the number of benefit periods a patient may have for hospital and skilled nursing facilities.
4. There is no limit to the number of days a beneficiary may claim payment for during a benefit period.
   A. 1, 3
   B. 2, 4
   C. 1, 2, 3
   D. All of the above
   E. None of the above

158) Which of the following is (are) true regarding Medicare benefits?
1. Medicare recipients still have to pay Medicare coinsurance.
2. Medicare recipients have no out-of-pocket financial obligations to providers.
3. Medicare recipients still have to pay Medicare deductibles.
4. Medicare recipients pay no Medicare deductibles after their 65th birthday.
   A. 1, 3
   B. 2, 4
   C. 1, 2, 3
   D. All of the above
   E. None of the above

159) Which of the following is (are) not true regarding Medicare benefits?
1. Medicare recipients still have to pay Medicare coinsurance.
2. Medicare recipients have no out-of-pocket financial obligations to providers.
3. Medicare recipients still have to pay Medicare deductibles.
4. Medicare recipients pay no Medicare deductibles after their 65th birthday.
   A. 1, 3
   B. 2, 4
   C. 1, 2, 3
   D. All of the above
   E. None of the above

160) Which of the following is (are) true regarding coverage for Medicare benefits?
1. There are many medical services that Medicare does not cover.
2. Beneficiaries are not responsible for paying for medical services not covered by Medicare.
3. A Medicare supplemental insurance policy (Medigap) is sometimes purchased by beneficiaries to pay for services not covered by Medicare.
4. Medicare pays for all medically necessary care.
   A. 1, 3
   B. 2, 4
   C. 1, 2, 3
   D. All of the above
   E. None of the above

Healthcare Reimbursement   277

161) **Which of the following statements is (are) not true regarding coverage for Medicare benefits?**
   1. There are many medical services that Medicare does not cover.
   2. Beneficiaries are not responsible for paying for medical services not covered by Medicare.
   3. A Medicare supplemental insurance policy (Medigap) is sometimes purchased by beneficiaries to pay for services not covered by Medicare.
   4. Medicare pays for all medically necessary care.
      A. 1, 3
      B. 2, 4
      C. 1, 2, 3
      D. All of the above
      E. None of the above

162) **Which of the following statements is (are) true regarding Medigap policies?**
   1. Medigap is private insurance.
   2. Medigap is designed to help pay for Medicare cost-sharing amounts.
   3. Medigap has at least 10 standard policies, each with different combinations of benefits.
   4. The best time to purchase a Medigap policy is during the open enrollment period.
      A. 1, 3
      B. 2, 4
      C. 1, 2, 3
      D. All of the above
      E. None of the above

163) **Which of the following statements is (are) not true regarding Medigap policies?**
   1. Medigap is federal insurance.
   2. Medigap is designed to help pay for Medicare cost-sharing amounts.
   3. Medigap has a single policy with a single group of benefits.
   4. The best time to purchase a Medigap policy is during the open enrollment period.
      A. 1, 3
      B. 2, 4
      C. 1, 2, 3
      D. All of the above
      E. None of the above

164) **Which of the following statements is (are) true regarding the purchase of a Medigap policy during the open enrollment period?**
   1. The best time for a beneficiary to buy a policy is during the open enrollment period.
   2. During the open enrollment period, the beneficiary has the right to buy the Medigap policy of his or her choice.
   3. During the open enrollment period, the beneficiary cannot be turned down for a Medigap policy.
   4. During the open enrollment period, the beneficiary cannot be charged a higher premium for a Medigap policy because of poor health.
      A. 1, 3
      B. 2, 4
      C. 1, 2, 3
      D. All of the above
      E. None of the above

165) Which of the following statements is (are) not true regarding the purchase of a Medigap policy during the open enrollment period?
1. The best time for a beneficiary to buy a policy is after 36 months of Medicare enrollment.
2. During the open enrollment period, the beneficiary has the right to buy the Medigap policy of his or her choice.
3. The beneficiary can be turned down for a Medigap policy if he or she is a particularly high health risk.
4. During the open enrollment period, the beneficiary cannot be charged a higher premium for a Medigap policy because of poor health.
    A. 1, 3
    B. 2, 4
    C. 1, 2, 3
    D. All of the above
    E. None of the above

166) Which of the following statements is (are) true regarding the purchase of a Medigap policy during the open enrollment period?
1. The best time for a beneficiary to buy a policy is after 36 months of Medicare enrollment.
2. During the open enrollment period, the beneficiary has the right to buy the Medigap policy of his or her choice.
3. The beneficiary can be turned down for a Medigap policy if he or she is a particularly high health risk.
4. During the open enrollment period, the beneficiary cannot be charged a higher premium for a Medigap policy because of poor health.
    A. 1, 3
    B. 2, 4
    C. 1, 2, 3
    D. All of the above
    E. None of the above

167) Which of the following statements defines Medicare's open enrollment period?
    A. It is a period that begins the date the person who is 65 or older first enrolls in Medicare and ends 6 months later.
    B. It is a period that begins the date the person who is 75 or older first enrolls in Medicare and ends 4 months later.
    C. It is a period that begins the date the person who is 65 or older first enrolls in Medicare and ends 36 months later.
    D. It is a period that begins the date the person who is 55 or older first enrolls in Medicare and ends 6 months later.
    E. It is a period that begins the date the person who is 45 or older first enrolls in Medicare and ends 12 months later.

168) Which of the following statements is (are) true regarding a Medicare beneficiary's open enrollment period?
1. The beneficiary must be 65 years of age or older.
2. The open enrollment period begins the first day of Medicare enrollment.
3. The open enrollment period lasts for 6 months.
4. Outside the continental United States, the period lasts for 12 months.

A. 1, 3
B. 2, 4
C. 1, 2, 3
D. All of the above
E. None of the above

169) Which of the following statements is (are) not true regarding a Medicare beneficiary's open enrollment period?
1. The beneficiary must be 65 years of age or older.
2. The open enrollment period begins after 6 months of Medicare enrollment.
3. The open enrollment period lasts for 6 months.
4. Outside the continental United States, the period lasts for 12 months.
    A. 1, 3
    B. 2, 4
    C. 1, 2, 3
    D. All of the above
    E. None of the above

170) Which of the following statements is (are) true regarding Medicare Select?
1. It is another type of Medicare supplemental health insurance.
2. Insurance companies and HMOs sell it.
3. It offers benefits similar to Medigap.
4. It limits treatment to specific hospitals and physicians except in emergencies.
    A. 1, 3
    B. 2, 4
    C. 1, 2, 3
    D. All of the above
    E. None of the above

171) Which of the following statements is (are) not true regarding Medicare Select?
1. It is more expensive than Medigap insurance.
2. It offers benefits similar to Medigap.
3. It is sold by the federal government.
4. It limits treatment to specific hospitals and physicians except in emergencies.
    A. 1, 3
    B. 2, 4
    C. 1, 2, 3
    D. All of the above
    E. None of the above

172) Medicare benefits under the Part A program include all except which of the following?
1. Inpatient hospital services
2. Hemodialysis (outpatient)
3. Home health services
4. Ambulatory surgery
    A. 1, 3
    B. 2, 4
    C. 1, 2, 3
    D. All of the above
    E. None of the above

173) Other insurance companies will pay before Medicare when which of the following occur?
1. The individual is 65 or older and is covered by a group health insurance.
2. The individual is younger than 65 and disabled and is covered by a group health insurance.
3. The individual has Medicare because of permanent kidney failure.
4. The individual has an illness or injury that is covered under workers' compensation, the federal black lung program, no-fault insurance, or any liability insurance.
   A. 1, 3
   B. 2, 4
   C. 1, 2, 3
   D. All of the above
   E. None of the above

174) The state may pay for an individual's Medicare costs when which of the following is (are) true?
1. The individual must be entitled to Medicare hospital insurance (Part A program).
2. The individual's income level must be at or below the national poverty guidelines.
3. The individual cannot have resources worth more than $6,680 (home and first car don't count).
4. The couple cannot have resources worth more than $10,020 (home and first car don't count).
   A. 1, 3
   B. 2, 4
   C. 1, 2, 3
   D. All of the above
   E. None of the above

175) The state may pay for an individual's Medicare costs when which of the following is (are) true?
1. The individual must be entitled to workers' compensation insurance.
2. The individual's income level must be at or below the national poverty guidelines.
3. The individual cannot have resources worth more than $10,000 (home and first car don't count).
4. The couple cannot have resources worth more than $10,020 (home and first car don't count).
   A. 1, 3
   B. 2, 4
   C. 1, 2, 3
   D. All of the above
   E. None of the above

176) Which of the following statements is (are) true regarding the Balanced Budget Act of 1997?
1. Medicare pays for yearly colorectal screening for people over the age of 50.
2. Medicare pays for screening mammograms for women over the age of 40.
3. Medicare pays for screening Pap smears every 3 years.
4. Medicare pays for diabetic educational programs aimed at self-management.
   A. 1, 3
   B. 2, 4
   C. 1, 2, 3
   D. All of the above
   E. None of the above

177) Which of the following statements is (are) true regarding the Balanced Budget Act of 1997?
   1. Medicare pays for one influenza vaccine per year, one pneumococcal vaccine per lifetime, and hepatitis B vaccine for those at medium to high risk for infection.
   2. Medicare pays for glucose test strips for diabetics who are not insulin dependent.
   3. Medicare pays for bone mass tests for those at risk for osteoporosis.
   4. Medicare pays for diabetic educational programs aimed at self-management.
      A. 1, 3
      B. 2, 4
      C. 1, 2, 3
      D. All of the above
      E. None of the above

178) Which of the following statements is (are) true regarding the Balanced Budget Act of 1997?
   1. Medicare pays for one cosmetic surgical procedure per year.
   2. Medicare pays for glucose test strips for diabetics who are not insulin dependent.
   3. Medicare pays for CT scans to rule out coronary artery disease.
   4. Medicare pays for diabetic educational programs aimed at self-management.
      A. 1, 3
      B. 2, 4
      C. 1, 2, 3
      D. All of the above
      E. None of the above

179) Which of the following statements is (are) not true regarding the Balanced Budget Act of 1997?
   1. Medicare pays for one cosmetic surgical procedure per year.
   2. Medicare pays for prostate screening for men over the age of 50.
   3. Medicare pays for CT scans to rule out coronary artery disease.
   4. Medicare pays for diabetic educational programs aimed at self-management.
      A. 1, 3
      B. 2, 4
      C. 1, 2, 3
      D. All of the above
      E. None of the above

180) Which of the following statements is (are) true regarding the Centers for Medicare & Medicaid Services (CMS)?
   1. It is a federal agency within the U.S. Department of Health and Human Services.
   2. It runs the Medicare and Medicaid programs.
   3. It helps to run the State Children's Health Insurance Program (SCHIP).
   4. It regulates all laboratory testing performed on humans in the United States.
      A. 1, 3
      B. 2, 4
      C. 1, 2, 3
      D. All of the above
      E. None of the above

181) Which of the following statements is (are) true regarding the CMS?
   1. It helps eliminate discrimination based on health status for people buying health insurance.
   2. It runs the Medicare and Medicaid programs.
   3. It helps to run the State Children's Health Insurance Program (SCHIP).
   4. It regulates research laboratory testing.
      A. 1, 3
      B. 2, 4
      C. 1, 2, 3
      D. All of the above
      E. None of the above

182) Which of the following statements is (are) true regarding the CMS?
   1. It is a state agency within the U.S. Department of Agriculture.
   2. It runs the Medicare and Medicaid programs.
   3. It helps to run the Social Security Administration.
   4. It regulates all laboratory testing (except research) performed on humans in the United States.
      A. 1, 3
      B. 2, 4
      C. 1, 2, 3
      D. All of the above
      E. None of the above

183) Which of the following statements is (are) not true regarding the CMS?
   1. It is a state agency within the U.S. Department of Agriculture.
   2. It runs the Medicare and Medicaid programs.
   3. It helps to run the Social Security Administration.
   4. It regulates all laboratory testing (except research) performed on humans in the United States.
      A. 1, 3
      B. 2, 4
      C. 1, 2, 3
      D. All of the above
      E. None of the above

184) A patient meets the following criteria:
   - Has a defined disability
   - Has filed an application for worker's benefits
   - Has achieved a minimum employment period covered by Social Security
   - Is younger than 65 years old
   - Has been disabled for 5 months

   This patient is entitled to
      A. SSI
      B. CHIP
      C. Social Security Disability Insurance (SSDI)
      D. Workers' compensation

185) In 1965 Medicare legislation provided health benefits to patients older than 65 and
      A. Veterans
      B. Disabled veterans
      C. Welfare recipients
      D. Disabled individuals

186) Which of the following statements is (are) true regarding Medicaid?
    1. It is a national health insurance program.
    2. It is aimed at serving the poor and needy.
    3. It was created by Title XIX of the Social Security Act.
    4. State welfare or state health departments operate it.
        A. 1, 3
        B. 2, 4
        C. 1, 2, 3
        D. All of the above
        E. None of the above

187) Which of the following statements is (are) true regarding Medicaid?
    1. It is a national health insurance program.
    2. It is operated within the guidelines set by CMS.
    3. It was created by Title XIX of the Social Security Act.
    4. There are no out-of-pocket expenses for patients covered by this program.
        A. 1, 3
        B. 2, 4
        C. 1, 2, 3
        D. All of the above
        E. None of the above

188) Which of the following statements is (are) true regarding Medicaid?
    1. It is a national health insurance program.
    2. It is aimed at providing medical insurance for the aged.
    3. It was created by Title XIX of the Social Security Act.
    4. It is operated by the CMS.
        A. 1, 3
        B. 2, 4
        C. 1, 2, 3
        D. All of the above
        E. None of the above

189) Which of the following statements is (are) not true regarding Medicaid?
    1. It is a national health insurance program.
    2. It is aimed at providing medical insurance for the aged.
    3. It was created by Title XIX of the Social Security Act.
    4. It is operated by the CMS.
        A. 1, 3
        B. 2, 4
        C. 1, 2, 3
        D. All of the above
        E. None of the above

190) Which of the following statements is (are) true regarding Medicaid?
1. It is a state health insurance program.
2. It is operated within the guidelines set by CMS.
3. It was created by Title XVI of the Social Security Act.
4. There are no out-of-pocket expenses for patients covered by this program.
    A. 1, 3
    B. 2, 4
    C. 1, 2, 3
    D. All of the above
    E. None of the above

191) Which of the following statements regarding Medicaid is (are) not true?
1. It is a state health insurance program.
2. It is operated within the guidelines set by CMS.
3. It was created by Title XVI of the Social Security Act.
4. There are no out-of-pocket expenses for patients covered by this program.
    A. 1, 3
    B. 2, 4
    C. 1, 2, 3
    D. All of the above
    E. None of the above

192) Which of the following services is (are) federally mandated by the Medicaid program?
1. Inpatient hospital care and outpatient services
2. Physician services
3. Skilled nursing home services for adults
4. Laboratory and x-ray services
    A. 1, 3
    B. 2, 4
    C. 1, 2, 3
    D. All of the above
    E. None of the above

193) Which of the following services is (are) federally mandated by the Medicaid program?
1. Inpatient hospital care and outpatient services
2. Carpentry services
3. Skilled nursing home services for adults
4. Electrician's services
    A. 1, 3
    B. 2, 4
    C. 1, 2, 3
    D. All of the above
    E. None of the above

194) Which of the following services is (are) not federally mandated by the Medicaid program?
1. Inpatient hospital care and outpatient services
2. Carpentry services
3. Skilled nursing home services for adults
4. Electrician's services

A. 1, 3
B. 2, 4
C. 1, 2, 3
D. All of the above
E. None of the above

195) Groups eligible for Medicaid under CMS standards include which of the following?
1. Categorically needy
2. Spiritually needy
3. Medically needy
4. Ethnically needy
    A. 1, 3
    B. 2, 4
    C. 1, 2, 3
    D. All of the above
    E. None of the above

196) Groups ineligible for Medicaid under CMS standards include which of the following?
1. Categorically needy
2. Spiritually needy
3. Medically needy
4. Ethnically needy
    A. 1, 3
    B. 2, 4
    C. 1, 2, 3
    D. All of the above
    E. None of the above

197) Which of the following statements regarding Medicaid eligibility is (are) true?
1. Eligibility standards are set by each state.
2. Minimum eligibility standards are set by CMS.
3. The categorically needy are usually eligible for Medicaid.
4. The medically needy are usually eligible for Medicaid.
    A. 1, 3
    B. 2, 4
    C. 1, 2, 3
    D. All of the above
    E. None of the above

198) Which of the following statements regarding Medicaid eligibility is (are) true?
1. Eligibility standards are set by each state.
2. Minimum eligibility standards are set by CMS.
3. The categorically needy are usually eligible for Medicaid.
4. The spiritually impoverished are usually eligible for Medicaid.
    A. 1, 3
    B. 2, 4
    C. 1, 2, 3
    D. All of the above
    E. None of the above

CHAPTER SIX

199) Which of the following statements regarding Medicaid eligibility is (are) not true?
1. Eligibility standards are set by each state.
2. Minimum eligibility standards for Medicaid are set by the Social Security Administration.
3. The categorically needy are usually eligible for Medicaid.
4. The spiritually impoverished are usually eligible for Medicaid.
    A. 1, 3
    B. 2, 4
    C. 1, 2, 3
    D. All of the above
    E. None of the above

200) Which of the following groups is (are) considered a "mandatory Medicaid eligibility group"?
1. Recipients of Aid to Families with Dependent Children (AFDC)
2. Recipients of Supplemental Security Income (SSI)
3. Infants born to Medicaid-eligible pregnant women
4. Children younger than age 6 and pregnant women who meet the state's AFDC financial re-quirements
    A. 1, 3
    B. 2, 4
    C. 1, 2, 3
    D. All of the above
    E. None of the above

201) Which of the following groups is (are) considered a "mandatory Medicaid eligibility group"?
1. Recipients of Aid to Families with Dependent Children (AFDC)
2. Recipients of workers' compensation insurance
3. Infants born to Medicaid-eligible pregnant women
4. Children younger than age 6 who are the beneficiaries of a no-fault tort action
    A. 1, 3
    B. 2, 4
    C. 1, 2, 3
    D. All of the above
    E. None of the above

202) Which of the following groups is (are) not considered a "mandatory Medicaid eligibility group"?
1. Recipients of Aid to Families with Dependent Children (AFDC)
2. Recipients of workers' compensation insurance
3. Infants born to Medicaid-eligible pregnant women
4. Children younger than age 6 who are the beneficiaries of a no-fault tort action
    A. 1, 3
    B. 2, 4
    C. 1, 2, 3
    D. All of the above
    E. None of the above

203) Which of the following asset transfers is (are) exempted from state-imposed penalties during a "look back" for inappropriately transferred assets?
1. Transfers to a spouse or to a third party for the sole benefit of the spouse
2. Transfers by a spouse to a third party for the sole benefit of the spouse
3. Transfers in which imposing a penalty would cause undue hardship
4. Transfers to a sibling for the sole benefit of the sibling
   A. 1, 3
   B. 2, 4
   C. 1, 2, 3
   D. All of the above
   E. None of the above

204) Which of the following asset transfers is (are) not exempted from state-imposed penalties during a "look back" for inappropriately transferred assets?
1. Transfers to a spouse or to a third party for the sole benefit of the spouse
2. Transfers by a spouse to a third party for the sole benefit of the third party
3. Transfers in which imposing a penalty would cause undue hardship
4. Transfers to a sibling for the sole benefit of the sibling
   A. 1, 3
   B. 2, 4
   C. 1, 2, 3
   D. All of the above
   E. None of the above

205) Which of the following asset transfers is (are) exempted from state-imposed penalties during a "look back" for inappropriately transferred assets?
1. Transfers to a spouse or to a third party for the sole benefit of the spouse
2. Transfers by a spouse to a third party for the sole benefit of the third party
3. Transfers in which imposing a penalty would cause undue hardship
4. Transfers to a sibling for the sole benefit of the sibling
   A. 1, 3
   B. 2, 4
   C. 1, 2, 3
   D. All of the above
   E. None of the above

206) Which of the following statements is (are) true regarding a "penalty period" imposed by the state?
1. It is the amount of time the state will withhold payment from nursing homes and other long-term care facilities.
2. There is no limit to the length of time in a penalty period.
3. Penalty periods are imposed by the state when an "inappropriate transfer of assets" has occurred.
4. The length of the penalty period is based on the fair market value of the transferred asset and the monthly cost of the long-term care facility.
   A. 1, 3
   B. 2, 4
   C. 1, 2, 3
   D. All of the above
   E. None of the above

207) Which of the following statements is (are) true regarding a "penalty period" imposed by the state?
1. It is the amount of time the state will withhold payment from nursing homes and other long-term care facilities.
2. There is a 2-year limit to the length of a penalty period.
3. Penalty periods are imposed by the state when an "inappropriate transfer of assets" has occurred.
4. The length of the penalty period is based on the fair market value of all the marital assets divided by the predicted length of stay in the long-term care facility.
   A. 1, 3
   B. 2, 4
   C. 1, 2, 3
   D. All of the above
   E. None of the above

208) Which of the following statements is (are) not true regarding a "penalty period" imposed by the state?
1. It is the amount of time the state will withhold payment from nursing homes and other long-term care facilities.
2. There is a 2-year limit to the length of a penalty period.
3. Penalty periods are imposed by the state when an "inappropriate transfer of assets" has occurred.
4. The length of the penalty period is based on the fair market value of all the marital assets divided by the predicted length of stay in the long-term care facility.
   A. 1, 3
   B. 2, 4
   C. 1, 2, 3
   D. All of the above
   E. None of the above

209) Which of the following statements is (are) true regarding the "look back" or financial evaluation of an individual's eligibility for Medicaid?
1. It is a financial evaluation undertaken by the state to establish Medicaid eligibility.
2. Recent transfers of assets are examined.
3. The look back commonly examines financial records for 60 months before the date of an individual's institutionalization.
4. Transfers of assets for less than fair market value may invoke penalties from the state.
   A. 1, 3
   B. 2, 4
   C. 1, 2, 3
   D. All of the above
   E. None of the above

210) Which of the following statements is (are) true regarding the "look back" or financial evaluation of an individual's eligibility for Medicaid?
1. It is a financial evaluation undertaken by the federal government to establish workers' compensation eligibility.
2. Recent transfers of assets are examined.
3. The look back commonly examines financial records for 6 months before the date of an individual's institutionalization.
4. Transfers of assets for less than fair market value may invoke penalties from the state.

A. 1, 3
B. 2, 4
C. 1, 2, 3
D. All of the above
E. None of the above

211) Which of the following statements is (are) not true regarding the "look back" or financial evaluation of an individual's eligibility for Medicaid?
1. It is a financial evaluation undertaken by the federal government to establish workers' compensation eligibility.
2. Recent transfers of assets are examined.
3. The look back commonly examines financial records for 6 months before the date of an individual's institutionalization.
4. Transfers of assets for less than fair market value may invoke penalties from the state.
    A. 1, 3
    B. 2, 4
    C. 1, 2, 3
    D. All of the above
    E. None of the above

212) The penalty period imposed by the state for inappropriate transfers of assets before Medicaid application is calculated by which of the following formulas?
    A. Fair market value of transferred asset / Average monthly cost of nursing facility in the state = Months of penalty period
    B. Medicaid approved value of transferred asset / Standard Monthly Medicaid Allowance (SMMA) for nursing homes in that state = Months of penalty period
    C. Average cost of an individual's assets / Standard Monthly Medicaid Allowance (SMMA) for nursing homes in that state = Months of penalty period
    D. Medicare approved value of transferred asset / Standard Monthly Medicaid Allowance (SMMA) for nursing homes in that state = Months of penalty period
    E. Medicare approved value of transferred asset / Standard Monthly Medicare Allowance (SMMA) for nursing homes in that state = Months of penalty period

213) Which of the following statements is (are) true regarding the term spousal impoverishment before Medicaid eligibility?
1. It refers to the depletion of a couple's life savings that occurs when one is paying the expenses associated with the institutionalization of the spouse.
2. It refers to the government protection from savings depletion that is granted only to those who are Medicare eligible.
3. It refers to amendments to the Social Security Act in 1988 that allow a couple to have Medicaid benefits without spending down their resources.
4. Federal Medicaid guidelines mandate the "community spouse" first reach 161% of the federal poverty level before the institutionalized spouse is eligible for Medicaid benefits.
    A. 1, 3
    B. 2, 4
    C. 1, 2, 3
    D. All of the above
    E. None of the above

214) Which of the following statements is (are) not true regarding the term spousal impoverishment before Medicaid eligibility?
1. It refers to the depletion of a couple's life savings that occurs when one is paying the expenses associated with the institutionalization of the spouse.
2. It refers to the government protection from savings depletion that is granted only to those who are Medicare eligible.
3. It refers to amendments to the Social Security Act in 1988 that allow a couple to have Medicaid benefits without spending down their resources.
4. Federal Medicaid guidelines mandate the "community spouse" first reach 161% of the federal poverty level before the institutionalized spouse is eligible for Medicaid benefits.
   A. 1, 3
   B. 2, 4
   C. 1, 2, 3
   D. All of the above
   E. None of the above

215) Which of the following statements is (are) true regarding the eligibility of an institutionalized spouse for Medicaid?
1. The institutionalized spouse must remain in the medical facility for at least 30 days.
2. The state must evaluate the couple's resources.
3. The spousal resource amount (SRA) must be calculated.
4. Spousal resource amounts (SRAs) that are above the state's minimum resource standard are depletable resources.
   A. 1, 3
   B. 2, 4
   C. 1, 2, 3
   D. All of the above
   E. None of the above

216) Which of the following statements is (are) true regarding the eligibility of an institutionalized spouse for Medicaid?
1. The institutionalized spouse must remain in the medical facility for at least 90 days.
2. The state must evaluate the couple's resources.
3. The spousal poverty depletion rate (SPDR) must be calculated.
4. Spousal resource amounts that are above the state's minimum resource standard are depletable resources.
   A. 1, 3
   B. 2, 4
   C. 1, 2, 3
   D. All of the above
   E. None of the above

217) Which of the following statements is (are) not true regarding the eligibility of an institutionalized spouse for Medicaid?
1. The institutionalized spouse must remain in the medical facility for at least 90 days.
2. The state must evaluate the couple's resources.
3. The spousal poverty depletion rate (SPDR) must be calculated.
4. Spousal resource amounts that are above the state's minimum resource standard are depletable resources.

A. 1, 3
B. 2, 4
C. 1, 2, 3
D. All of the above
E. None of the above

218) **Which of the following is (are) true regarding Medicaid eligibility for a couple with a spouse in a medical facility or nursing home?**
   1. The community spouse's income is not considered available to the spouse in the medical facility.
   2. For the purposes of Medicaid eligibility, the community spouse is considered to own all the matrimonial assets.
   3. The state will use the income eligibility standards for one person rather than two.
   4. For the purposes of Medicaid eligibility, the institutionalized spouse is considered to own all the matrimonial assets.
      A. 1, 3
      B. 2, 4
      C. 1, 2, 3
      D. All of the above
      E. None of the above

219) **Which of the following is (are) not true regarding Medicaid eligibility for a couple with a spouse in a medical facility or nursing home?**
   1. The community spouse's income is not considered available to the spouse in the medical facility.
   2. For the purposes of Medicaid eligibility, the community spouse is considered to own all the matrimonial assets.
   3. The state will use the income eligibility standards for one person rather than two.
   4. For the purposes of Medicaid eligibility, the institutionalized spouse is considered to own all the matrimonial assets.
      A. 1, 3
      B. 2, 4
      C. 1, 2, 3
      D. All of the above
      E. None of the above

220) **Which of the following statements regarding trusts is (are) true?**
   1. It is a legal title to property, held by one party for the benefit of another party.
   2. There are usually at least three parties involved in the establishment of a trust.
   3. A trust's grantor donates the assets of a trust.
   4. A trust's beneficiary is the recipient of some or all of the trust's assets.
      A. 1, 3
      B. 2, 4
      C. 1, 2, 3
      D. All of the above
      E. None of the above

221) Which of the following statements regarding trusts is (are) true?
1. It is a legal title to property, held by one party for the benefit of another party.
2. There are usually at least six parties involved in the establishment of a trust.
3. A trust's grantor donates the assets of a trust.
4. A trust's beneficiary is the entity that donates the trust's assets.
   A. 1, 3
   B. 2, 4
   C. 1, 2, 3
   D. All of the above
   E. None of the above

222) Which of the following statements regarding trusts is (are) true?
1. It is a legal title to property, held by one party for the benefit of another party.
2. A trust's trustee holds and manages the assets in the trust for the beneficiary.
3. A trust's grantor donates the assets of a trust.
4. A revocable trust is a trust whose terms or beneficiaries can be changed.
   A. 1, 3
   B. 2, 4
   C. 1, 2, 3
   D. All of the above
   E. None of the above

223) Which of the following statements regarding trusts is (are) not true?
1. It is a legal title to property, held by one party for the benefit of another party.
2. A trust's trustee holds and manages the assets in the trust for the beneficiary.
3. A trust's grantor donates the assets of a trust.
4. A revocable trust is a trust whose terms or beneficiaries can be changed.
   A. 1, 3
   B. 2, 4
   C. 1, 2, 3
   D. All of the above
   E. None of the above

224) Which of the following statements regarding trusts is (are) true?
1. It is a legal title to property, held by one party for the benefit of that party.
2. A trust's assets can exist in many forms, such as cash, real estate, businesses, or stocks.
3. A trust's trustee donates the assets of a trust.
4. An irrevocable trust is a trust whose terms or beneficiaries cannot be changed.
   A. 1, 3
   B. 2, 4
   C. 1, 2, 3
   D. All of the above
   E. None of the above

225) Which of the following statements regarding trusts is (are) true?
1. It is a legal title to property, held by one party for the benefit of another party.
2. A trust's assets can exist in many forms, such as cash, real estate, businesses, or stocks.
3. A trust's grantor donates the assets of a trust.
4. An irrevocable trust is a trust whose terms or beneficiaries cannot be changed.

A. 1, 3
B. 2, 4
C. 1, 2, 3
D. All of the above
E. None of the above

226) **Which of the following statements regarding trusts is (are) true?**
1. It is a legal title to property, held by one party for the benefit of another party.
2. A trust's assets can exist only as cash or stock.
3. A trust's grantor donates the assets of a trust.
4. An irrevocable trust is a trust whose terms or beneficiaries can be changed.
    A. 1, 3
    B. 2, 4
    C. 1, 2, 3
    D. All of the above
    E. None of the above

227) **Which of the following is (are) true regarding the treatment of trusts under CMS regulations?**
1. CMS would like to prevent the use of trusts created only to transfer assets to ensure Medicaid eligibility.
2. How CMS treats a trust depends on what type of trust it is.
3. Monies that are paid from a trust to an individual are treated as income to that individual.
4. Monies from a trust that could be paid to an individual, but are not, are treated as available resources.
    A. 1, 3
    B. 2, 4
    C. 1, 2, 3
    D. All of the above
    E. None of the above

228) **Which of the following is (are) true regarding the treatment of trusts under CMS regulations?**
1. CMS would like to encourage the use of trusts created only to transfer assets to ensure Medicaid eligibility.
2. How CMS treats a trust depends on what type of trust it is (revocable or irrevocable).
3. Monies that are paid from a trust to an individual are treated as protected assets.
4. Monies from a trust that could be paid to an individual, but are not, are treated as available resources.
    A. 1, 3
    B. 2, 4
    C. 1, 2, 3
    D. All of the above
    E. None of the above

229) Which of the following is (are) not true regarding the treatment of trusts under CMS regulations?
1. CMS would like to encourage the use of trusts created only to transfer assets to ensure Medicaid eligibility.
2. How CMS treats a trust depends on what type of trust it is (revocable or irrevocable).
3. Monies that are paid from a trust to an individual are treated as protected assets.
4. Monies from a trust that could be paid to an individual, but are not, are treated as available resources.
    A. 1, 3
    B. 2, 4
    C. 1, 2, 3
    D. All of the above
    E. None of the above

230) A local court establishes a trust for a severely disabled individual. The trust is funded by the individual's Social Security benefits. Which of the following statements describes how CMS will view these assets upon the individual's application for Medicaid benefits?
    A. The assets will be considered not available to the individual because they are placed in an irrevocable trust.
    B. The assets will be considered not available to the individual because the title to the assets is held by the trust.
    C. The assets will be considered available to the individual because the trust was established within the look-back period.
    D. The assets will not be considered available to the individual because he or she is disabled.
    E. The assets will be considered available to the individual because the assets are from Social Security.

231) When applying for SSI, it is important for the patient to know
    A. The criteria are state-specific and have explicit eligibility guidelines.
    B. SSI is based on low income and medical criteria.
    C. SSI is for children, the disabled, and elderly.
    D. All of the above
    E. None of the above

232) Under the Medicare program, the phrase assignment of benefits means
1. The patient or beneficiary directs Medicare to pay covered benefits directly to the provider of services.
2. The provider must accept Medicare's allowable charge as payment in full.
3. The patient assigns, or turns over, his or her benefits to a family member.
4. The Medicare patient has benefit coverage under Medicare.
    A. 1, 2
    B. 2, 3
    C. 3, 4
    D. All of the above
    E. None of the above

233) **Which of the following statements is (are) true regarding the Women's Health and Cancer Rights Act?**
1. It is a law enacted as part of the Defense Appropriations Bill.
2. It ensures coverage for surgery of the contralateral breast to provide a symmetrical appearance after mastectomy.
3. It amended ERISA to require both health plans and self-insured plans to provide coverage for mastectomies and certain reconstructive surgeries.
4. It ensures coverage for breast prostheses after mastectomy.
    A. 1, 3
    B. 2, 3, 4
    C. 1, 2, 3
    D. All of the above
    E. None of the above

234) **Which of the following statements is (are) true regarding the Women's Health and Cancer Rights Act?**
1. It is a law enacted as part of the Omnibus Appropriations Bill.
2. It ensures coverage for surgery of the contralateral breast to provide a symmetrical appearance after mastectomy.
3. It amended ERISA to require both health plans and self-insured plans to provide coverage for abdominoplasty and rhinoplasty surgeries.
4. It ensures coverage for breast prostheses after mastectomy.
    A. 1, 3
    B. 2, 4
    C. 1, 2, 4
    D. All of the above
    E. None of the above

235) **Which of the following statements is (are) true regarding the Women's Health and Cancer Rights Act?**
1. It was instituted as part of an Amendment to the Civil Rights Act of 1963.
2. It ensures coverage for surgery of the contralateral breast to provide a symmetrical appearance after mastectomy.
3. It amended ERISA to require only healthcare plans to provide coverage for mastectomies and certain reconstructive surgeries; self-insured plans are excluded from the mandates of this Act.
4. It ensures coverage for breast prostheses after mastectomy.
    A. 1, 3
    B. 2, 4
    C. 1, 2, 3
    D. All of the above
    E. None of the above

236) Which of the following statements is (are) not true regarding the Women's Health and Cancer Rights Act?
1. It ensures coverage for purely cosmetic surgery of the breast after mastectomy is not allowed.
2. It ensures coverage for surgery of the contralateral breast to provide a symmetrical appearance after mastectomy.
3. It amended ERISA to require only healthcare plans to provide coverage for mastectomies and certain reconstructive surgeries; self-insured plans are excluded from the mandates of this Act.
4. It ensures coverage for breast prostheses after mastectomy.
   A. 1, 3
   B. 2, 4
   C. 1, 2, 3
   D. All of the above
   E. None of the above

237) Which of the following statements is (are) true regarding the Women's Health and Cancer Rights Act?
1. Costs associated with a plan's coinsurance are waived by this Act.
2. It ensures coverage for surgery of the contralateral breast to provide a symmetrical appearance after mastectomy.
3. Costs associated with a plan's deductibles are waived by this Act.
4. It ensures coverage for breast prostheses after mastectomy.
   A. 1, 3
   B. 2, 4
   C. 1, 2, 3
   D. All of the above
   E. None of the above

238) Which of the following statements is (are) not true regarding the Women's Health and Cancer Rights Act?
1. Costs associated with a plan's coinsurance are waived by this Act.
2. It ensures coverage for surgery of the contralateral breast to provide a symmetrical appearance after mastectomy.
3. Costs associated with a plan's deductibles are waived by this Act.
4. It ensures coverage for breast prostheses after mastectomy.
   A. 1, 3
   B. 2, 4
   C. 1, 2, 3
   D. All of the above
   E. None of the above

239) Which of the following statements is (are) true regarding the Women's Health and Cancer Rights Act?
1. A group health plan is prohibited from denying a patient eligibility to enroll or renew coverage solely for the purpose of avoiding the requirements of the Act.
2. A group health plan is prohibited from inducing an attending physician to limit the care that is required under the Act.
3. The Act specifically states that its provisions shall not be construed to prevent a group health plan from negotiating the level and type of reimbursement with a provider for care provided in accordance with the Act.
4. A group health plan may penalize, reduce, or limit the reimbursement to physicians who provide women health care in order to reduce the utilization of services associated with this Act.

A. 1, 3
B. 2, 4
C. 1, 2, 3
D. All of the above
E. None of the above

240) Which of the following statements is (are) true regarding the Women's Health and Cancer Rights Act?
1. A group health plan may deny a patient eligibility to enroll or renew coverage solely for the purpose of avoiding the requirements of the Act.
2. A group health plan may induce an attending physician to limit the care that is required under the Act.
3. A group health plan may penalize, reduce, or limit the reimbursement to physicians who provide women's health care to reduce the utilization of services associated with this Act.
4. The Act specifically states that its provisions shall be construed to prevent a group health plan from negotiating the level and type of reimbursement with a provider for care provided in accordance with the Act.
    A. 1, 3
    B. 2, 4
    C. 1, 2, 3
    D. All of the above
    E. None of the above

241) Which of the following statements is (are) not true regarding the Women's Health and Cancer Rights Act?
1. A group health plan may not deny a patient eligibility to enroll or renew coverage solely for the purpose of avoiding the requirements of the Act.
2. A group health plan may induce an attending physician to limit the care that is required under the Act.
3. A group health plan may not penalize, reduce, or limit the reimbursement to physicians who provide women's health care to reduce the utilization of services associated with this Act.
4. The Act specifically states that its provisions shall be construed to prevent a group health plan from negotiating the level and type of reimbursement with a provider for care provided in accordance with the Act.
    A. 1, 3
    B. 2, 4
    C. 1, 2, 3
    D. All of the above
    E. None of the above

242) Which of the following plan types is (are) bound by the requirements of the Women's Health and Cancer Rights Act?
1. Private employer plans
2. Public employer plans
3. Health insurance companies
4. Nonfederal government, self-insured plans
    A. 1
    B. 2
    C. 1, 2, 3
    D. All of the above
    E. None of the above

243) Which of the following plan types is (are) not bound by the requirements of the Women's Health and Cancer Rights Act?
    1. Private employer plans
    2. Self-insured automotive manufacturers
    3. Health insurance companies
    4. Self-insured pharmaceutical manufacturers
        A. 1, 3
        B. 2, 4
        C. 1, 2, 3
        D. All of the above
        E. None of the above

244) All the following statements are true regarding the Mental Health Parity Act (MHPA), except which one?
    A. It is a federal law enacted to protect the rights of individuals with mental health problems.
    B. It prohibits employers or plans from setting annual dollar limits on mental health treatment benefits, unless similar limits are set on medical and surgical care.
    C. It prohibits employers or plans from setting lifetime dollar limits on mental health treatment benefits, unless similar limits are set on medical and surgical care.
    D. It requires all plans to provide mental health benefits.
    E. None of the above

245) All employers are bound under the MHPA, except
    1. Airlines
    2. Employers with 50 or fewer employees
    3. Munitions and weapons manufacturers
    4. Employers that can demonstrate that compliance will cause financial hardship
    5. Employers with 100 or fewer employees
        A. 1, 3
        B. 2, 4
        C. 1, 2, 3
        D. All of the above
        E. None of the above

246) The MHPA requires nonexempt employers to offer their employees all of the following benefits, except
    1. Mental health benefits equal to medical and surgical benefits
    2. Mental health copayments equal to those of the medical and surgical benefits
    3. Parity in the number of outpatient visits for mental health care as offered in medical and surgical benefits
    4. Parity in the number of inpatient days for mental health care as offered in medical or surgical benefits
    5. Parity in the number of inpatient days for chemical dependency as offered in medical or surgical benefits
        A. 1, 3
        B. 2, 4
        C. 1, 2, 3
        D. All of the above
        E. None of the above

247) Which of the following individual(s) is (are) protected under the Pregnancy Discrimination Act (PDA)?
1. An employee's spouse
2. A pregnant but unwed employee
3. A part-time employee
4. An independent contractor
5. Employee of a successor corporation
   A. 1, 2
   B. 3, 4
   C. 1, 2, 3
   D. All of the above
   E. None of the above

248) Although employers must provide maternity benefits along with healthcare benefits under the Pregnancy Discrimination Act, they are permitted to recoup some of their cost by which of the following?
1. Limiting the terms of reimbursement, including maximal reimbursable amount
2. Increasing the deductibles for maternity-related benefits
3. Increasing the copayments for maternity-related benefits
4. Limiting the choice of physicians and hospitals to those that offer steep discounts for network participation
5. Limiting the number of plans available to employees that offer maternity benefits
   A. 1, 2
   B. 2, 4
   C. 1, 2, 3
   D. All of the above
   E. None of the above

249) The wife of an eligible part-time employee requests payment from her husband's employer for a termination of pregnancy. This is the wife's second abortion, and the fetus is in its 12th week. Under the Pregnancy Discrimination Act the employer may legally refuse, because
1. Wives of eligible employees are not covered under PDA regulations.
2. Wives of part-time employees are not covered under PDA regulations.
3. First-trimester pregnancies are not covered under PDA regulations.
4. Terminations of pregnancies (abortions) are not covered under PDA regulations.
5. The Pregnancy Discrimination Act's lifetime limit on the number of abortions is one.
   A. 1, 3
   B. 2, 4
   C. 1, 2, 3
   D. 4
   E. None of the above

250) A female employee is out of work for 3 months secondary to complications of pregnancy and childbirth. Under the policies of the PDA, her employer can legally deny her disability benefits if
1. Disability benefits are not available to other employees for disabilities related to medical and surgical treatment.
2. She is not a full-time employee.
3. The employer has fewer than 50 employees.
4. The employee is not married.
5. The employee has not worked for at least 18 months for that employer.
   A. 1
   B. 2, 4
   C. 3, 5
   D. All of the above
   E. None of the above

251) Which of the following terms refers to an intentional deception on the part of a person that could result in some unauthorized benefit to himself or some other person(s)?
   A. Abuse
   B. Inappropriate utilization
   C. Collusion
   D. Fraud
   E. Fiscal affirmation

252) Which of the following statements is (are) true regarding the Mental Health Parity Act of 1996?
1. It is a federal law.
2. It is aimed at protecting the rights of individuals with mental health problems.
3. It forbids lifetime or annual dollar limits on mental health care (unless comparable limits apply to medical and/or surgical treatment).
4. Its definition of mental illness excludes chemical dependency.
   A. 1, 3
   B. 2, 4
   C. 1, 2, 3
   D. All of the above
   E. None of the above

253) Which of the following statements is (are) true regarding the Mental Health Parity Act of 1996?
1. It is a county law.
2. It is aimed at protecting the rights of individuals with mental health problems.
3. It ensures lifetime or annual dollar limits on mental health care.
4. Its definition of mental illness excludes chemical dependency.
   A. 1, 3
   B. 2, 4
   C. 1, 2, 3
   D. All of the above
   E. None of the above

254) Which of the following statements is (are) not true regarding the Mental Health Parity Act of 1996?
1. It is a county law.
2. It mandates that insurance plans cover mental health treatments.
3. It ensures lifetime or annual dollar limits on mental health care.
4. Its definition of mental illness excludes chemical dependency.
    A. 1, 3
    B. 2, 4
    C. 1, 2, 3
    D. All of the above
    E. None of the above

255) Which of the following types of employers is (are) bound under the tenets of the Mental Health Parity Act?
1. Airlines
2. Employers with 50 or fewer employees
3. Munitions and weapons manufacturers
4. Employers that can demonstrate that compliance will cause financial hardship
    A. 1, 3
    B. 2, 4
    C. 1, 2, 3
    D. All of the above
    E. None of the above

256) Which of the following types of employers is (are) not bound under the tenets of the Mental Health Parity Act?
1. Airlines
2. Employers with 50 or fewer employees
3. Munitions and weapons manufacturers
4. Employers that can demonstrate that compliance will cause financial hardship
    A. 1, 3
    B. 2, 4
    C. 1, 2, 3
    D. All of the above
    E. None of the above

257) Which of the following mental health benefit limitations is (are) allowable under the tenets of the Mental Health Parity Act?
1. Limited number of annual outpatient visits
2. Limited number of inpatient days annually
3. A per-visit fee limit
4. Higher deductibles and copayments for mental health treatments than for medical and surgical treatments
    A. 1, 3
    B. 2, 4
    C. 1, 2, 3
    D. All of the above
    E. None of the above

258) Which of the following mental health benefit limitations is (are) allowable under the tenets of the Mental Health Parity Act?
1. Per-visit fee limit
2. Limited number of annual outpatient visits
3. Limited number of inpatient days annually
4. No mental health benefits
    A. 1, 3
    B. 2, 4
    C. 1, 2, 3
    D. All of the above
    E. None of the above

259) Which of the following mental health benefit limitations is (are) allowable under the tenets of the Mental Health Parity Act?
1. Annual dollar limit for mental health care
2. Limited number of annual outpatient visits
3. Lifetime dollar limit on mental health care
4. Limited number of inpatient days annually
    A. 1, 3
    B. 2, 4
    C. 1, 2, 3
    D. All of the above
    E. None of the above

260) Which of the following mental health benefit limitations is (are) not allowable under the tenets of the Mental Health Parity Act?
1. Annual dollar limit for mental health care
2. Limited number of annual outpatient visits
3. Lifetime dollar limit on mental health care
4. Limited number of inpatient days annually
    A. 1, 3
    B. 2, 4
    C. 1, 2, 3
    D. All of the above
    E. None of the above

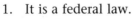
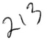

261) Which of the following statements is (are) true regarding the Pregnancy Discrimination Act?
1. It is a federal law.
2. It extends to pregnant individuals the same rights and benefits extended to those with medical problems.
3. It is an amendment to the Civil Rights Act of 1964.
4. It extends to pregnant individuals the same rights and benefits extended to those with surgical problems.
    A. 1, 3
    B. 2, 4
    C. 1, 2, 3
    D. All of the above
    E. None of the above

262) Which of the following statements is (are) true regarding the Pregnancy Discrimination Act?
1. It is a state law.
2. It extends to pregnant individuals the same rights and benefits extended to those with medical problems.
3. It is an amendment to the Social Security Act.
4. It extends to pregnant individuals the same rights and benefits extended to those with surgical problems.
   A. 1, 3
   B. 2, 4
   C. 1, 2, 3
   D. All of the above
   E. None of the above

263) Which of the following statements is (are) not true regarding the Pregnancy Discrimination Act?
1. It is a state law.
2. It extends to pregnant individuals the same rights and benefits extended to those with medical problems.
3. It is an amendment to the Social Security Act.
4. It extends to pregnant individuals the same rights and benefits extended to those with surgical problems.
   A. 1, 3
   B. 2, 4
   C. 1, 2, 3
   D. All of the above
   E. None of the above

264) Under the terms of the Pregnancy Discrimination Act, in which of the following categories is (are) a pregnant patient to be treated the same as a patient with medical and surgical problems?
1. Health insurance benefits
2. Short-term sick leave
3. Disability benefits
4. Employment policies (such as seniority, leave extensions, and reinstatement)
   A. 1, 3
   B. 2, 4
   C. 1, 2, 3
   D. All of the above
   E. None of the above

265) Under the terms of the Pregnancy Discrimination Act, in which of the following categories is (are) a pregnant patient to be treated the same as a patient with medical and surgical problems?
1. Health insurance benefits
2. "Leadoff hitter status" in company softball league
3. Disability benefits
4. Car insurance benefits
   A. 1, 3
   B. 2, 4
   C. 1, 2, 3
   D. All of the above
   E. None of the above

266) Which of the following types of limitations is (are) prohibited under the terms of the Pregnancy Discrimination Act?
1. Provider choice
2. Provider access
3. Cost of providers or services
4. Quality of providers or services
    A. 1, 3
    B. 2, 4
    C. 1, 2, 3
    D. All of the above
    E. None of the above

267) Which of the following limitations is (are) prohibited under the terms of the Pregnancy Discrimination Act?
1. Limiting the number of physicians or hospitals that provide maternity care when medical and surgical care providers are limited
2. Limiting the number of plans that offer maternity care without corresponding limits on medical and surgical care
3. Limiting the reimbursement for maternity care when there are corresponding limits on medical and surgical care
4. Exacting higher deductibles, copayments, or out-of-pocket maximums for maternity care than for medical and surgical care
    A. 1, 3
    B. 2, 4
    C. 1, 2, 3
    D. All of the above
    E. None of the above

268) Which of the following limitations is (are) prohibited under the terms of the Pregnancy Discrimination Act?
1. Limiting the number of physicians or hospitals that provide maternity care when medical and surgical care providers are not limited
2. Limiting the number of plans that offer maternity care without corresponding limits on medical and surgical care
3. Limiting the reimbursement for maternity care when there are no corresponding limits on medical and surgical care
4. Exacting higher deductibles, copayments, or out-of-pocket maximums for maternity care than for medical and surgical care
    A. 1, 3
    B. 2, 4
    C. 1, 2, 3
    D. All of the above
    E. None of the above

269) Which of the following limitations is (are) prohibited under the terms of the Pregnancy Discrimination Act?
1. Limiting the number of physicians or hospitals that provide maternity care when medical and surgical care providers are not limited
2. Limiting the number of plans that offer maternity care with corresponding limits on medical and surgical care
3. Limiting the reimbursement for maternity care when there are no corresponding limits on medical and surgical care
4. Exacting deductibles, copayments, or out-of-pocket maximums for maternity care
   A. 1, 3
   B. 2, 4
   C. 1, 2, 3
   D. All of the above
   E. None of the above

270) Who of the following is (are) not protected under the Pregnancy Discrimination Act?
1. A pregnant but unwed employee
2. A part-time employee
3. An independent contractor
4. Employee of a successor corporation
   A. 1, 2
   B. 3, 4
   C. 1, 2, 3
   D. All of the above
   E. None of the above

271) Which of the following benefits is (are) excluded under the terms of the Pregnancy Discrimination Act?
1. Home health care
2. Abortions
3. Home physical therapy care
4. Mandatory maternity leave
   A. 1, 3
   B. 2, 4
   C. 1, 2, 3
   D. All of the above
   E. None of the above

272) Which of the following benefits is (are) usually included under the terms of the Pregnancy Discrimination Act?
1. Home health care
2. Abortions
3. Home physical therapy care
4. Mandatory maternity leave
   A. 1, 3
   B. 2, 4
   C. 1, 2, 3
   D. All of the above
   E. None of the above

306 CHAPTER SIX

273) Which of the following statements is (are) true regarding the Tax Equity and Fiscal Responsibility Act (TEFRA)?
1. It established a case-based reimbursement system called diagnosis-related groups, or DRGs.
2. It amended the Social Security Act and made Medicare secondary to employer group health plans for active employees 65 to 69 years old and their spouses in the same age group.
3. It established peer review organizations (PROs).
4. It revised the Age Discrimination in Employment Act.
    A. 1, 3
    B. 2, 4
    C. 1, 2, 3
    D. All of the above
    E. None of the above

274) Which of the following statements is (are) true regarding TEFRA?
1. It established a case-based reimbursement system called diagnosis-related groups, or DRGs.
2. It amended the Social Security Act and made Medicare secondary to employer group health plans for active employees 65 to 69 years old and their spouses in the same age group.
3. It established peer review organizations (PROs).
4. It revised the Mental Health Parity Act.
    A. 1, 3
    B. 2, 4
    C. 1, 2, 3
    D. All of the above
    E. None of the above

275) Which of the following statements is (are) true regarding TEFRA?
1. It established a reimbursement system called health maintenance organizations, or HMOs.
2. It amended the Social Security Act and made Medicare secondary to employer group health plans for active employees 65 to 69 years old and their spouses in the same age group.
3. It revised the Mental Health Parity Act.
4. It established peer review organizations (PROs).
    A. 1, 3
    B. 2, 4
    C. 1, 2, 3
    D. All of the above
    E. None of the above

276) Under TEFRA of 1982, which of the following statements is (are) true regarding diagnosis-related groups?
1. It is a case-based reimbursement system.
2. It is a prospective payment program.
3. It places limits on the rate increases in hospital revenues.
4. It is a cost-containment system.
    A. 1, 3
    B. 2, 4
    C. 1, 2, 3
    D. All of the above
    E. None of the above

277) Under the terms of TEFRA of 1982, which of the following statements is (are) true regarding diagnosis-related groups?
1. It is a case-based reimbursement system.
2. It is a retrospective payment program.
3. It places limits on the rate increases in hospital revenues.
4. It is a clinical quality improvement system.
   A. 1, 3
   B. 2, 4
   C. 1, 2, 3
   D. All of the above
   E. None of the above

278) Under the terms of TEFRA of 1982, which of the following statements is (are) not true regarding diagnosis-related groups?
1. It is a case-based reimbursement system.
2. It is a retrospective payment program.
3. It places limits on the rate increases in hospital revenues.
4. It is a clinical quality improvement system.
   A. 1, 3
   B. 2, 4
   C. 1, 2, 3
   D. All of the above
   E. None of the above

279) Under the terms of TEFRA of 1982, which of the following medical specialties is exempted from the diagnosis-related groups (DRGs) program?
   A. Cardiology
   B. Endocrinology
   C. Rehabilitation medicine
   D. Radiation oncology
   E. Family medicine

280) Which of the following was (were) amended or revised under TEFRA?
1. The Mental Health Parity Act
2. The Social Security Act
3. The Tuberculosis Containment Act
4. The Age Discrimination in Employment Act
   A. 1, 3
   B. 2, 4
   C. 1, 2, 3
   D. All of the above
   E. None of the above

281) Which of the following was (were) not amended or revised under TEFRA?
   1. The Mental Health Parity Act
   2. The Social Security Act
   3. The Tuberculosis Containment Act
   4. The Age Discrimination in Employment Act
      A. 1, 3
      B. 2, 4
      C. 1, 2, 3
      D. All of the above
      E. None of the above

282) Which of the following was (were) established under the terms of TEFRA?
   1. Peer review organizations (PROs)
   2. HMOs
   3. Diagnosis-related groups (DRGs)
   4. Independent practice organizations (IPAs)
      A. 1, 3
      B. 2, 4
      C. 1, 2, 3
      D. All of the above
      E. None of the above

283) Which of the following was (were) not established under the terms of TEFRA?
   1. Peer review organizations (PROs)
   2. HMOs
   3. Diagnosis-related groups (DRGs)
   4. Independent practice organizations (IPAs)
      A. 1, 3
      B. 2, 4
      C. 1, 2, 3
      D. All of the above
      E. None of the above

284) Which of the following is (are) true regarding peer review organizations (PROs)?
   1. They were established under the Tax Equity and Fiscal Responsibility Act.
   2. They are entities selected by CMS to reduce medical costs.
   3. They are entities selected by CMS to ensure quality of care and appropriateness of admissions, readmissions, and discharges.
   4. PROs concern themselves with the care of Medicare and Medicaid patients.
      A. 1, 3
      B. 2, 4
      C. 1, 2, 3
      D. All of the above
      E. None of the above

285) Which of the following is (are) true regarding peer review organizations (PROs)?
   1. They were established under the Social Security Act.
   2. They are entities selected by CMS to reduce medical costs.
   3. They are entities selected by the Social Security Administration to ensure that cost of care is reduced, regardless of consequences to the quality of care.
   4. They concern themselves with the care of Medicare and Medicaid patients.

A. 1, 3
B. 2, 4
C. 1, 2, 3
D. All of the above
E. None of the above

286) Which of the following is (are) not true regarding peer review organizations (PROs)?
1. They were established under the Social Security Act.
2. They are entities selected by CMS to reduce medical costs.
3. They are entities selected by the Social Security Administration to ensure that cost of care is reduced regardless of consequences to the quality of care.
4. They concern themselves with the care of Medicare and Medicaid patients.
    A. 1, 3
    B. 2, 4
    C. 1, 2, 3
    D. All of the above
    E. None of the above

287) All the following statements regarding Medicare Part D coverage are true, except which ones?
1. It is a plan to help subsidize prescription drug costs.
2. It is a plan available to all elderly people in the United States.
3. The plan includes additional subsidies for eligible recipients with low income and assets.
4. It covers 100% of the costs of prescription drugs for eligible recipients.
    A. 1, 3
    B. 2, 4
    C. 1, 2, 3
    D. All of the above
    E. None of the above

288) All the following statements regarding Medicare Part D coverage are true, except which ones?
1. It is a plan to help subsidize the cost of hospital and clinic visits.
2. It is a plan available to all elderly people in the United States.
3. The plan is free to undocumented alien workers in the United States.
4. It covers 100% of the costs of prescription drugs for eligible recipients.
    A. 1, 3
    B. 2, 4
    C. 1, 2, 3
    D. All of the above
    E. None of the above

289) Which of the following statements regarding Medicare Part D coverage is (are) true?
1. It is a plan to help subsidize prescription drug costs.
2. It is a plan available to Medicare recipients.
3. The plan includes additional subsidies for eligible recipients with low income and assets.
4. The plan pays for only part of the costs of prescription drugs; the patient is responsible for a portion also.
    A. 1, 3
    B. 2, 4
    C. 1, 2, 3
    D. All of the above
    E. None of the above

NOTES

Appendix 6-B

Healthcare Reimbursement Answers

1) **ANSWER: A**
   The sentinel effect is a hypothesis that was extrapolated from the research principle called the Hawthorne effect. The hypothesis is the basis for the impact of utilization review on hospital admissions.

2) **ANSWER: C**
   The Case Manager should always seek approval, benefit information, and preferred provider information before putting equipment into place.

3) **ANSWER: B**
   Price alone should never be the determining factor. The goal of case management is to meet the patient's needs in a safe and cost-effective manner so that quality is maintained.

4) **ANSWER: C**

5) **ANSWER: C**
   One of the aims of HIPAA legislation is to streamline claims submission and reduce paperwork.

6) **ANSWER: D**
   All healthcare organizations are affected by HIPAA regulations and must be compliant with the regulations concerning the safety and security of patient information. This includes all healthcare providers, even one-physician offices; health plans; employers; public health authorities; life insurers; clearinghouses; billing agencies; information systems vendors; service organizations; and universities.

7) **ANSWER: A**
   States can modify the portability requirements of HIPAA.

8) **ANSWER: D**
   Under the HIPAA provisions, plans may not require an individual to pay a premium or contribution greater than that for a similarly situated individual based on a health status–related factor.

9) **ANSWER: D**
   There is no requirement for any employer to offer health insurance coverage. The provision of health coverage by an employer is voluntary. HIPAA neither requires specific benefits nor prohibits a plan from restricting the amount or nature of benefits for similarly situated individuals. If a person's new employer does not offer health insurance, he or she may be able to continue coverage under the previous employer's plan under COBRA continuation coverage. Finally, HIPAA does not set premium rates, but it does prohibit plans and issuers from charging an

individual more than similarly situated individuals in the same plan because of health status. Plans may offer premium discounts or rebates for participation in wellness programs.

10) **ANSWER: B**
Under HIPAA, the only preexisting conditions that may be excluded under a preexisting condition exclusion are those for which medical advice, diagnosis, care, or treatment was recommended or received within the 6-month period ending on a subscriber's enrollment date. If a subscriber had a medical condition in the past but had not received any medical advice, diagnosis, care, or treatment within the 6 months before his or her enrollment date in the plan, the old condition is not a preexisting condition for which an exclusion can be applied.

11) **ANSWER: D**
Preexisting condition exclusions cannot be applied to pregnancy, regardless of whether the woman had previous coverage. In addition, a preexisting condition exclusion cannot be applied to a newborn, an adopted child younger than age 18, or a child younger than 18 placed for adoption as long as the child became covered under the health plan within 30 days of birth, adoption, or placement for adoption and provided the child does not incur a subsequent 63-day or longer break in coverage.

12) **ANSWER: D**
Creditable coverage refers to a period of time during which a person was covered under a health insurance policy. Most health coverage is creditable coverage, such as coverage under a group health plan (including COBRA continuation coverage), HMO, individual health insurance policy, Medicaid, or Medicare. Creditable coverage does not include coverage consisting solely of "excepted benefits," such as coverage solely for dental or vision benefits.

13) **ANSWER: C**
Creditable coverage refers to a period of time during which a person was covered under a health insurance policy. Most health coverage is creditable coverage, such as coverage under a group health plan (including COBRA continuation coverage), HMO, individual health insurance policy, Medicaid, or Medicare. Creditable coverage does not include coverage consisting solely of "excepted benefits," such as coverage solely for dental or vision benefits.

14) **ANSWER: D**
Utilization review can be performed in all the categories mentioned, plus inpatient or on selected procedures.

15) **ANSWER: D**
Preadmission/precertification is commonly known as prospective review. Concurrent review occurs during the event, as in concurrent hospital review. Retrospective review is after the event, as in chart review or claims review.

16) **ANSWER: C**

17) **ANSWER: A**
An indemnity health insurance plan is a legal entity licensed by the state insurance department. It exists to provide health insurance to its enrollees. An indemnity health insurer "indemnifies" or reimburses the enrollee for the costs of healthcare claims that are medically necessary and appropriate for his or her care. Indemnity insurers historically had not spent money or time on utilization or quality management. Now, because of savings demonstrated by the managed care companies, some indemnity companies have adopted these cost-saving approaches.

18) **ANSWER: B**
An indemnity health insurance plan is a legal entity licensed by the state insurance department. It exists to provide health insurance to its enrollees. An indemnity health insurer "indemnifies" or reimburses the enrollee for the costs of healthcare claims that are medically necessary and appropriate for his or her care. Indemnity insurers historically had not spent money or time on utilization or quality management. Now, because of savings demonstrated by the managed care companies, some indemnity companies have adopted these cost-saving approaches.

19) **ANSWER: B**
A well-run self-insurance program can achieve the following benefits for an employer: reduced service costs that are usually incurred by conventional insurers, exemption from providing benefits mandated by ERISA, elimination of the costs of premium taxes, and improved cash flow.

20) **ANSWER: A**
A well-run self-insurance program can achieve the following benefits for an employer: reduced service costs that are usually incurred by conventional insurers, exemption from providing benefits mandated by ERISA, elimination of the costs of premium taxes, and improved cash flow.

21) **ANSWER: E**
Large employers (greater than 500 employees) tend to self-insure. Conversely, employers with fewer than 500 employees find it difficult to self-insure, because they lack the cash reserves necessary to handle large claims losses. An employer's decision to self-insure should be based on the size of its employee base, its cash reserves, group claims experience, employee health status, and the ability to find reinsurance for its catastrophic losses.

22) **ANSWER: E**
Third-party administrators (TPAs) usually operate in the environment of the self-insured employer. Although they may act as an agent of the insurer, the TPA is not party to the insurance contract between the employer and the employee. The TPA does not incur any risk for employer or employee losses. A TPA's sole function is to perform insurance-type administrative services for self-insured employers. These services include, but are not limited to, performing claims adjudication and payment, maintaining all records, providing utilization and quality management, case management, and managing the provider network.

23) **ANSWER: C**
TPAs are neither paid premiums nor traditionally invest money. These activities are more characteristic of indemnity insurers.

24) **ANSWER: B**
TPAs are neither paid premiums nor traditionally invest money. These activities are more characteristic of indemnity insurers. TPAs are not licensed to practice medicine or render medical care.

25) **ANSWER: A**
TPAs do not share risk or bear liability in the insurance contract between the employer and the employee, and they do not traditionally collect premiums or invest money.

26) **ANSWER: B**
TPAs do not share risk or bear liability in the insurance contract between the employer and the employee, and they do not traditionally collect premiums or invest money.

27) **ANSWER: A**
The car owner and his or her car insurance company are financially responsible for injury and property damage caused by car accidents.

28) **ANSWER: A**
Each state determines what the minimum level of liability insurance will be for drivers in that state. Although the costs of car insurance premiums may vary by the cost of the automobile, the community accident experience, or the driving record of the owner, the minimum policy limits for personal injury protection do not.

29) **ANSWER: B**
Each state determines what the minimum level of liability insurance will be for drivers in that state. Although the costs of car insurance premiums may vary by the cost of the automobile, the community accident experience, or the driving record of the owner, the minimum policy limits for personal injury protection do not.

30) **ANSWER: B**
Automobile accident victims are characterized by their youth and the seriousness of their injuries, which include closed head trauma, spinal trauma, and permanent disability.

31) **ANSWER: A**
Automobile accident victims are characterized by their youth and the seriousness of their injuries, which include closed head trauma, spinal trauma, and permanent disability.

32) **ANSWER: C**
PIP refers to the part of an auto insurance policy that covers medical claims for injuries sustained in an auto accident.

33) **ANSWER: A**
PIP refers to the part of an auto insurance policy that covers medical claims for injuries sustained in an auto accident.

34) **ANSWER: A**
PIP refers to the part of an auto insurance policy that covers medical claims for injuries sustained in an auto accident.

35) **ANSWER: B**
PIP refers to the part of an auto insurance policy that covers medical claims for injuries sustained in an auto accident.

36) **ANSWER: D**

37) **ANSWER: C**
PIP is the part of the automobile insurance policy responsible for coverage of bodily injury of drivers, passengers, and pedestrians.

38) **ANSWER: E**
No-fault insurance implies no blame is assigned to accidents. All parties injured during the accident are covered, regardless of blame, when a no-fault policy is purchased.

39) **ANSWER: C**
The point of service (POS) plan evolved from a PPO, which has provider choice and a network but no gatekeeper, and an HMO, which has a network and gatekeeper but limits provider choice. An indemnity plan has provider choice but no network or gatekeeper.

40) **ANSWER: B**

41) **ANSWER: D**
The scope of coverage under workers' compensation varies by state, with respect to benefits payable in case of death, total disability, and partial disability due to specific injuries or continuing during specified periods.

42) **ANSWER: B**
Managed care comprises systems and mechanisms striving to control, direct, and approve access to a wide range of services and costs within the healthcare delivery system. Case management is one of those mechanisms. Workers' compensation is a benefit program for injured or ill employees.

43) **ANSWER: C**

44) **ANSWER: D**

45) **ANSWER: B**
Although Case Managers make recommendations, actual claims processing is done by a claims examiner.

46) **ANSWER: C**

47) **ANSWER: D**

48) **ANSWER: E**
Currently, definitions of medical necessity contained in health insurance contracts are characterized by ambiguity and inconsistency. They do not clearly cover all clinical eventualities.

49) **ANSWER: E**
In the standard health insurance contract, when medical necessity is defined, it is often defined in terms of what is appropriate, reasonable, and acceptable. These terms are rarely, if ever, explained. Further, investigational, experimental, and custodial care are usually specifically excluded in the definition; however, they also are rarely, if ever, defined.

50) **ANSWER: B**
The issue of what is medically necessary is an important one, and it affects the payment of every claim for health services. A longer and more inclusive wording of the contract does not solve the problem of defining what is medically necessary; rather, a methodological or procedural approach to the definition is necessary. This procedural approach describes the steps that should be taken when determining what is medically necessary.

51) **ANSWER: D**
When determining what is medically necessary for a particular case, the reviewer should take into account the contents of the patient's medical record, the opinion of the treating physician, the opinion of an objective physician who is a specialist in the field of medicine in question, and the reasonable expectation of the patient.

52) **ANSWER: E**
When determining what is medically necessary for a particular case, it is important that the reviewer take into account the contents of the patient's medical record, the opinion of the treating physician, the opinion of an objective physician who is a specialist in the field of medicine in question, and the reasonable expectations of the patient.

53) **ANSWER: D**

54) **ANSWER: B**
The intent of medical necessity determinations is to protect the subscribers from irregular, dangerous, or unnecessary medical procedures. Perverse incentives for lowering medical utilization, such as year-end bonuses linked to medical loss ratios, should have no place in medical necessity determinations.

55) **ANSWER: D**
The decision-making process for medical necessity determinations should be supervised by the medical director and should be characterized by fairness, reproducibility, and utilization of the best available information.

56) **ANSWER: D**
Only the medical director should make a denial of claim payment for lack of medical necessity. Although the Case Manager is involved in the case presentation and subsequent discussion, the responsibility for making the final decision rests with the medical director. The claims personnel should have no say in medical decision making.

57) **ANSWER: E**
Only the medical director should be authorized to make claims denials for lack of medical necessity.

58) **ANSWER: D**
An indemnity health insurance plan is a legal entity licensed by the state insurance department. It exists to provide health insurance to its enrollees. An indemnity health insurer "indemnifies" or reimburses the enrollee for the costs of healthcare claims. Indemnity insurers historically had not spent money or time on utilization or quality management. Now, because of savings demonstrated by the managed care companies, some indemnity companies have adopted these cost-savings approaches. These companies are referred to as "managed indemnity" companies.

59) **ANSWER: E**
These activities characterize managed care rather than indemnity insurance companies.

60) **ANSWER: D**

61) **ANSWER: D**
Large employers (greater than 500 employees) tend to self-insure. Conversely, employers with fewer than 500 employees find it difficult to self-insure because they lack the cash reserves necessary to handle large claims losses. An employer's decision to self-insure should be based on the size of its employee base, its cash reserves, group claims experience, employee health status, and the ability to find reinsurance for its catastrophic losses.

62) **ANSWER: B**
The car owner and his or her car insurance company are financially responsible for injury and property damage caused by car accidents.

63) **ANSWER: C**
No-fault insurance asks the insurance company of each of the parties involved to contribute to paying for damages or costs of injuries, regardless of who caused the accident.

64) **ANSWER: C**
Each state determines what its minimum allowable insurance policy limits for medical expenses and lost wages will be.

Healthcare Reimbursement 317

65) **ANSWER: A**
COB is a process designed by insurance companies to limit payments made to claimants. The COB process is structured such that payments made to the claimant do not exceed the expenses incurred.

66) **ANSWER: B**
COB rules are voluntary; however, compliance is high among insurers. There is no federal mandate for compliance with COB rules.

67) **ANSWER: B**
Under the COB rules adopted by the National Association of Insurance Commissioners (NAIC), the insurance plan that covers the individual as an employee pays first.

68) **ANSWER: A**
Under the COB rules adopted by the National Association of Insurance Commissioners (NAIC), the insurance plan that covers the individual as a dependent pays second.

69) **ANSWER: B**
Under the COB rules adopted by the National Association of Insurance Commissioners (NAIC), the insurance plan that covers the individual as an employee pays first.

70) **ANSWER: A**
Under the COB rules adopted by the National Association of Insurance Commissioners (NAIC), the insurance plan that covers the individual as a dependent pays second.

71) **ANSWER: B**
The birthday rule is invoked when two married parents have named the same dependent child in their health insurance policies. The rule can only be invoked when both insurance companies have adopted the birthday rule to settle COB disputes.

72) **ANSWER: C**
The birthday rule is invoked when there are two or more policies that cover the claimant as a dependent and the insurance companies have both adopted the birthday rule. The order of payment is based on the order of birthdays of the parents who have the dependent on their policies.

73) **ANSWER: B**
In the case of a dependent carried on two or more insurance policies, the birthday rule is invoked first. If one or both of the insurers of the dependent do not ascribe to the birthday rule, then the male/female rule is invoked. The male/female rule states that the insurer of the father (male parent or guardian) pays first.

74) **ANSWER: A**
The divorce decree usually designates a primary insurance carrier for the child from one of the parents' policies. If the court has not determined a primary insurance carrier, the parent with custody of the child pays first. The birthday rule is not invoked in cases of divorce.

75) **ANSWER: B**
According to COB rules adopted by the National Association of Insurance Commissioners, the insurance carrier of the parent with custody pays first.

76) **ANSWER: A**
According to COB rules adopted by the National Association of Insurance Commissioners, the insurance carrier of the parent with custody pays first. The insurance carrier of the custodial

parent's spouse pays second. If the custodial parent is not married, the noncustodial parent's carrier pays second.

77) **ANSWER: A**

The insurance plan of the mother pays first. COB rules state that the plan of the parent with custody pays first.

78) **ANSWER: C**

The insurance plan of the mother's spouse pays second. According to the COB rules, the plan of the spouse of the parent with custody pays second.

79) **ANSWER: D**

The plan of the spouse of the noncustodial parent pays last.

80) **ANSWER: B**

According to the COB rules adopted by the National Association of Insurance Commissioners (NAIC), the plan covering the individual as an active employee pays first. Workers' compensation insurance would be primary only if the nurse made medical claims stemming from a job-related injury.

81) **ANSWER: B**

According to the COB rules adopted by the National Association of Insurance Commissioners (NAIC), the plan covering the individual as an active employee pays first, and the plan covering that individual as an inactive employee (such as a retiree or laid-off employee) pays second. Workers' compensation insurance would be primary only if the employee made medical claims stemming from a job-related injury.

82) **ANSWER: C**

According to the COB rules adopted by the National Association of Insurance Commissioners (NAIC), the plan covering the individual as an active employee pays first, and the plan covering that individual as an inactive employee (such as a retiree or laid-off employee) pays second. Workers' compensation insurance would be primary only if the employee made medical claims stemming from a job-related injury. His unemployment insurance benefit pays for salary replacement, not healthcare bills.

83) **ANSWER: A**

According to the COB rules adopted by the National Association of Insurance Commissioners (NAIC), the plan covering the individual as an active employee pays first, and the plan covering that individual as an inactive employee (such as a retiree or laid-off employee) pays second. Workers' compensation insurance would be primary only if the employee made medical claims stemming from a job-related injury. His unemployment insurance benefit pays for salary replacement, not healthcare bills.

84) **ANSWER: A**

According to the COB rules adopted by the National Association of Insurance Commissioners (NAIC), the plan covering the individual as an active employee pays first, and the plan covering that individual as an inactive employee (such as a retiree or laid-off employee) pays second. Workers' compensation insurance would be primary only if the nurse made medical claims stemming from a job-related injury.

85) **ANSWER: C**

According to the COB rules adopted by the National Association of Insurance Commissioners, the plan covering an individual as a COBRA continuee is secondary to a plan covering that

86) **ANSWER: B**
According to the COB rules adopted by the National Association of Insurance Commissioners, the plan covering an individual as a COBRA continuee is secondary to a plan covering that individual as an employee, a member, or a dependent. Unemployment insurance benefits only cover salary replacement, not healthcare costs. When working for an employer who does not pay health insurance benefits, the employee cannot successfully sue for benefits when he gets ill.

87) **ANSWER: D**
Automobile accident victims are characterized by their youth and the seriousness of their injuries, which include closed head trauma, spinal trauma, and permanent disability.

88) **ANSWER: B**
PIP policy minimums are set by the state insurance department. These minimums may not be sufficient to cover the medical costs of more severe injuries.

89) **ANSWER: C**
Medical bill review and review for reasonable and customary charges are components of retrospective review, not utilization review.

90) **ANSWER: D**
A claims edit is logic within the standard claims processing system (or program safeguard contractor supplemental edit software) that selects certain claims; evaluates or compares information on the selected claims or other accessible source; and, depending on the evaluation, takes action on the claims, such as pay in full, pay in part, or suspend for manual review.

91) **ANSWER: A**
A claims edit is logic within the standard claims processing system (or program safeguard contractor supplemental edit software) that selects certain claims; evaluates or compares information on the selected claims or other accessible source; and, depending on the evaluation, takes action on the claims, such as pay in full, pay in part, or suspend for manual review.

92) **ANSWER: B**
A claims edit is logic within the standard claims processing system (or program safeguard contractor supplemental edit software) that selects certain claims; evaluates or compares information on the selected claims or other accessible source; and, depending on the evaluation, takes action on the claims, such as pay in full, pay in part, or suspend for manual review.

93) **ANSWER: D**
Authoritative evidence is written medical or scientific conclusions demonstrating the medical effectiveness of a service. It is produced by at least one of the following:
- Controlled clinical trials published in peer-reviewed medical or scientific journals
- Controlled clinical trials completed and accepted for publication in peer-reviewed medical or scientific journals
- Assessments initiated by CMS
- Evaluations or studies initiated by Medicare contractors
- Case studies published in peer-reviewed medical or scientific journals that present treatment protocols

320 CHAPTER SIX

94) **ANSWER: B**

95) **ANSWER: A**

Health insurance does not coordinate benefits with workers' compensation. COB assures insurers that benefit payment will not exceed 100% of the charges billed.

96) **ANSWER: A**

Currently, definitions of medical necessity contained in health insurance contracts are characterized by ambiguity and inconsistency. They do not clearly cover all clinical eventualities.

97) **ANSWER: B**

Currently, definitions of medical necessity contained in health insurance contracts are characterized by ambiguity and inconsistency. They do not clearly cover all clinical eventualities.

98) **ANSWER: D**

In the standard health insurance contract, when medical necessity is defined, it is often defined in terms of what is appropriate, reasonable, and acceptable. These terms are rarely, if ever, explained. Further, investigational, experimental treatments, and custodial care are usually mentioned as specific exclusions in the definition; however, they also are rarely, if ever, defined.

99) **ANSWER: A**

The issue of what is medically necessary is an important one, and it affects the payment of every claim for health services. A longer and more inclusive wording of the contract does not solve the problem of defining what is medically necessary; rather, a methodological or procedural approach to the definition is necessary. This procedural approach describes the steps that should be taken when determining what is medically necessary.

100) **ANSWER: B**

When determining what is medically necessary for a particular case, the reviewer should take into account the contents of the patient's medical record, the opinion of the treating physician, and the opinion of an objective physician who is a specialist in the field of medicine in question.

101) **ANSWER: A**

The decision-making process for medical necessity determinations should be supervised by the medical director and should be characterized by fairness, reproducibility, and utilization of the best available information. Arbitrary and capricious behavior is a violation of legal and ethical standards.

102) **ANSWER: B**

When cases of medical necessity are litigated, the courts place significant weight on the reasonable expectations of a layperson in the position of a patient. The court implies that if "reasonable laypersons" could expect a certain medical benefit under their contract, then they may be entitled to it. This expectation principle is used by the courts to justify granting a wide range of benefits to the subscriber that the insurer's policy language appears to exclude. In the *Ponder* case the insurer denied treatment for temporomandibular joint syndrome because it was excluded by the contract. The fairness of the contract was questioned, however, because the purchaser of the insurance did not understand the meaning of the exclusionary criteria in the contract. As the court stated, subscribers "could only discover what they had bought with their premiums as their diseases were diagnosed, and they found out to their sorrow, the true meaning of those mysterious words in their insurance contracts."

Healthcare Reimbursement 321

103) ANSWER: A
When cases of medical necessity are litigated, the courts place significant weight on the reasonable expectations of a layperson in the position of a patient. The court implies that if "reasonable laypersons" could expect a certain medical benefit under their contract, then they may be entitled to it. This expectation principle is used by the courts to justify granting a wide range of benefits to the subscriber that the insurer's policy language appears to exclude. In the *Ponder* case the insurer denied treatment for temporomandibular joint syndrome because it was excluded by the contract. The fairness of the contract was questioned, however, because the purchaser of the insurance did not understand the meaning of the exclusionary criteria in the contract. As the court stated, subscribers "could only discover what they had bought with their premiums as their diseases were diagnosed, and they found out to their sorrow, the true meaning of those mysterious words in their insurance contracts."

104) ANSWER: C
When cases of medical necessity are litigated, the courts place significant weight on the reasonable expectations of a layperson in the position of a patient. The court implies that if "reasonable laypersons" could expect a certain medical benefit under their contract, then they may be entitled to it. This expectation principle is used by the courts to justify granting a wide range of benefits to the subscriber that the insurer's policy language appears to exclude. In the *Ponder* case the insurer denied treatment for temporomandibular joint syndrome because it was excluded by the contract. The fairness of the contract was questioned, however, because the purchaser of the insurance did not understand the meaning of the exclusionary criteria in the contract. As the court stated, subscribers "could only discover what they had bought with their premiums as their diseases were diagnosed, and they found out to their sorrow, the true meaning of those mysterious words in their insurance contracts."

105) ANSWER: B
Utilization review reviews services for medical necessity, appropriateness, and efficiency. It includes review for medical necessity of an admission, length of stay review, discharge planning, and all services ordered. It can be done prospectively, concurrently, and retrospectively. Although dollar amounts may be used to establish the types of services reviewed, care is not denied based on cost but on lack of medical necessity, appropriateness, or a contractual exclusion. Utilization review compares treatment rendered with nationally recognized and accepted standards of care and protocols.

106) ANSWER: A
PIP policy minimums are set by the state insurance department. These minimums may not be sufficient to cover the medical costs of more severe injuries.

107) ANSWER: E
No-fault insurance implies no blame is assigned to auto accidents. All parties injured during an accident are covered, regardless of blame, when a no-fault policy is purchased.

108) ANSWER: E
State financing and benefit laws vary widely. In general, unemployment compensation benefits under state laws are intended to replace about 50% of an average worker's previous wages. Maximum weekly benefits provisions, however, result in benefits of less than 50% for most higher-earning workers. All states pay benefits to some unemployed persons for 26 weeks. In some states the duration of benefits depends on the amount earned and the number of weeks worked in a previous year. In other states all recipients are entitled to benefits

322 CHAPTER SIX

for the same length of time. During periods of heavy unemployment, federal law authorizes extended benefits, in some cases up to 39 weeks; in 1975 extended benefits were payable for up to 65 weeks. Extended benefits are financed in part by federal employer taxes.

109) ANSWER: A
State financing and benefit laws vary widely. In general, unemployment compensation benefits under state laws are intended to replace about 50% of an average worker's previous wages. Maximum weekly benefits provisions, however, result in benefits of less than 50% for most higher-earning workers. All states pay benefits to some unemployed persons for 26 weeks. In some states the duration of benefits depends on the amount earned and the number of weeks worked in a previous year. In other states all recipients are entitled to benefits for the same length of time. During periods of heavy unemployment federal law authorizes extended benefits, in some cases up to 39 weeks; in 1975 extended benefits were payable for up to 65 weeks. Extended benefits are financed in part by federal employer taxes.

110) ANSWER: B
State financing and benefit laws vary widely. In general, unemployment compensation benefits under state laws are intended to replace about 50% of an average worker's previous wages. Maximum weekly benefits provisions, however, result in benefits of less than 50% for most higher-earning workers. All states pay benefits to some unemployed persons for 26 weeks. In some states the duration of benefits depends on the amount earned and the number of weeks worked in a previous year. In other states all recipients are entitled to benefits for the same length of time. During periods of heavy unemployment federal law authorizes extended benefits, in some cases up to 39 weeks; in 1975 extended benefits were payable for up to 65 weeks. Extended benefits are financed in part by federal employer taxes.

111) ANSWER: B
State financing and benefit laws vary widely. In general, unemployment compensation benefits under state laws are intended to replace about 50% of an average worker's previous wages. Maximum weekly benefits provisions, however, result in benefits of less than 50% for most higher-earning workers. All states pay benefits to some unemployed persons for 26 weeks. In some states the duration of benefits depends on the amount earned and the number of weeks worked in a previous year. In other states all recipients are entitled to benefits for the same length of time. During periods of heavy unemployment federal law authorizes extended benefits, in some cases up to 39 weeks; in 1975 extended benefits were payable for up to 65 weeks. Extended benefits are financed in part by federal employer taxes.

112) ANSWER: C
State financing and benefit laws vary widely. In general, unemployment compensation benefits under state laws are intended to replace about 50% of an average worker's previous wages. Maximum weekly benefits provisions, however, result in benefits of less than 50% for most higher-earning workers. All states pay benefits to some unemployed persons for 26 weeks. In some states the duration of benefits depends on the amount earned and the number of weeks worked in a previous year. In other states all recipients are entitled to benefits for the same length of time. During periods of heavy unemployment federal law authorizes extended benefits, in some cases up to 39 weeks; in 1975 extended benefits were payable for up to 65 weeks. Extended benefits are financed in part by federal employer taxes.

113) ANSWER: C
Transfers to a sibling are not exempted by the state, and this asset transfer would be assessed a penalty period. See Section 1917(c) of the Social Security Act; U.S. Code Reference 42 U.S.C.1396p(c).

114) **ANSWER: A**
The penalty period is calculated by using this formula: Fair market value of the asset / Average monthly cost for the facility in that state = Penalty period in months. In the previous example this is calculated as $100,000 / $2,000 per month = 50-month penalty period. See Section 1917(c) of the Social Security Act; U.S. Code Reference 42 U.S.C.1396p(c).

115) **ANSWER: D**
There is no limit to the penalty period imposed during a look back on asset transfers. See Section 1917(c) of the Social Security Act; U.S. Code Reference 42 U.S.C.1396p(c).

116) **ANSWER: D**
The look-back period is 60 months before the date the individual applies for Medicaid or is institutionalized. See Section 1917(c) of the Social Security Act; U.S. Code Reference 42 U.S.C.1396p(c).

117) **ANSWER: C**
An asset transferred at less than the fair market value will prompt the imposition of a penalty period. Some exceptions to this rule are transfers to the spouse, a trust fund set up to care for the individual, or for a reason other than to qualify for Medicaid. See Section 1917(c) of the Social Security Act; U.S. Code Reference 42 U.S.C. 1396p(c).

118) **ANSWER: C**
Assets put in irrevocable trusts within 60 months of application for Medicaid or admission to nursing facility are considered transfers of assets below fair market value and are, therefore, considered available to the individual.

119) **ANSWER: A**
Assets placed in trusts established by a parent, grandparent, guardian, or court for the benefit of an individual who is disabled and under the age of 65, using the individual's own funds, are not counted as being available by CMS.

120) **ANSWER: B**
COBRA, the Consolidated Omnibus Budget Reconciliation Act of 1986.

121) **ANSWER: A**
Although benefits can vary from state to state, in general, unemployment benefits are designed to replace about 50% of an average worker's previous wages. The minimum duration of benefits mandated by the federal government is 26 weeks.

122) **ANSWER: B**
Unemployment benefits were established by the Social Security Act of 1935. Although benefits can vary from state to state, in general, unemployment benefits are designed to replace about 50% of an average worker's previous wages. The minimum duration of benefits mandated by the federal government is 26 weeks.

123) **ANSWER: A**
SCHIP is a federal program to provide health coverage to uninsured children. Although individual states set their own eligibility criteria, they must follow federal guidelines. Eligibility guidelines include a low income, lack of insurance, and lack of eligibility for Medicaid. There is no lower age limit to eligibility.

124) **ANSWER: D**

125) **ANSWER: A**
CMS defines inappropriate utilization as "utilization of services that are in excess of a beneficiary's medical needs and condition (overutilization) or receiving a capitated Medicare payment and failing to provide services to meet a beneficiary's medical needs and condition (underutilization)."

126) **ANSWER: C**
The Medicare program was created by Title XVIII of the Social Security Act. The program, which went into effect in 1966, was first administered by the Social Security Administration; in 1977 the Medicare program was transferred to the newly created Health Care Financing Administration, now known as the Centers for Medicare & Medicaid Services (CMS). Medicare was created to help the elderly and disabled, not underutilized physicians, although that may seem the case today.

127) **ANSWER: D**
Medicare is divided into two parts, Part A and Part B. Part A is the hospital insurance program, is funded by Social Security taxes, and is provided to eligible individuals at no personal expense. As one might suspect, Part A provides a basic hospital insurance plan covering hospital care, extended care, home health services, and hospice care for terminally ill patients.

128) **ANSWER: C**
Medicare provides health insurance to persons 65 years old; generally, people over the age of 65 are eligible for Medicare benefits on their own or their spouse's employment. Any one of the following must be true: the patient must receive benefits under the Social Security or Railroad Retirement systems, the patient must be eligible for benefits under Social Security or Railroad Retirement System but has not filed for them, or the patient's spouse has Medicare-covered government employment.

129) **ANSWER: C**
Medicare was enacted under Title XIX of the Social Security Act and is divided into two parts, Part A and Part B. Part A is the hospital insurance program, is funded by Social Security taxes, and is provided to eligible individuals at no personal expense. As one might suspect, Part A provides a basic hospital insurance plan covering hospital care, extended care, home health services, and hospice care for terminally ill patients.

130) **ANSWER: E**
Medicare provides health insurance to persons 65 years old; generally, people over the age of 65 are eligible for Medicare benefits on their own or their spouse's employment. Any one of the following must be true: the patient must receive benefits under the Social Security or Railroad Retirement systems, the patient must be eligible for benefits under Social Security or Railroad Retirement System but has not filed for them, or the patient's spouse has Medicare-covered government employment.

131) **ANSWER: B**
The Medicare program was created by Title XVIII of the Social Security Act. The program, which went into effect in 1966, was first administered by the Social Security Administration; in 1977 the Medicare program was transferred to the newly created Health Care Financing Administration, now known as the Centers for Medicare & Medicaid Services (CMS). Medicare was created to help the elderly and disabled, not underutilized physicians, although that may seem the case today.

132) **ANSWER: A**
A person becomes entitled to Medicare on the basis of disability after he or she has been entitled to Social Security disability benefits for 24 months. An individual has a 5-month waiting period before receiving Social Security disability payments, which means that, in most instances, there is a 29-month period before the individual becomes entitled to Medicare. Those who have served active duty in the armed forces are entitled to Veterans benefits, which include care in Veterans Administration hospitals.

133) **ANSWER: C**
A person is considered to have end-stage renal disease if he or she has irreparable kidney damage that requires a transplant or dialysis to maintain life. A person becomes eligible for Medicare if he or she requires regular dialysis or has a kidney transplant and meets the following requirements: has worked the required amount of time under Social Security, the Railroad Retirement Board, or is a government employee; or the beneficiary is receiving or is eligible for Social Security or Railroad Retirement case benefits; or the patient is a spouse or a dependent child of a person who has worked the required amount of time, or who is receiving Social Security or Railroad Retirement case benefits.

134) **ANSWER: A**
A person is considered to have end-stage renal disease if he or she has irreparable kidney damage that requires a transplant or dialysis to maintain life. A person becomes eligible for Medicare if he or she requires regular dialysis or has a kidney transplant and meets the following requirements: has worked the required amount of time under Social Security, the Railroad Retirement Board, or is a government employee; or the beneficiary is receiving or is eligible for Social Security or Railroad Retirement case benefits; or the patient is a spouse or a dependent child of a person who has worked the required amount of time, or who is receiving Social Security or Railroad Retirement case benefits.

135) **ANSWER: C**
A person becomes entitled to Medicare on the basis of disability after he or she has been entitled to Social Security disability benefits for 24 months. An individual has a 5-month waiting period before receiving Social Security disability payments, which means that, in most instances, there is a 29-month period before the individual becomes entitled to Medicare. Those who have served active duty in the armed forces are entitled to Veterans benefits, which include care in Veterans Administration hospitals.

136) **ANSWER: C**
If a person becomes entitled to Medicare solely because of end-stage renal disease, he or she has a 3-month wait until he or she is covered (or the 3rd month after the month in which a regular course of dialysis starts).

137) **ANSWER: D**

138) **ANSWER: B**
For those beneficiaries entitled to Medicare solely because of end-stage renal disease, Medicare protection ends 12 months after the month the patient no longer requires maintenance dialysis treatments, or 36 months after a successful kidney transplant.

139) **ANSWER: B**
If a person becomes entitled to Medicare solely because of end-stage renal disease, he or she has a 3-month wait until he or she is covered (or the 3rd month after the month in

which a regular course of dialysis starts). For those beneficiaries entitled to Medicare solely because of end-stage renal disease, Medicare protection ends 12 months after the month the patient no longer requires maintenance dialysis treatments, or 36 months after a successful kidney transplant.

140) **ANSWER: D**

141) **ANSWER: A**
The Medicare Part A benefit provides coverage for the following: inpatient hospital services, skilled nursing facilities, home health services, and hospice care. Physician fees and outpatient care are covered under Medicare Part B.

142) **ANSWER: A**
The Medicare Part A benefit provides coverage for the following: inpatient hospital services, skilled nursing facilities, home health services, and hospice care. Hemodialysis and ambulatory surgery are outpatient procedures and are covered under Medicare Part B.

143) **ANSWER: B**
Medicare Select is another type of Medicare supplemental health insurance sold by insurance companies and HMOs throughout most of the country. Medicare Select is the same as standard Medigap insurance in nearly all respects. The only difference between Medicare Select and standard Medigap insurance is that each insurer has specific hospitals and, in some cases, specific doctors that a patient must use, except in an emergency, to be eligible for full benefits. Medicare Select policies generally have lower premiums than other Medigap policies because of this requirement.

144) **ANSWER: A**

145) **ANSWER: C**

146) **ANSWER: D**

147) **ANSWER: C**
Only medically necessary care is covered in the Medicare program.

148) **ANSWER: B**
Medicare will help pay for 100 days of care in a skilled nursing facility. Only medically necessary care is covered in the Medicare program.

149) **ANSWER: C**
Medicare Part B helps pay for the cost of physician services, outpatient hospital services, medical equipment and supplies, and other health services and supplies. Inpatient hospital stays are covered under the Part A program.

150) **ANSWER: B**
Medicare Part B helps pay for the cost of physician services, outpatient hospital services, medical equipment and supplies, and other health services and supplies. Inpatient hospital stays and hospice care are covered under the Part A program.

151) **ANSWER: A**
If a person younger than 65 years old becomes eligible for Medicare due to end-stage renal disease, the benefits extended to the patient by Medicare cover only those medical expenses that are attendant to the treatment of the end-stage renal disease. Arthroscopic and retinal surgeries are not treatments for end-stage renal disease and are therefore not covered.

Healthcare Reimbursement **327**

152) ANSWER: B
If a person younger than 65 years old becomes eligible for Medicare due to end-stage renal disease, the benefits extended to the patient by Medicare cover only those medical expenses that are attendant to the treatment of the end-stage renal disease. Speech therapy and neurosurgery are not treatments for end-stage renal disease and are therefore not covered.

153) ANSWER: D
A reserve day is one of 60 extra days of hospital care that Medicare pays for during the lifetime of a beneficiary. Medicare Part A includes an extra 60 hospital days that can be used if the patient has a prolonged illness necessitating a hospital stay of longer than 90 days. A Medicare beneficiary has only 60 nonrenewable reserve days in a lifetime. The beneficiary has the right to choose when to use these reserve days.

154) ANSWER: A
A reserve day is one of 60 extra days of hospital care that Medicare pays for during the lifetime of a beneficiary. Medicare Part A includes an extra 60 hospital days that can be used if the patient has a prolonged illness necessitating a hospital stay of longer than 90 days. A Medicare beneficiary has only 60 nonrenewable reserve days in a lifetime. The beneficiary has the right to choose when to use these reserve days.

155) ANSWER: C
Medicare defines a benefit period as that period of time that begins the first day of a patient's admission to a hospital, skilled nursing facility, or hospice and ends after he or she has been discharged for 60 contiguous days. There is no limit to the number of benefit periods a beneficiary may have for hospital and skilled nursing care. But there is a limit to the number of days of care for which a beneficiary may claim payment.

156) ANSWER: B
Medicare defines a benefit period as that period of time that begins the first day of a patient's admission to a hospital, skilled nursing facility, or hospice and ends after he or she has been discharged for 60 contiguous days. There is no limit to the number of benefit periods a beneficiary may have for hospital and skilled nursing care. But there is a limit to the number of days of care for which a beneficiary may claim payment.

157) ANSWER: A
Medicare defines a benefit period as that period of time that begins the first day of a patient's admission to a hospital, skilled nursing facility, or hospice and ends after he or she has been discharged for 60 contiguous days. There is no limit to the number of benefit periods a beneficiary may have for hospital and skilled nursing care. But there is a limit to the number of days of care for which a beneficiary may claim payment.

158) ANSWER: A
Medicare recipients are responsible for Medicare coinsurance and deductibles.

159) ANSWER: B
Medicare recipients are responsible for Medicare coinsurance and deductibles. Age does not change a member's financial obligations.

160) ANSWER: A
Although Medicare covers many healthcare costs, recipients still have to pay Medicare's coinsurance and deductibles. There are also many medical services that Medicare does not cover; because of this, Medicare recipients sometimes buy a Medicare supplemental insurance (Medigap) policy.

161) **ANSWER: B**
Although Medicare covers many healthcare costs, recipients still have to pay Medicare's coinsurance and deductibles. There are also many medical services that Medicare does not cover; because of this, Medicare recipients sometimes buy a Medicare supplemental insurance (Medigap) policy.

162) **ANSWER: D**
Medigap is private insurance designed to help pay for Medicare cost-sharing amounts. There are 10 standard Medigap policies, and each offers a different combination of benefits. The best time to buy a policy is during the Medigap open enrollment period. For a period of 6 months from the date the patient is first enrolled in Medicare Part B and is age 65 or older, he or she has a right to buy the Medigap policy of his or her choice. That is the open enrollment period. Patients cannot be turned down or charged higher premiums because of poor health if they buy a policy during this period. Once the Medigap open enrollment period ends, patients may not be able to buy the policy of their choice. Patients may have to accept whatever Medigap policy an insurance company is willing to sell them.

163) **ANSWER: A**
Medigap is private insurance designed to help pay for Medicare cost-sharing amounts. There are 10 standard Medigap policies, and each offers a different combination of benefits. The best time to buy a policy is during the Medigap open enrollment period. For a period of 6 months from the date the patient is first enrolled in Medicare Part B and is age 65 or older, he or she has a right to buy the Medigap policy of his or her choice. That is the open enrollment period. Patients cannot be turned down or charged higher premiums because of poor health if they buy a policy during this period. Once the Medigap open enrollment period ends, patients may not be able to buy the policy of their choice. Patients may have to accept whatever Medigap policy an insurance company is willing to sell them.

164) **ANSWER: D**
The best time to buy a policy is during the Medigap open enrollment period. For a period of 6 months from the date the patient is first enrolled in Medicare Part B and is age 65 or older, he or she has a right to buy the Medigap policy of his or her choice. That is the open enrollment period. Patients cannot be turned down or charged higher premiums because of poor health if they buy a policy during this period. Once the Medigap open enrollment period ends, patients may not be able to buy the policy of their choice. Patients may have to accept whatever Medigap policy an insurance company is willing to sell them.

165) **ANSWER: A**
The best time to buy a policy is during the Medigap open enrollment period. For a period of 6 months from the date the patient is first enrolled in Medicare Part B and is age 65 or older, he or she has a right to buy the Medigap policy of his or her choice. That is the open enrollment period. Patients cannot be turned down or charged higher premiums because of poor health if they buy a policy during this period. Once the Medigap open enrollment period ends, patients may not be able to buy the policy of their choice. Patients may have to accept whatever Medigap policy an insurance company is willing to sell them.

166) **ANSWER: B**
The best time to buy a policy is during the Medigap open enrollment period. For a period of 6 months from the date the patient is first enrolled in Medicare Part B and is age 65 or older, he or she has a right to buy the Medigap policy of his or her choice. That is the open enrollment period. Patients cannot be turned down or charged higher premiums because of poor

Healthcare Reimbursement **329**

health if they buy a policy during this period. Once the Medigap open enrollment period ends, patients may not be able to buy the policy of their choice. Patients may have to accept whatever Medigap policy an insurance company is willing to sell them.

167) **ANSWER: A**
The open enrollment period is a period of 6 months from the date the patient is first enrolled in Medicare Part B and is age 65 or older.

168) **ANSWER: C**
The open enrollment period is a period of 6 months from the date the patient is first enrolled in Medicare Part B and is age 65 or older. Geography does not affect the Medicare open enrollment period.

169) **ANSWER: B**
The open enrollment period is a period of 6 months from the date the patient is first enrolled in Medicare Part B and is age 65 or older. Geography does not affect the Medicare open enrollment period.

170) **ANSWER: D**
Medicare Select is another type of Medicare supplemental health insurance sold by insurance companies and HMOs throughout most of the country. Medicare Select is the same as standard Medigap insurance in nearly all respects. The only difference between Medicare Select and standard Medigap insurance is that each insurer has specific hospitals and, in some cases, specific doctors that a patient must use, except in an emergency, to be eligible for full benefits. Medicare Select policies generally have lower premiums than other Medigap policies because of this requirement.

171) **ANSWER: A**
Medicare Select is another type of Medicare supplemental health insurance sold by insurance companies and HMOs throughout most of the country. Medicare Select is the same as standard Medigap insurance in nearly all respects. The only difference between Medicare Select and standard Medigap insurance is that each insurer has specific hospitals and, in some cases, specific doctors that a patient must use, except in an emergency, to be eligible for full benefits. Medicare Select policies generally have lower premiums than other Medigap policies because of this requirement.

172) **ANSWER: B**
The Medicare Part A benefit provides coverage for the following: inpatient hospital services, skilled nursing facilities, home health services, and hospice care. Hemodialysis and ambulatory surgery are outpatient procedures and are covered under Medicare Part B.

173) **ANSWER: D**
Other health insurance policies may have to pay before Medicare pays its share of a patient's bill. For those patients who have other health insurance policies and are eligible for Medicare (not including Medigap policies), the other insurance pays first if the patient is 65 or older; if the patient or his or her spouse is currently working for an employer with 20 or more employees and has group health insurance based on that employment; if the patient is under age 65 and is disabled; if the patient or any member of his or her family is currently working for an employer with 100 or more employees and has group health insurance based on that employment; if the patient has Medicare because of permanent kidney failure; or if the patient has an illness or injury that is covered under workers' compensation, the federal black lung program, no-fault insurance, or any liability insurance.

330 CHAPTER SIX

174) ANSWER: D
For individuals who have a low income and limited resources, the state may pay for Medicare costs, including premiums, deductibles, and coinsurance. To qualify, the individual must be entitled to Medicare hospital insurance (Part A), his or her annual income level must be at or below the national poverty guidelines, and he or she cannot have resources such as bank accounts or stocks and bonds worth more than $6,680 for one person or $10,020 for a couple (home and first car don't count).

175) ANSWER: B
For individuals who have a low income and limited resources, the state may pay for Medicare costs, including premiums, deductibles, and coinsurance. To qualify, the individual must be entitled to Medicare hospital insurance (Part A), his or her annual income level must be at or below the national poverty guidelines, and he or she cannot have resources such as bank accounts or stocks and bonds worth more than $6,680 for one person or $10,020 for a couple (home and first car don't count).

176) ANSWER: D
An awareness of the cost efficiency of preventive care over restorative treatments has prompted the federal government to add to the Medicare benefits package. The following changes in Medicare coverage have been made by the Balanced Budget Act of 1997:

- *Vaccine outreach:* Currently, Medicare pays for one influenza vaccination per year, hepatitis B vaccine for medium to high-risk patients, and one pneumococcal vaccine per lifetime.
- *Breast cancer screening:* Medicare pays for yearly screening mammograms for women over age 40. The Part B deductible is waived for this procedure.
- *Cervical cancer screening:* Medicare pays for screening Pap smears every 3 years and covers screening pelvic exams every 3 years or yearly for women at high risk. The Part B deductible is waived.
- *Colorectal cancer screening:* Medicare pays for yearly colorectal screening for people over age 50.
- *Diabetic education:* Medicare covers educational programs aimed at outpatient self-management.
- *Glucose test strips:* Medicare pays for glucose test strips for diabetics who are not insulin dependent.
- *Osteoporosis screening:* Medicare covers the costs of bone mass tests for beneficiaries who are at clinical risk for osteoporosis.
- *Prostate cancer screening:* Medicare pays for yearly prostate cancer screening for men over the age of 50.

177) ANSWER: D
An awareness of the cost efficiency of preventive care over restorative treatments has prompted the federal government to add to the Medicare benefits package. The following changes in Medicare coverage have been made by the Balanced Budget Act of 1997:

- *Vaccine outreach:* Currently, Medicare pays for one influenza vaccination per year and one pneumococcal vaccine per lifetime and hepatitis B vaccine for people of medium to high risk for the disease.
- *Breast cancer screening:* Medicare pays for yearly screening mammograms for women over age 40. The Part B deductible is waived for this procedure.

- *Cervical cancer screening:* Medicare pays for screening Pap smears every 3 years and covers screening pelvic exams every 3 years or yearly for women at high risk. The Part B deductible is waived.
- *Colorectal cancer screening:* Medicare pays for yearly colorectal screening for people over age 50.
- *Diabetic education:* Medicare covers educational programs aimed at outpatient self-management.
- *Glucose test strips:* Medicare pays for glucose test strips for diabetics who are not insulin dependent.
- *Osteoporosis screening:* Medicare covers the costs of bone mass tests for beneficiaries who are at clinical risk for osteoporosis.
- *Prostate cancer screening:* Medicare pays for yearly prostate cancer screening for men over the age of 50.

178) **ANSWER: B**

An awareness of the cost efficiency of preventive care over restorative treatments has prompted the federal government to add to the Medicare benefits package. The following changes in Medicare coverage have been made by the Balanced Budget Act of 1997:

- *Vaccine outreach:* Currently, Medicare pays for one influenza vaccination per year and one pneumococcal vaccine per lifetime and hepatitis B vaccine for those at medium to high risk for infection.
- *Breast cancer screening:* Medicare pays for yearly screening mammograms for women over age 40. The Part B deductible is waived for this procedure.
- *Cervical cancer screening:* Medicare pays for screening Pap smears every 3 years and covers screening pelvic exams every 3 years or yearly for women at high risk. The Part B deductible is waived.
- *Colorectal cancer screening:* Medicare pays for yearly colorectal screening for people over age 50.
- *Diabetic education*: Medicare covers educational programs aimed at outpatient self-management.
- *Glucose test strips:* Medicare pays for glucose test strips for diabetics who are not insulin dependent.
- *Osteoporosis screening:* Medicare covers the costs of bone mass tests for beneficiaries who are at clinical risk for osteoporosis.
- *Prostate cancer screening:* Medicare pays for yearly prostate cancer screening for men over the age of 50.

179) **ANSWER: A**

An awareness of the cost efficiency of preventive care over restorative treatments has prompted the federal government to add to the Medicare benefits package. The following changes in Medicare coverage have been made by the Balanced Budget Act of 1997:

- *Vaccine outreach:* Currently, Medicare pays for one influenza vaccination per year and one pneumococcal vaccine per lifetime and hepatitis B vaccine for those at medium to high risk for infection.
- *Breast cancer screening:* Medicare pays for yearly screening mammograms for women over age 40. The Part B deductible is waived for this procedure.

- *Cervical cancer screening:* Medicare pays for screening Pap smears every 3 years and covers screening pelvic exams every 3 years or yearly for women at high risk. The Part B deductible is waived.
- *Colorectal cancer screening:* Medicare pays for yearly colorectal screening for people over age 50.
- *Diabetic education:* Medicare covers educational programs aimed at outpatient self-management.
- *Glucose test strips:* Medicare pays for glucose test strips for diabetics who are not insulin dependent.
- *Osteoporosis screening:* Medicare covers the costs of bone mass tests for beneficiaries who are at clinical risk for osteoporosis.
- *Prostate cancer screening:* Medicare pays for yearly prostate cancer screening for men over the age of 50.

180) **ANSWER: D**
The Centers for Medicare & Medicaid Services (CMS) is a federal agency within the U.S. Department of Health and Human Services. CMS runs the Medicare and Medicaid programs—two national healthcare programs that benefit about 75 million Americans. With the Health Resources and Services Administration, CMS runs the State Children's Health Insurance Program, a program that is expected to cover many of the approximately 10 million uninsured children in the United States. CMS also regulates all laboratory testing (except research) performed on humans in the United States. Approximately 158,000 laboratory entities fall within CMS regulatory responsibility. CMS, with the U.S. Departments of Labor and Treasury, helps millions of Americans and small companies get and keep health insurance coverage and helps eliminate discrimination based on health status for people buying health insurance.

181) **ANSWER: C**
The Centers for Medicare & Medicaid Services (CMS) is a federal agency within the U.S. Department of Health and Human Services. CMS runs the Medicare and Medicaid programs—two national healthcare programs that benefit about 75 million Americans. With the Health Resources and Services Administration, CMS runs the State Children's Health Insurance Program, a program that is expected to cover many of the approximately 10 million uninsured children in the United States. CMS also regulates all laboratory testing (except research) performed on humans in the United States. Approximately 158,000 laboratory entities fall within CMS regulatory responsibility. CMS, with the U.S. Departments of Labor and Treasury, helps millions of Americans and small companies get and keep health insurance coverage and helps eliminate discrimination based on health status for people buying health insurance.

182) **ANSWER: B**
The Centers for Medicare & Medicaid Services (CMS) is a federal agency within the U.S. Department of Health and Human Services. CMS runs the Medicare and Medicaid programs—two national healthcare programs that benefit about 75 million Americans. With the Health Resources and Services Administration, CMS runs the State Children's Health Insurance Program, a program that is expected to cover many of the approximately 10 million uninsured children in the United States. CMS also regulates all laboratory testing (except research) performed on humans in the United States. Approximately 158,000 laboratory entities fall within CMS regulatory responsibility. CMS, with the U.S. Departments of Labor and Treasury, helps

millions of Americans and small companies get and keep health insurance coverage and helps eliminate discrimination based on health status for people buying health insurance.

183) **ANSWER: A**
The Centers for Medicare & Medicaid Services (CMS) is a federal agency within the U.S. Department of Health and Human Services. CMS runs the Medicare and Medicaid programs—two national healthcare programs that benefit about 75 million Americans. With the Health Resources and Services Administration, CMS runs the State Children's Health Insurance Program, a program that is expected to cover many of the approximately 10 million uninsured children in the United States. CMS also regulates all laboratory testing (except research) performed on humans in the United States. Approximately 158,000 laboratory entities fall within CMS regulatory responsibility. CMS, with the U.S. Departments of Labor and Treasury, helps millions of Americans and small companies get and keep health insurance coverage and helps eliminate discrimination based on health status for people buying health insurance.

184) **ANSWER: C**
This monthly benefit is available in the first month the patient meets the previous criteria.

185) **ANSWER: D**

186) **ANSWER: D**
Medicaid is a national insurance program aimed at serving the poor and the needy. All 50 states, the District of Columbia, Guam, Puerto Rico, and the Virgin Islands operate Medicaid plans. It was created by Title XIX of the Social Security Act and is part of the federal and state welfare system. State welfare or health departments usually operate the Medicaid program, within the guidelines issued by the CMS, and are funded by the general tax revenues of the federal and state governments. Patients covered by the Medicaid program have no out-of-pocket expense for coverage.

187) **ANSWER: D**
Medicaid is a national insurance program aimed at serving the poor and the needy. All 50 states, the District of Columbia, Guam, Puerto Rico, and the Virgin Islands operate Medicaid plans. It was created by Title XIX of the Social Security Act and is part of the federal and state welfare system. State welfare or health departments usually operate the Medicaid program, within the guidelines issued by the CMS, and are funded by the general tax revenues of the federal and state governments. Patients covered by the Medicaid program have no out-of-pocket expense for coverage.

188) **ANSWER: A**
Medicaid is a national insurance program aimed at serving the poor and the needy. All 50 states, the District of Columbia, Guam, Puerto Rico, and the Virgin Islands operate Medicaid plans. It was created by Title XIX of the Social Security Act and is part of the federal and state welfare system. State welfare or health departments usually operate the Medicaid program, within the guidelines issued by the CMS, and are funded by the general tax revenues of the federal and state governments. Patients covered by the Medicaid program have no out-of-pocket expense for coverage. Providing medical insurance for the aged is the purpose of the Medicare program.

189) **ANSWER: B**
Medicaid is a national insurance program aimed at serving the poor and the needy. All 50 states, the District of Columbia, Guam, Puerto Rico, and the Virgin Islands operate Medicaid plans. It

334 CHAPTER SIX

was created by Title XIX of the Social Security Act and is part of the federal and state welfare system. State welfare or health departments usually operate the Medicaid program, within the guidelines issued by the CMS, and are funded by the general tax revenues of the federal and state governments. Patients covered by the Medicaid program have no out-of-pocket expense for coverage. Providing medical insurance for the aged is the aim of the Medicare program.

190) **ANSWER: B**
Medicaid is a national insurance program aimed at serving the poor and the needy. All 50 states, the District of Columbia, Guam, Puerto Rico, and the Virgin Islands operate Medicaid plans. It was created by Title XIX of the Social Security Act and is part of the federal and state welfare system. State welfare or health departments usually operate the Medicaid program, within the guidelines issued by the CMS, and are funded by the general tax revenues of the federal and state governments. Patients covered by the Medicaid program have no out-of-pocket expense for coverage.

191) **ANSWER: A**
Medicaid is a national insurance program aimed at serving the poor and the needy. All 50 states, the District of Columbia, Guam, Puerto Rico, and the Virgin Islands operate Medicaid plans. It was created by Title XIX of the Social Security Act and is part of the federal and state welfare system. State welfare or health departments usually operate the Medicaid program, within the guidelines issued by the CMS, and are funded by the general tax revenues of the federal and state governments. Patients covered by the Medicaid program have no out-of-pocket expense for coverage.

192) **ANSWER: D**
Although Medicaid benefits can vary from state to state, the program must furnish the federally mandated services that include inpatient hospital care, outpatient services, physicians' services, skilled nursing home services for adults, laboratory and x-ray services, family planning services, and early and periodic screening, diagnosis, and treatment for children under age 21 (EPSDT).

193) **ANSWER: A**
Although Medicaid benefits can vary from state to state, the program must furnish the federally mandated services that include inpatient hospital care, outpatient services, physicians' services, skilled nursing home services for adults, laboratory and x-ray services, family planning services, and early and periodic screening, diagnosis, and treatment for children under age 21 (EPSDT).

194) **ANSWER: B**
Although Medicaid benefits can vary from state to state, the program must furnish the federally mandated services that include inpatient hospital care, outpatient services, physicians' services, skilled nursing home services for adults, laboratory and x-ray services, family planning services, and early and periodic screening, diagnosis, and treatment for children under age 21 (EPSDT).

195) **ANSWER: A**
Eligibility requirements for Medicaid benefits are set by each state, although CMS has set some minimum standards. The people who are eligible under these standards are as follows:
- *Categorically needy:* Families and certain children who qualify for public assistance; that is, they are eligible for Aid to Families with Dependent Children (AFDC) or

Healthcare Reimbursement **335**

Supplemental Security Income (SSI). Examples are the aged, blind, and physically disabled adults and children.
- *Medically needy:* Those people who earn enough to meet their basic needs but have inadequate resources to pay healthcare bills. For example, TB-infected persons who are financially eligible for Medicaid at the SSI level (only for TB-related ambulatory services and TB drugs).

196) **ANSWER: B**
Eligibility requirements for Medicaid benefits are set by each state, although CMS has set some minimum standards. The people who are eligible under these standards are as follows:
- *Categorically needy:* Families and certain children who qualify for public assistance; that is, they are eligible for Aid to Families with Dependent Children (AFDC) or Supplemental Security Income (SSI). Examples are the aged, blind, and physically disabled adults and children.
- *Medically needy:* Those people who earn enough to meet their basic needs but have inadequate resources to pay healthcare bills. For example, TB-infected persons who are financially eligible for Medicaid at the SSI level (only for TB-related ambulatory services and TB drugs).

197) **ANSWER: D**
Eligibility requirements for Medicaid benefits are set by each state, although CMS has set some minimum standards. The people who are eligible under these standards are as follows:
- *Categorically needy:* Families and certain children who qualify for public assistance; that is, they are eligible for Aid to Families with Dependent Children (AFDC) or Supplemental Security Income (SSI). Examples are the aged, blind, and physically disabled adults and children.
- *Medically needy:* Those people who earn enough to meet their basic needs but have inadequate resources to pay healthcare bills. For example, TB-infected persons who are financially eligible for Medicaid at the SSI level (only for TB-related ambulatory services and TB drugs).

198) **ANSWER: C**
Eligibility requirements for Medicaid benefits are set by each state, although CMS has set some minimum standards. The people who are eligible under these standards are as follows:
- *Categorically needy:* Families and certain children who qualify for public assistance; that is, they are eligible for Aid to Families with Dependent Children (AFDC) or Supplemental Security Income (SSI). Examples are the aged, blind, and physically disabled adults and children.
- *Medically needy:* Those people who earn enough to meet their basic needs but have inadequate resources to pay healthcare bills. For example, TB-infected persons who are financially eligible for Medicaid at the SSI level (only for TB-related ambulatory services and TB drugs).

199) **ANSWER: B**
Eligibility requirements for Medicaid benefits are set by each state, although CMS has set some minimum standards. The people who are eligible under these standards are as follows:
- *Categorically needy:* Families and certain children who qualify for public assistance; that is, they are eligible for Aid to Families with Dependent Children (AFDC) or

Supplemental Security Income (SSI). Examples are the aged, blind, and physically disabled adults and children.
- *Medically needy:* Those people who earn enough to meet their basic needs but have inadequate resources to pay healthcare bills. For example, TB-infected persons who are financially eligible for Medicaid at the SSI level (only for TB-related ambulatory services and TB drugs).

200) **ANSWER: D**
To be eligible for federal funds, states are required to provide Medicaid coverage for most individuals who receive federally assisted income maintenance payments, as well as for related groups not receiving cash payments. Some examples of the mandatory Medicaid eligibility groups are as follows:

- Recipients of Aid to Families with Dependent Children (AFDC)
- Supplemental Security Income (SSI) recipients (or, in states using more restrictive criteria, aged, blind, and disabled individuals who meet criteria that are more restrictive than those of the SSI program and that were in place in the state's approved Medicaid plan as of January 1, 1972)
- Infants born to Medicaid-eligible pregnant women
- Children under age 6 and pregnant women who meet the state's AFDC financial requirements or whose family income is at or below 133% of the federal poverty level (The minimum mandatory income level for pregnant women and infants in certain states may be higher than 133% if, as of certain dates, the state had established a higher percentage for covering those groups.)
- Recipients of adoption assistance and foster care under Title IV-E of the Social Security Act

201) **ANSWER: A**
To be eligible for federal funds, states are required to provide Medicaid coverage for most individuals who receive federally assisted income maintenance payments, as well as for related groups not receiving cash payments. Some examples of the mandatory Medicaid eligibility groups are as follows:

- Recipients of Aid to Families with Dependent Children (AFDC)
- Supplemental Security Income (SSI) recipients (or, in states using more restrictive criteria, aged, blind, and disabled individuals who meet criteria that are more restrictive than those of the SSI program and that were in place in the state's approved Medicaid plan as of January 1, 1972)
- Infants born to Medicaid-eligible pregnant women
- Children under age 6 and pregnant women who meet the state's AFDC financial requirements or whose family income is at or below 133% of the federal poverty level (The minimum mandatory income level for pregnant women and infants in certain states may be higher than 133% if, as of certain dates, the state had established a higher percentage for covering those groups.)
- Recipients of adoption assistance and foster care under Title IV-E of the Social Security Act

202) **ANSWER: B**
To be eligible for federal funds, states are required to provide Medicaid coverage for most individuals who receive federally assisted income maintenance payments, as well as for

related groups not receiving cash payments. Some examples of the mandatory Medicaid eligibility groups are as follows:

- Recipients of Aid to Families with Dependent Children (AFDC)
- Supplemental Security Income (SSI) recipients (or, in states using more restrictive criteria, aged, blind, and disabled individuals who meet criteria that are more restrictive than those of the SSI program and that were in place in the state's approved Medicaid plan as of January 1, 1972)
- Infants born to Medicaid-eligible pregnant women
- Children under age 6 and pregnant women who meet the state's AFDC financial requirements or whose family income is at or below 133% of the federal poverty level (The minimum mandatory income level for pregnant women and infants in certain states may be higher than 133% if, as of certain dates, the state had established a higher percentage for covering those groups.)
- Recipients of adoption assistance and foster care under Title IV-E of the Social Security Act

203) **ANSWER: C**
Transfers to a sibling are not exempted by the state, and this asset transfer would be assessed a penalty period. See Section 1917(c) of the Social Security Act; U.S. Code Reference 42 U.S.C.1396p(c).

204) **ANSWER: B**
Transfers to a sibling or a friend are not exempted by the state, and this asset transfer would be assessed a penalty period. See Section 1917(c) of the Social Security Act; U.S. Code Reference 42 U.S.C.1396p(c).

205) **ANSWER: A**
Transfers to a sibling or a friend are not exempted by the state, and this asset transfer would be assessed a penalty period. See Section 1917(c) of the Social Security Act; U.S. Code Reference 42 U.S.C.1396p(c).

206) **ANSWER: D**
A penalty period is the amount of time that a state will withhold payment for a nursing facility and certain other long-term care services. There is no limit to the length of the penalty period. The penalty period is calculated by determining the fair market value of the transferred asset and dividing the value of the asset by the average monthly private pay rate of a nursing facility in that state. For example, if an asset worth $120,000 has been transferred and the average cost of a nursing facility in that state is $2,000 per month, then the penalty period is calculated as $120,000 / $2,000 per month = 60-month penalty period.

207) **ANSWER: A**
A penalty period is the amount of time that a state will withhold payment for a nursing facility and certain other long-term care services. There is no limit to the length of the penalty period. The penalty period is calculated by determining the fair market value of the transferred asset and dividing the value of the asset by the average monthly private pay rate of a nursing facility in that state. For example, if an asset worth $120,000 has been transferred and the average cost of a nursing facility in that state is $2,000 per month, then the penalty period is calculated as $120,000 / $2,000 per month = 60-month penalty period.

208) ANSWER: B
A penalty period is the amount of time that a state will withhold payment for a nursing facility and certain other long-term care services. There is no limit to the length of the penalty period. The penalty period is calculated by determining the fair market value of the transferred asset and dividing the value of the asset by the average monthly private pay rate of a nursing facility in that state. For example, if an asset worth $120,000 has been transferred and the average cost of a nursing facility in that state is $2,000 per month, then the penalty period is calculated as $120,000 / $2,000 per month = 60-month penalty period.

209) ANSWER: D
States look back into an individual's financial records during the evaluation of eligibility for Medicaid. The state looks to find transfers of assets for 60 months before the date the individual is institutionalized or, if later, the date he or she applies for Medicaid. If a transfer of assets for less than fair market value is found, the state will impose a penalty period.

210) ANSWER: B
States look back into an individual's financial records during the evaluation of eligibility for Medicaid. Employment status, rather than financial status, determines workers' compensation eligibility. The state looks to find transfers of assets for 60 months before the date the individual is institutionalized or, if later, the date he or she applies for Medicaid. If a transfer of assets for less than fair market value is found, the state will impose a penalty period.

211) ANSWER: A
States look back into an individual's financial records during the evaluation of eligibility for Medicaid. Employment status, rather than financial status, determines workers' compensation eligibility. The state looks to find transfers of assets for 60 months before the date the individual is institutionalized or, if later, the date he or she applies for Medicaid. If a transfer of assets for less than fair market value is found, the state will impose a penalty period.

212) ANSWER: A
The penalty period is calculated by determining the fair market value of the transferred asset and dividing the value of the asset by the average monthly private pay rate of a nursing facility in that state. For example, if an asset worth $120,000 has been transferred and the average cost of a nursing facility in that state is $2,000 per month, then the penalty period is calculated as $120,000 / $2,000 per month = 60-month penalty period.

213) ANSWER: A
Placing a spouse in a nursing home can be a very expensive proposition. With monthly expenses running $2,000 to $3,000, these bills can quickly wipe out a lifetime of savings, leaving the community-based spouse (community spouse) destitute. This situation is referred to as spousal impoverishment. In an attempt to prevent this, Congress enacted provisions in 1988 that allow a couple to have Medicaid benefits without "spending down" their resources. These provisions help ensure that spousal impoverishment will not occur and that community spouses are able to live out their lives with independence and dignity (Section 1924 of the Social Security Act; U.S. Code Reference 42 U.S.C.1396r-5). Medicare eligibility is not necessary for Medicaid benefits.

214) ANSWER: B
Placing a spouse in a nursing home can be a very expensive proposition. With monthly expenses running $2,000 to $3,000, these bills can quickly wipe out a lifetime of savings, leaving the community-based spouse (community spouse) destitute. This situation is referred

Healthcare Reimbursement 339

to as spousal impoverishment. In an attempt to prevent this, Congress enacted provisions in 1988 that allow a couple to have Medicaid benefits without "spending down" their resources. These provisions help ensure that spousal impoverishment will not occur and that community spouses are able to live out their lives with independence and dignity (Section 1924 of the Social Security Act; U.S. Code Reference 42 U.S.C. 1396r-5). Medicare eligibility is not necessary for Medicaid benefits.

215) **ANSWER: D**
To be eligible for Medicaid under this provision, the member of the couple who is in a nursing facility or medical institution must be expected to remain there for at least 30 days. The state then evaluates the couple's resources. After the state's evaluation, it determines the spousal resource amount, or SRA. The SRA is the number the state measures against its minimum resource standard for an institutionalized patient to receive Medicaid. An institutionalized spouse who has less than this amount is eligible for Medicaid. The SRA is equal to the following: the combined spousal assets, minus the house, car, household goods, and burial costs, divided by two. It is described in the following formula:

$$SRA = \frac{(\text{Combined spousal assets}) - (\text{Protected assets: house, car, etc.})}{2}$$

To determine whether the spouse residing in a medical facility is eligible for Medicaid, the SRA must be less than the state's minimum resource standard. This number was $109,560 in 2011. If the SRA is greater than the state's minimum resource standard, the remainder becomes attributable to the spouse who is residing in a medical institution as countable or depletable resources.

216) **ANSWER: B**
To be eligible for Medicaid under this provision, the member of the couple who is in a nursing facility or medical institution must be expected to remain there for at least 30 days. The state then evaluates the couple's resources. After the state's evaluation, it determines the spousal resource amount, or SRA. The SRA is the number the state measures against its minimum resource standard for an institutionalized patient to receive Medicaid. An institutionalized spouse who has less than this amount is eligible for Medicaid. The SRA is equal to the following: the combined spousal assets, minus the house, car, household goods, and burial costs, divided by two. It is described in the following formula:

$$SRA = \frac{(\text{Couple's combined assets}) - (\text{Protected assets: house, car, etc.})}{2}$$

To determine whether the spouse residing in a medical facility is eligible for Medicaid, the SRA must be less than the state's minimum resource standard. This number was $109,560 in 2011. If the SRA is greater than the state's minimum resource standard, the remainder becomes attributable to the spouse who is residing in a medical institution as countable or depletable resources. There is no spousal poverty depletion rate (SPDR).

217) **ANSWER: A**
To be eligible for Medicaid under this provision, the member of the couple who is in a nursing facility or medical institution must be expected to remain there for at least 30 days. The state then evaluates the couple's resources. After the state's evaluation, it determines the spousal resource amount, or SRA. The SRA is the number the state measures against its minimum resource standard for an institutionalized patient to receive Medicaid. An institutionalized spouse who has less than this amount is eligible for Medicaid. The SRA is equal to the

following: the combined spousal assets, minus the house, car, household goods, and burial costs, divided by two. It is described in the following formula:

$$SRA = \frac{(\text{Combined spousal assets}) - (\text{Protected assets: house, car, etc.})}{2}$$

To determine whether the spouse residing in a medical facility is eligible for Medicaid, the SRA must be less than the state's minimum resource standard. This number was $109,560 in 2011. If the SRA is greater than the state's minimum resource standard, the remainder becomes attributable to the spouse that is residing in a medical institution as countable or depletable resources. There is no spousal poverty depletion rate (SPDR).

218) **ANSWER: A**
The community spouse's income is not considered available to the spouse who is in the medical facility, and the two individuals are not considered a couple for these purposes. The state uses the income eligibility standards for one person rather than two. Therefore, the standard income eligibility process for Medicaid is used.

219) **ANSWER: B**
The community spouse's income is not considered available to the spouse who is in the medical facility, and the two individuals are not considered a couple for these purposes. The state uses the income eligibility standards for one person rather than two. Therefore, the standard income eligibility process for Medicaid is used.

220) **ANSWER: D**
A trust is a legal title to property, held by one party, for the benefit of another. There are usually three parties involved in a trust. The first is the grantor, the person or entity who establishes the trust and donates the assets. A trustee is a person or qualified trust company who holds and manages the assets for the benefit of another. The beneficiary is the recipient of some or all of the trust's assets. The assets held by a trust can exist in many forms, for example, money, real estate, art, businesses, stocks, bonds, and many other tangible assets. Trusts usually come in two varieties: revocable trusts, those trusts whose terms or beneficiaries can be changed, and irrevocable trusts, those trusts whose terms and beneficiaries are unchangeable. Putting an asset in a trust transfers that asset from the individual's ownership to that of the trustee, who holds the property for the beneficiary(ies).

221) **ANSWER: A**
A trust is a legal title to property, held by one party, for the benefit of another. There are usually three parties involved in a trust. The first is the grantor, the person or entity who establishes the trust and donates the assets. A trustee is a person or qualified trust company who holds and manages the assets for the benefit of another. The beneficiary is the recipient of some or all of the trust's assets. The assets held by a trust can exist in many forms, for example, money, real estate, art, businesses, stocks, bonds, and many other tangible assets. Trusts usually come in two varieties: revocable trusts, those trusts whose terms or beneficiaries can be changed, and irrevocable trusts, those trusts whose terms and beneficiaries are unchangeable. Putting an asset in a trust transfers that asset from the individual's ownership to that of the trustee, who holds the property for the beneficiary(ies).

222) **ANSWER: D**
A trust is a legal title to property, held by one party, for the benefit of another. There are usually three parties involved in a trust. The first is the grantor, the person or entity who establishes the trust and donates the assets. A trustee is a person or qualified trust company

who holds and manages the assets for the benefit of another. The beneficiary is the recipient of some or all of the trust's assets. The assets held by a trust can exist in many forms, for example, money, real estate, art, businesses, stocks, bonds, and many other tangible assets. Trusts usually come in two varieties: revocable trusts, those trusts whose terms or beneficiaries can be changed, and irrevocable trusts, those trusts whose terms and beneficiaries are unchangeable. Putting an asset in a trust transfers that asset from the individual's ownership to that of the trustee, who holds the property for the beneficiary(ies).

223) **ANSWER: E**
A trust is a legal title to property, held by one party, for the benefit of another. There are usually three parties involved in a trust. The first is the grantor, the person or entity who establishes the trust and donates the assets. A trustee is a person or qualified trust company who holds and manages the assets for the benefit of another. The beneficiary is the recipient of some or all of the trust's assets. The assets held by a trust can exist in many forms, for example, money, real estate, art, businesses, stocks, bonds, and many other tangible assets. Trusts usually come in two varieties: revocable trusts, those trusts whose terms or beneficiaries can be changed, and irrevocable trusts, those trusts whose terms and beneficiaries are unchangeable. Putting an asset in a trust transfers that asset from the individual's ownership to that of the trustee, who holds the property for the beneficiary(ies).

224) **ANSWER: B**
A trust is a legal title to property, held by one party, for the benefit of another. There are usually three parties involved in a trust. The first is the grantor, the person or entity who establishes the trust and donates the assets. A trustee is a person or qualified trust company who holds and manages the assets for the benefit of another. The beneficiary is the recipient of some or all of the trust's assets. The assets held by a trust can exist in many forms, for example, money, real estate, art, businesses, stocks, bonds, and many other tangible assets. Trusts usually come in two varieties: revocable trusts, those trusts whose terms or beneficiaries can be changed, and irrevocable trusts, those trusts whose terms and beneficiaries are unchangeable. Putting an asset in a trust transfers that asset from the individual's ownership to that of the trustee, who holds the property for the beneficiary(ies).

225) **ANSWER: D**
A trust is a legal title to property, held by one party, for the benefit of another. There are usually three parties involved in a trust. The first is the grantor, the person or entity who establishes the trust and donates the assets. A trustee is a person or qualified trust company who holds and manages the assets for the benefit of another. The beneficiary is the recipient of some or all of the trust's assets. The assets held by a trust can exist in many forms, for example, money, real estate, art, businesses, stocks, bonds, and many other tangible assets. Trusts usually come in two varieties: revocable trusts, those trusts whose terms or beneficiaries can be changed, and irrevocable trusts, those trusts whose terms and beneficiaries are unchangeable. Putting an asset in a trust transfers that asset from the individual's ownership to that of the trustee, who holds the property for the beneficiary(ies).

226) **ANSWER: A**
A trust is a legal title to property, held by one party, for the benefit of another. There are usually three parties involved in a trust. The first is the grantor, the person or entity who establishes the trust and donates the assets. A trustee is a person or qualified trust company who holds and manages the assets for the benefit of another. The beneficiary is the recipient of some or all of the trust's assets. The assets held by a trust can exist in many forms, for example, money, real estate, art, businesses, stocks, bonds, and many other tangible assets.

342 CHAPTER SIX

Trusts usually come in two varieties: revocable trusts, those trusts whose terms or beneficiaries can be changed, and irrevocable trusts, those trusts whose terms and beneficiaries are unchangeable. Putting an asset in a trust transfers that asset from the individual's ownership to that of the trustee, who holds the property for the beneficiary(ies).

227) **ANSWER: D**
How a trust is treated by CMS depends to some extent on the type of trust it is, for example, whether it is revocable or irrevocable, and what specific requirements and conditions the trust contains. In general, payments from a trust actually made to, or for the benefit of, the individual are treated as income to the individual. CMS considers monies that could be paid to an individual or for the benefit of the individual, but are not, as available resources. Further, amounts that could be paid to, or for the benefit of, the individual but are paid to someone else are treated as transfers of assets for less than fair market value. Amounts transferred into a trust, which cannot, in any way, be paid to or for the benefit of the individual, are also treated as transfers of assets for less than fair market value.

228) **ANSWER: B**
How a trust is treated by CMS depends to some extent on the type of trust it is, for example, whether it is revocable or irrevocable, and what specific requirements and conditions the trust contains. In general, payments from a trust actually made to, or for the benefit of, the individual are treated as income to the individual. CMS considers monies that could be paid to an individual or for the benefit of the individual, but are not, as available resources. Further, amounts that could be paid to, or for the benefit of, the individual but are paid to someone else are treated as transfers of assets for less than fair market value. Amounts transferred into a trust, which cannot, in any way, be paid to or for the benefit of the individual, are also treated as transfers of assets for less than fair market value.

229) **ANSWER: A**
How a trust is treated by CMS depends to some extent on the type of trust it is, for example, whether it is revocable or irrevocable, and what specific requirements and conditions the trust contains. In general, payments from a trust actually made to, or for the benefit of, the individual are treated as income to the individual. CMS considers monies that could be paid to an individual or for the benefit of the individual, but are not, as available resources. Further, amounts that could be paid to, or for the benefit of, the individual but are paid to someone else are treated as transfers of assets for less than fair market value. Amounts transferred into a trust, which cannot, in any way, be paid to or for the benefit of the individual, are also treated as transfers of assets for less than fair market value.

230) **ANSWER: A**
Assets placed in trusts established by a parent, grandparent, guardian, or court for the benefit of an individual who is disabled and under the age of 65, using the individual's own funds, are not counted as being available by CMS. The Social Security benefits are counted as an individual's own contribution to the trust.

231) **ANSWER: D**

232) **ANSWER: A**
The patient usually signs a form, before care being rendered, directing Medicare to pay the provider of services directly, and the provider must accept Medicare's allowable charge as payment in full.

233) **ANSWER: B**
The Women's Health and Cancer Rights Act is a law that was enacted as part of an Omnibus Appropriations Bill, and it became effective for plan years beginning on or after October 21, 1998. This Act amended ERISA to require group health plans, including self-insured plans that provide coverage for mastectomies, to provide certain reconstructive and related services after mastectomies. The services mandated by the Act include the following:

- Reconstruction of the breast upon which the mastectomy has been performed
- Surgery and reconstruction of the other breast to produce a symmetrical appearance
- Prosthesis and treatment for physical complications attendant to the mastectomy, for example, lymphedema

234) **ANSWER: C**
The Women's Health and Cancer Rights Act is a law that was enacted as part of an Omnibus Appropriations Bill, and it became effective for plan years beginning on or after October 21, 1998. This Act amended ERISA to require group health plans, including self-insured plans that provide coverage for mastectomies, to provide certain reconstructive and related services after mastectomies. The services mandated by the Act include the following:

- Reconstruction of the breast upon which the mastectomy has been performed
- Surgery and reconstruction of the other breast to produce a symmetrical appearance
- Prosthesis and treatment for physical complications attendant to the mastectomy, for example, lymphedema

235) **ANSWER: B**
The Women's Health and Cancer Rights Act is a law that was enacted as part of an Omnibus Appropriations Bill, and it became effective for plan years beginning on or after October 21, 1998. This Act amended ERISA to require group health plans, including self-insured plans that provide coverage for mastectomies, to provide certain reconstructive and related services after mastectomies. The services mandated by the Act include the following:

- Reconstruction of the breast upon which the mastectomy has been performed
- Surgery and reconstruction of the other breast to produce a symmetrical appearance
- Prosthesis and treatment for physical complications attendant to the mastectomy, for example, lymphedema

236) **ANSWER: A**
The Women's Health and Cancer Rights Act is a law that was enacted as part of an Omnibus Appropriations Bill, and it became effective for plan years beginning on or after October 21, 1998. This Act amended ERISA to require group health plans, including self-insured plans that provide coverage for mastectomies, to provide certain reconstructive and related services after mastectomies. The services mandated by the Act include the following:

- Reconstruction of the breast upon which the mastectomy has been performed
- Surgery and reconstruction of the other breast to produce a symmetrical appearance
- Prosthesis and treatment for physical complications attendant to the mastectomy, for example, lymphedema

237) **ANSWER: B**

238) **ANSWER: A**
The Women's Health and Cancer Rights Act is a law that was enacted as part of an Omnibus Appropriations Bill, and it became effective for plan years beginning on or after October 21, 1998. This Act amended ERISA to require group health plans, including self-insured plans that provide coverage for mastectomies, to provide certain reconstructive and related services after mastectomies. The services mandated by the Act include the following:

- Reconstruction of the breast upon which the mastectomy has been performed
- Surgery and reconstruction of the other breast to produce a symmetrical appearance
- Prosthesis and treatment for physical complications attendant to the mastectomy, for example, lymphedema

It should be noted that the law specifically states these services may be subject to annual deductibles and coinsurance under the plan's normal terms.

239) **ANSWER: C**
This Act imposes prohibitions on the insurers that include the following: A group health plan is prohibited from denying a patient eligibility to enroll or renew coverage solely for the purpose of avoiding the requirements of the Act, and a group health plan is prohibited from inducing an attending physician to limit the care that is required under the Act, whether that takes the form of penalty, reducing, or limiting the reimbursement to such physician. This prohibition should not be thought of as an impediment to effective price negotiation. The Act specifically states that its provisions shall not be construed to prevent a group health plan from negotiating the level and type of reimbursement with a provider for care provided in accordance with the Act.

240) **ANSWER: E**
This Act imposes prohibitions on the insurers that include the following: A group health plan is prohibited from denying a patient eligibility to enroll or renew coverage solely for the purpose of avoiding the requirements of the Act, and a group health plan is prohibited from inducing an attending physician to limit the care that is required under the Act, whether that takes the form of penalty, reducing, or limiting the reimbursement to such physician. This prohibition should not be thought of as an impediment to effective price negotiation. The Act specifically states that its provisions shall not be construed to prevent a group health plan from negotiating the level and type of reimbursement with a provider for care provided in accordance with the Act.

241) **ANSWER: B**
This Act imposes prohibitions on the insurers that include the following: A group health plan is prohibited from denying a patient eligibility to enroll or renew coverage solely for the purpose of avoiding the requirements of the Act, and a group health plan is prohibited from inducing an attending physician to limit the care that is required under the Act, whether that takes the form of penalty, reducing, or limiting the reimbursement to such physician. This prohibition should not be thought of as an impediment to effective price negotiation. The Act specifically states that its provisions shall not be construed to prevent a group health plan from negotiating the level and type of reimbursement with a provider for care provided in accordance with the Act.

242) **ANSWER: C**
This law applies to private and public employer plans and health insurance issuers. Nonfederal governmental, self-insured plans may elect to opt out of this Act's requirements, in the

Healthcare Reimbursement **345**

same manner as they may opt out of the requirements of HIPAA, the Mental Health Parity Act, and the Newborns' and Mothers' Health Protection Act.

243) **ANSWER: B**
This law applies to private and public employer plans and health insurance issuers. Nonfederal governmental, self-insured plans may elect to opt out of this Act's requirements, in the same manner as they may opt out of the requirements of HIPAA, the Mental Health Parity Act, and the Newborns' and Mothers' Health Protection Act.

244) **ANSWER: D**
The MHPA does not require a plan to offer mental health benefits, but if it does, those benefits must have the same financial limitations as medical and surgical care.

245) **ANSWER: B**
The MHPA exempts employers with 50 or fewer workers and those employers or plans that can demonstrate that parity would cause at least a 1% increase in healthcare benefits. Specific industries are not addressed in the legislation.

246) **ANSWER: E**
The MHPA does not require health plans or employers to offer mental health benefits. It does not require that those benefits be the same as medical or surgical benefits, nor does it require parity in copayments, annual number of outpatient visits, or inpatient days. The MHPA does not recognize chemical dependency as a mental health issue and does not require employers or group health plans to cover its treatment.

247) **ANSWER: D**

248) **ANSWER: E**
The employer is not permitted to recoup its losses on maternity care. Exacting higher copayments or larger deductibles for maternity-related benefits constitutes discrimination, as would any limitation in quality, access, or cost above those offered for general medical and surgical benefits.

249) **ANSWER: D**
Abortions are not a mandated benefit under Pregnancy Discrimination Act regulations. This does not prevent employers from offering abortion services as a benefit. Wives of eligible, part-time employees are covered under the Pregnancy Discrimination Act.

250) **ANSWER: A**
The PDA requires equal treatment between employees treated for maternity-related complications and those treated for medical and surgical complications. This does not imply that individuals with maternity-related complications are given superior benefits. In the extant case, if disability leave is not available for medical problems, it is not available for maternity-related problems. Full-time and part-time workers are covered under PDA as well as independent contractors. Married and unmarried workers are equally covered under PDA. Employers with fewer than 15 workers are exempt from the PDA regulations.

251) **ANSWER: D**
CMS defines fraud as "the intentional deception or misrepresentation that an individual knows, or should know, to be false, or does not believe to be true, and makes, knowing the deception could result in some unauthorized benefit to himself or some other person(s)."

252) ANSWER: D

The MHPA of 1996 is a federal law that protects individuals with mental health problems against discrimination by prohibiting lifetime or annual dollar limits on mental health care, unless comparable limits apply to medical or surgical treatment. Enforcement began during plan years beginning on or after January 1, 1998. The MHPA's definition of mental health excludes chemical dependency. Therefore, plans can have separate limits for the treatment of substance abuse.

253) ANSWER: B

The MHPA of 1996 is a federal law that protects individuals with mental health problems against discrimination by prohibiting lifetime or annual dollar limits on mental health care, unless comparable limits apply to medical or surgical treatment. Enforcement began during plan years beginning on or after January 1, 1998. The MHPA's definition of mental health excludes chemical dependency. Therefore, plans can have separate limits for the treatment of substance abuse.

254) ANSWER: C

The MHPA of 1996 is a federal law that protects individuals with mental health problems against discrimination by prohibiting lifetime or annual dollar limits on mental health care, unless comparable limits apply to medical or surgical treatment. Enforcement began during plan years beginning on or after January 1, 1998. The MHPA's definition of mental health excludes chemical dependency. Therefore, plans can have separate limits for the treatment of substance abuse. Under the MHPA, plans are not required to cover mental health treatment. However, if a plan does have mental health coverage, it cannot set separate dollar limits from medical care.

255) ANSWER: A

The MHPA exempts employers with 50 or fewer workers and those employers or plans that can demonstrate that parity would cause at least a 1% increase in healthcare benefits. Specific industries are not addressed in the legislation.

256) ANSWER: B

The MHPA exempts employers with 50 or fewer workers and those employers or plans that can demonstrate that parity would cause at least a 1% increase in healthcare benefits. Employers in specific industries are not addressed in the legislation.

257) ANSWER: D

Although annual or lifetime dollar limits cannot be set under the provisions of the Mental Health Parity Act, other limits are allowed. Examples of other allowable limits are as follows:

- Limited number of annual outpatient visits
- Limited number of inpatient days annually
- Per-visit fee limit
- Higher deductibles and copayments—allowed in mental health benefits under MHPA, without parity in medical and surgical benefits

258) ANSWER: D

Although annual or lifetime dollar limits cannot be set under the provisions of the Mental Health Parity Act, other limits are allowed. Examples of other allowable limits are as follows:

- Limited number of annual outpatient visits
- Limited number of inpatient days annually

- Per-visit fee limit
- Higher deductibles and copayments—allowed in mental health benefits under MHPA, without parity in medical and surgical benefits

If an employer does not offer medical benefits, it does not have to offer mental health benefits. Said differently, if an employer chooses not to offer mental health benefits, it must also choose not to offer medical benefits.

259) **ANSWER: B**
Although annual or lifetime dollar limits cannot be set under the provisions of the Mental Health Parity Act, other limits are allowed. Examples of other allowable limits are as follows:

- Limited number of annual outpatient visits
- Limited number of inpatient days annually
- Per-visit fee limit
- Higher deductibles and copayments—allowed in mental health benefits under MHPA, without parity in medical and surgical benefits

260) **ANSWER: A**
Although annual or lifetime dollar limits cannot be set under the provisions of the Mental Health Parity Act, other limits are allowed. Examples of other allowable limits are:

- Limited number of annual outpatient visits
- Limited number of inpatient days annually
- Per-visit fee limit
- Higher deductibles and copayments—allowed in mental health benefits under MHPA, without parity in medical and surgical benefits

If an employer does not offer medical benefits, it does not have to offer mental health benefits. Said differently, if an employer chooses not to offer mental health benefits, it must also choose not to offer medical benefits.

261) **ANSWER: D**
The Pregnancy Discrimination Act is a federal law that extends to disabilities associated with pregnancies and childbirth the same rights and benefits offered to employees with other medical disabilities. This federal law was created as an amendment to Title VII of the Civil Rights Act of 1964.

262) **ANSWER: B**
The Pregnancy Discrimination Act is a federal law that extends to disabilities associated with pregnancies and childbirth the same rights and benefits offered to employees with other medical disabilities. This federal law was created as an amendment to Title VII of the Civil Rights Act of 1964.

263) **ANSWER: A**
The Pregnancy Discrimination Act is a federal law that extends to disabilities associated with pregnancies and childbirth the same rights and benefits offered to employees with other medical disabilities. This federal law was created as an amendment to Title VII of the Civil Rights Act of 1964.

264) **ANSWER: D**
The Pregnancy Discrimination Act expects employers to treat equally individuals with disabilities attendant to medical and surgical conditions as they do disabilities associated with

pregnancy and childbirth. This same treatment includes the following categories: health insurance benefits, short-term sick leave, disability benefits, and employment policies (such as seniority, leave extensions, and reinstatement).

265) **ANSWER: A**
The Pregnancy Discrimination Act expects employers to treat equally individuals with disabilities attendant to medical and surgical conditions as they do disabilities associated with pregnancy and childbirth. This same treatment includes the following categories: health insurance benefits, short-term sick leave, disability benefits, and employment policies (such as seniority, leave extensions, and reinstatement).

266) **ANSWER: D**
The same treatment in the Pregnancy Discrimination Act means that in regard to choice, access, cost, and quality, maternity benefits will be the equal of medical benefits.

267) **ANSWER: B**
Under the terms of the Pregnancy Discrimination Act, all of the following are prohibited:
- Limiting the number of physicians or hospitals that provide maternity care when medical and surgical care providers are not limited
- Limiting the number of plans that offer maternity care without corresponding limits on medical and surgical care
- Limiting the reimbursement for maternity care when there are no corresponding limits on medical and surgical care
- Exacting higher deductibles, copayments, or out-of-pocket maximums for maternity care than for medical and surgical care

268) **ANSWER: D**

269) **ANSWER: A**
Under the terms of the Pregnancy Discrimination Act, all of the following are prohibited:
- Limiting the number of physicians or hospitals that provide maternity care when medical and surgical care providers are not limited
- Limiting the number of plans that offer maternity care without corresponding limits on medical and surgical care
- Limiting the reimbursement for maternity care when there are no corresponding limits on medical and surgical care
- Exacting higher deductibles, copayments, or out-of-pocket maximums for maternity care than for medical and surgical care

270) **ANSWER: E**
All the individuals listed are covered under the Pregnancy Discrimination Act.

271) **ANSWER: B**
Although its scope is large, the Pregnancy Discrimination Act does exclude some benefits. Those benefits are abortions and mandatory maternity leave.

272) **ANSWER: A**
Although its scope is large, the Pregnancy Discrimination Act does exclude some benefits. Those benefits are abortions and mandatory maternity leave. When home health and home physical therapy are allowed under medical benefits, they are included under maternity benefits also.

Healthcare Reimbursement **349**

273) **ANSWER: D**
TEFRA:
- Established the diagnosis-related groups or DRGs, a case-based reimbursement system. This prospective payment system determined the cost of care for selected diagnoses, while also placing limits on rate increases in hospital revenues.
- Exempted medical rehabilitation from DRGs. Rehabilitation would continue as a cost-based reimbursement system, subject to certain limits.
- Amended the Social Security Act and made Medicare secondary to employer group health plans for active employees 65 to 69 years old and their spouses in the same age group.
- Revised the Age Discrimination in Employment Act (ADEA) of 1967 by requiring employers to offer active employees age 65 to 69 and their spouses the same health benefits as those made available to younger employees.
- Established peer review organizations (PROs). A PRO is an entity that is selected by CMS to reduce costs associated with the hospital stays of Medicare and Medicaid patients. Further, they are charged with conducting reviews of hospital-based care on these patients to ensure quality of care and appropriateness of admissions, readmissions, and discharges. Through this review procedure, PROs can maintain and/or lower admission rates and reduce lengths of stay while ensuring against inadequate treatment.

274) **ANSWER: C**
TEFRA:
- Established the diagnosis-related groups or DRGs, a case-based reimbursement system. This prospective payment system determined the cost of care for selected diagnosis, while also placing limits on rate increases in hospital revenues.
- Exempted medical rehabilitation from DRGs. Rehabilitation would continue as a cost-based reimbursement system, subject to certain limits.
- Amended the Social Security Act and made Medicare secondary to employer group health plans for active employees 65 to 69 years old and their spouses in the same age group.
- Revised the Age Discrimination in Employment Act (ADEA) of 1967 by requiring employers to offer active employees age 65 to 69 and their spouses the same health benefits as those made available to younger employees.
- Established peer review organizations (PROs). A PRO is an entity that is selected by CMS to reduce costs associated with the hospital stays of Medicare and Medicaid patients. Further, they are charged with conducting reviews of hospital-based care on these patients to ensure quality of care and appropriateness of admissions, readmissions, and discharges. Through this review procedure, PROs can maintain and/or lower admission rates and reduce lengths of stay while ensuring against inadequate treatment.

275) **ANSWER: B**
TEFRA:
- Established the diagnosis-related groups or DRGs, a case-based reimbursement system. This prospective payment system determined the cost of care for selected diagnosis, while also placing limits on rate increases in hospital revenues.
- Exempted medical rehabilitation from DRGs. Rehabilitation would continue as a cost-based reimbursement system, subject to certain limits.

350 CHAPTER SIX

- Amended the Social Security Act, and made Medicare secondary to employer group health plans for active employees 65 to 69 years old and their spouses in the same age group.
- Revised the Age Discrimination in Employment Act (ADEA) of 1967 by requiring employers to offer active employees age 65 to 69 and their spouses the same health benefits as those made available to younger employees.
- Established peer review organizations (PROs). A PRO is an entity that is selected by CMS to reduce costs associated with the hospital stays of Medicare and Medicaid patients. Further, they are charged with conducting reviews of hospital-based care on these patients to ensure quality of care and appropriateness of admissions, readmissions, and discharges. Through this review procedure, PROs can maintain and/or lower admission rates and reduce lengths of stay while ensuring against inadequate treatment.

276) **ANSWER: D**
The TEFRA legislation of 1982 was designed to provide incentives for cost containment. Under TEFRA, the diagnosis-related groups, or DRGs, program was established. A case-based reimbursement system, this prospective payment system determined the cost of care for selected diagnoses, while also placing limits on rate increases in hospital revenues.

277) **ANSWER: A**
The TEFRA legislation of 1982 was designed to provide incentives for cost containment. Under TEFRA, the diagnosis-related groups, or DRGs, program was established. A case-based reimbursement system, this prospective payment system determined the cost of care for selected diagnoses, while also placing limits on rate increases in hospital revenues.

278) **ANSWER: B**
The TEFRA legislation of 1982 was designed to provide incentives for cost containment. Under TEFRA, the diagnosis-related groups, or DRGs, program was established. A case-based reimbursement system, this prospective payment system determined the cost of care for selected diagnoses, while also placing limits on rate increases in hospital revenues.

279) **ANSWER: C**
Under TEFRA, medical rehabilitation was exempted from the DRGs. Rehabilitation would continue to be a cost-based reimbursement system, subject to certain limits.

280) **ANSWER: B**
TEFRA amended the Social Security Act and made Medicare secondary to employer group health plans for active employees 65 to 69 years old and their spouses in the same age group. It also revised the Age Discrimination in Employment Act (ADEA) of 1967 by requiring employers to offer active employees age 65 to 69 and their spouses the same health benefits as those made available to younger employees.

281) **ANSWER: A**
TEFRA amended the Social Security Act and made Medicare secondary to employer group health plans for active employees 65 to 69 years old and their spouses in the same age group. It also revised the Age Discrimination in Employment Act (ADEA) of 1967 by requiring employers to offer active employees age 65 to 69 and their spouses the same health benefits as those made available to younger employees.

Healthcare Reimbursement 351

282) **ANSWER: A**
Under the terms of TEFRA, diagnosis-related groups and peer review organizations were created. DRGs are a prospective payment system that determines the cost of care for selected diagnoses, while also placing limits on rate increases in hospital revenues. A PRO is an entity that is selected by CMS to reduce costs associated with the hospital stays of Medicare and Medicaid patients. Further, they are charged with conducting reviews of hospital-based care on these patients to ensure quality of care and appropriateness of admissions, readmissions, and discharges. Through this review procedure, PROs can maintain and/or lower admission rates and reduce lengths of stay while ensuring against inadequate treatment.

283) **ANSWER: B**
Under the terms of TEFRA, diagnosis-related groups and peer review organizations were created. DRGs are a prospective payment system that determines the cost of care for selected diagnoses, while also placing limits on rate increases in hospital revenues. A PRO is an entity that is selected by CMS to reduce costs associated with the hospital stays of Medicare and Medicaid patients. Further, they are charged with conducting reviews of hospital-based care on these patients to ensure quality of care and appropriateness of admissions, readmissions, and discharges. Through this review procedure, PROs can maintain and/or lower admission rates and reduce lengths of stay while ensuring against inadequate treatment. HMOs and IPAs developed independent of federal legislation.

284) **ANSWER: D**
Under TEFRA, peer review organizations (PROs) were established. A PRO is an entity that is selected by CMS to reduce costs associated with the hospital stays of Medicare and Medicaid patients. Further, they are charged with conducting reviews of hospital-based care on these patients to ensure quality of care and appropriateness of admissions, readmissions, and discharges. Through this review procedure, PROs can maintain and/or lower admission rates and reduce lengths of stay while ensuring against inadequate treatment.

285) **ANSWER: B**
Under TEFRA, peer review organizations (PROs) were established. A PRO is an entity that is selected by CMS to reduce costs associated with the hospital stays of Medicare and Medicaid patients. Further, they are charged with conducting reviews of hospital-based care on these patients to ensure quality of care and appropriateness of admissions, readmissions, and discharges. Through this review procedure, PROs can maintain and/or lower admission rates and reduce lengths of stay while ensuring against inadequate treatment.

286) **ANSWER: A**
Under TEFRA, peer review organizations (PROs) were established. A PRO is an entity that is selected by CMS to reduce costs associated with the hospital stays of Medicare and Medicaid patients. Further, they are charged with conducting reviews of hospital-based care on these patients to ensure quality of care and appropriateness of admissions, readmissions, and discharges. Through this review procedure, PROs can maintain and/or lower admission rates and reduce lengths of stay while ensuring against inadequate treatment.

287) **ANSWER: B**
Medicare Part D is available to Medicare recipients only. This plan helps to subsidize costs but requires that the patient pay a share of the drug cost too.

288) ANSWER: E
Medicare Part D is a plan to subsidize prescription drug costs and is available to Medicare recipients only. This plan helps to subsidize costs but requires that the patient pay a share of the drug cost too.

289) ANSWER: D
Medicare Part D is available to Medicare recipients only. This plan helps to subsidize costs but requires that the patient pay a share of the drug cost too.

CHAPTER 7

Rehabilitation

WORKERS' COMPENSATION INSURANCE

Workers' compensation is a type of insurance that provides payments to employees for injuries and disabilities incurred in the course of employment in exchange for relinquishing their right to sue the employer for negligence. Before the enactment of legislation compelling employers to insure their employees for any injuries sustained in the course of their employment, the employee had the right to sue his or her employer to obtain damages for such injuries. The employee had an uphill battle in proving that he or she was not responsible for the accident, that no fellow worker was responsible, and that the accident was not a normal risk of the industry. The worker also had to prove the nature and extent of the injury. The employers aggressively defended themselves against these suits, and countersuits were advanced, claiming employee negligence. The workers' legal forays were expensive, time-consuming, and resulted in a very small number of successful suits. Injured workers and their families suffered serious financial, social, and psychological consequences in this system.

Nevertheless, the number of injuries and subsequent lawsuits increased to a point where governmental intervention encouraged the employers to adopt some form of compulsory workers' compensation insurance. Workers' compensation insurance was designed as a contract between the employer and employee to provide a no-fault source of insurance for work-related injuries.

Workers' compensation legislation was first enacted in the state of New York in 1910. By 1949 it was adopted by all states.[1] Under workers' compensation legislation scales of compensation are established for accidental injuries arising out of and in the course of employment, that is, the injury or illness occurred while the employee was at work and was caused by a work-related task. Workers' compensation benefits are awarded to the worker regardless of who was responsible for the accident.

The benefits payable in case of death, of total disability, and of partial disability vary by state. Although benefits vary among states, these benefits generally include the cost of medical bills attendant to treating the illness or injury as well as some percentage of lost wages. The compensation benefits, set forth by the state, take precedence over the funding source. Employees are entitled to the level of benefits mandated by the state without regard to the financial status or desires of the employers. Therefore, even if the employer is self-funded or self-administered, he or she is bound to offer the full level of benefits required by the state's workers' compensation commission. Self-funded group health insurance plans may be exempt from state-mandated benefits under ERISA (Employee Retirement Income Security Act) guidelines but are not exempt under workers' compensation regulations.

Administrative requirements compel the reporting of all accidents to a public board that is charged with the responsibility of making compensation awards to injured workers or, in case of death, to their families. In recent years coverage for occupational diseases has been added to state workers' compensation statutes.

Workers' compensation is the exclusive remedy to a worker's entitlements. If the worker is covered by workers' compensation insurance, he or she is excluded from claiming benefits for a covered injury under a group insurance policy and, further, is precluded from bringing suit against his or her employer for work-related injuries.

In many states the compensation laws are not compulsory but elective, such as in Texas. In such states the employer may elect to be governed by the provisions of the act or not. An employer electing not to be so governed is liable to suit by injured workers. This employer cannot assert as a defense to an action for damages that the employee's negligence was a contributing factor, that the accident was due to the actions of a fellow employee, or that the accident was a normal risk of the business.

Workers' compensation insurance premiums are paid by the employer, with no contribution by the employee. The authors of the workers' compensation legislation intended that the significant cost of this compulsory insurance would provide an incentive to employers to increase workers' safety programs and result in decreased work-related injuries. Stringent safety programs instituted by the major corporations have, nevertheless, failed to stop the rise in industrial accident rates. It is estimated that industrial accidents have cost U.S. manufacturers more than $11 billion per year.

Employees of the federal government are also covered under workers' compensation benefits. The federal government has its own workers' compensation program, and federal employers are subject to this system's requirements, statutory constraints, and benefit schedule. The Federal Employees' Compensation Act provides workers' compensation coverage to 3 million federal and postal workers around the world for employment-related injuries and occupational diseases. Benefits include wage replacement, payment for medical care, and, when necessary, medical and vocational rehabilitation assistance in returning to work.

Railroad workers and seafarers have workers' compensation programs that differ from state and federal programs. Railroad employees are covered under the Federal Employers' Liability Act (FELA). This Act provides that a carrier (railroad company) "shall be liable" to an employee who is injured by the negligence of that carrier. The FELA remedy is based on ordinary negligence law, not the no-fault law typical of state workers' compensation programs. FELA allows payments for pain and suffering. The amount of the payments is decided by a jury and is based on comparative negligence rather than a predetermined benefits schedule under workers' compensation.

In 1920 the federal government passed the Merchant Marine Act, more commonly known as the Jones Act, named after the legislation's sponsor, Senator Wesly L. Jones of Washington. It regulates maritime commerce in U.S. waters and between U.S. ports and affirms the rights of seamen and women working on U.S. vessels. Under the Jones

Act seamen and women employed on U.S. vessels are able to sue their ship owner when they are injured because of the owner's or the operator's negligence or if they are injured as a result of the vessel being unseaworthy. This right to sue the ship owner is unique to seamen and women on U.S. vessels. International maritime law does not allow seafarers the right to sue the ship owner.

AMERICANS WITH DISABILITIES ACT OF 1990

The Americans with Disabilities Act (ADA) is a federal law that prohibits discrimination against individuals with disabilities. The scope of the ADA is broad, and its goals include the elimination of discrimination against persons with disabilities in the following areas:

- Employment
- Education
- Recreation
- Transportation
- Telecommunication
- Access to public facilities (such as theatres, stores, banks, restaurants, places of employment, and senior centers)
- Access to public services (especially state and local government services and programs)

Organizations Exempt from ADA

Although this law is broad and its goals far-reaching, the ADA does have some exceptions:

- Religious organizations or private membership clubs (except when these organizations sponsor a public event)
- The federal government or corporations owned by the federal government
- Native American tribes
- Small employers (Compliance with this Act can prove a hardship for small employers. Therefore, employers with fewer than 15 employees are exempt. However, just because an accommodation is expensive for an employer does not automatically make it a "hardship" in the view of the government.)
- Housing (This aspect of discrimination is covered by the Fair Housing Amendments Act.)

Defining Disability

Federal legislators defined disability as follows:

1. Any physiological disorder or condition, cosmetic disfigurement, or anatomical loss affecting one or more systems of the body, including the following: the neurological system; the musculoskeletal system; the special sense organs and respiratory organs, including speech organs; the cardiovascular system; the reproductive system; the digestive system; the genitourinary system; the skin; and the endocrine system.
2. Any mental or psychological disorder, such as mental retardation, organic brain syndrome, emotional or mental illness, and specific learning disabilities.

Excluded Populations

Although the federal government hopes to end all discrimination against U.S. citizens, certain conditions do not qualify as disabilities under the ADA. Therefore, individuals with these conditions are not entitled to protection under the ADA:

- Transvestism
- Transsexualism
- Homosexuality and bisexuality
- Pedophilia, exhibitionism, and voyeurism
- Gender identity disorders (unless there is a physical cause)
- Compulsive gambling
- Pyromania
- Kleptomania
- Current alcohol or drug abuse (illegal or prescription)
- A communicable disease that can be transmitted through food handling (Persons in this category may be denied employment in a job involving food handling if there is no reasonable accommodation to eliminate that risk.)

One should note an apparent disparity in the law as it relates to drugs and alcohol. To wit, an employee currently using illegal drugs is never protected under the ADA. However, an employee with a history of drug abuse is protected. In contradistinction, the current use of alcohol is protected, as long as the alcohol does not impair the employee's job performance. Employees with alcohol dependence can be held to the same performance and conduct standards as their nondisabled coworkers. Prescription drug use is protected under the ADA, but the illegal use of prescription drugs is not.

Qualified Employee Criteria Under ADA

The employment provisions of the ADA do not pertain to all individuals of working age who meet the legal definition of disability. The ADA's provisions only apply to "qualified individuals." A person is considered qualified for a job if he or she has the requisite skill, experience, education, and the ability to perform the essential functions of the job as determined by the employer, with or without reasonable accommodation. The ADA does not require that the essential functions of the job be changed to make a "reasonable accommodation."

Essential Functions of a Job

The definition of essential functions of the job is critical to any ADA discrimination action. An employer can claim that although he or she is willing to make accommodations, the disabled candidate is unable to perform the essential functions of the job and, therefore, is not qualified. The candidate can claim that what the employer is demanding are not essential functions of the job. Although job analysis of essential functions can be a very complex determination, there are a few rules of thumb to guide you:

- Essential job functions recorded in the written job descriptions, prepared before advertising for the job or interviewing candidates, are considered evidential when determining the essential functions of the job.
- The job function in question takes up the majority of the job's time.

- The job function in question is considered "essential" to the jobs of others in the same or similar job.
- The job function is described in a collective bargaining agreement.

Reasonable Accommodation

The employer is obligated to make "reasonable accommodations" to an individual's disability that allows the employee to perform his or her job. Reasonable accommodations in employment may include the following:

- Making existing facilities readily accessible to and usable by an individual with disabilities
- Offering job restructuring, part time, or modified work schedules; reassignment to a vacant position; acquisition or modification of equipment or devices; appropriate adjustment or modification of examinations, training materials, or policies; the provision of qualified readers or interpreters; and other similar accommodations for individuals with disabilities

Difficulties in Returning to Work After an Injury

After a significant injury or illness a worker can have pain, muscular weakness, and lack of cardiovascular endurance, even after he or she is fully "recovered." Further, the worker may suffer from depression, anger, or hostility toward his or her employer or fellow workers. Significant injuries or illnesses can result in profound fear of returning to work. Needless to say, these situations all comprise significant obstacles to the worker returning to his or her job.

Take, as a more specific example, a construction worker who suffers severe leg and pelvic fractures after a fall at a construction site. When the worker has finally left the hospital after 8 weeks of confinement and his fractures have healed, is he ready to return to a physically demanding job? Let's consider the extent of his disabilities. We could expect that this worker would have a limited range of motion in his hip and knee joints. His muscular strength and cardiovascular endurance would undoubtedly be poor after his long confinement. The worker may be very angry at his employer for failing to supply adequate safety gear or for making the worker labor in an unsafe environment. Further, the worker may suffer from fear and anxiety that he will be injured again or that he will not be able to do the work he used to do. Finally, the worker may have continued pain from his injuries that limits his ability to work or even to exercise lightly. In the past a worker like this, with his many physical and psychological barriers to therapy, might never return to gainful employment. In this situation some believe work hardening programs can be useful in returning this worker to full employment.

WHAT IS A WORK HARDENING PROGRAM?

Work hardening programs (also called work conditioning and functional restoration programs) are multidisciplinary therapy programs aimed at returning a worker to an improved work status and function. These programs are highly structured and individualized. They use real or simulated work activities in addition to graded conditioning exercises and psychosocial support to restore a worker's physical, behavioral, and vocational functioning. Work hardening programs are neither aimed at treating the underlying condition that led to the disability nor at returning a patient to full independent functioning, but rather they exist to fill the gap between acute medical therapy and return to work.

Work hardening programs are historically an extension of physical and occupational therapy programs. Through a more mature understanding of the complexities of returning a patient to the workforce, they have encouraged the participation of more therapeutic specialties in the work hardening team. Members of the work hardening "multidisciplinary team" include

- Occupational therapists
- Physical therapists
- Vocational therapists
- Psychologists
- Orthotic and prosthetic services
- Ergonomic services

Eligibility for a Work Hardening Program

Not all workers are suitable for work hardening programs. Some may be so permanently disabled they can no longer return to their previous jobs. Some may be in too much physical or psychological pain to meaningfully participate in therapy. Others may not be well enough to safely participate (e.g., patients after a myocardial infarction who may have continued chest pain). Finally, some may not be interested in participating in therapy.

Patient eligibility criteria for work hardening programs are as follows:

- The principal illness or injury that resulted in disability must be resolved enough for therapy to be safely tolerated.
- Because work hardening therapy is job-oriented, there must be both a job available and a plan to return to that specific job.
- The full range of deficits that interfere with work must be identified (including physical, psychological, and vocational deficits).
- The patient must have a willingness to participate in the therapy.

Constituents of Typical Work Hardening Programs

Work hardening programs are individualized, both by the nature of the individual patient characteristics and by the demands of the job. Therefore, there is no "typical" work hardening program. A person who suffered a foot injury while working as an electronic part assembler at a computer factory has different therapeutic needs than an obese construction worker who suffered a heart attack while on the job. Each of these situations has different physical and emotional disabilities and so requires different physical and emotional therapies. Therefore, the duration of work hardening programs can last a few weeks or take several months. They can use only physical therapists to increase strength and endurance or require psychologists, physical therapists, an ergonomic expert, and orthotic specialists to retrain a worker to accommodate his or her new prosthesis.

Because of these inherent differences in both underlying disabilities and therapeutic goals, the medical literature on the subject of work hardening is complex and often contradictory. There are methodological variabilities, heterogeneous groups of study subjects, variable definitions of disability and employment, and limited outcome measures. Despite these difficulties, in most parts of the United States employers find that work hardening programs are an effective way to return workers to full employment.

ASSESSING THE PATIENT'S LEVEL OF PHYSICAL AND MENTAL IMPAIRMENT

The rehabilitation Case Manager seeks to promote optimal outcomes for his or her patients. He or she is responsible for implementing a quality care plan that is cost effective, realistic, and optimal for the patient. Although rehabilitation Case Managers are often found in institutions such as acute care facilities, rehabilitation facilities, and skilled nursing facilities, they also may be agency based, insurance based, or independent. To effectively collaborate with the patient, family, and other healthcare providers, the Case Manager must start by clinically assessing the patient. This assessment identifies problems that might hinder the patient's return to health and full function. Common problems found in these assessments are as follows:

- Temporary or permanent functional changes
- Physiological impairments
- Psychological or social problems
- Difficulties integrating back into the community
- Educational deficits of the patient or family
- Cognitive deficits of the patient or family

Assessment Tools

The Case Manager can use several tools in assessing patients with central nervous system injuries. One of these tools is the Ranchos Los Amigos Levels of Cognitive Functioning (Exhibit 7-1), which divides a patient's cognitive abilities into eight levels of increasing complexity and functionality. Level I corresponds to a patient with "no response to stimuli," and level VIII corresponds to a patient who is alert and oriented with purposeful and appropriate responses but less so than in his or her premorbid condition. In general, patients in levels I, II, and III require skilled nursing placement and are not appropriate for rehabilitation. If the patient's clinical status improves, he or she can be reassessed for rehabilitation. Levels IV through VIII are recognized as usually appropriate for rehabilitation.

Another tool frequently used to assess comatose/recovering patients is the Glasgow coma scale (Exhibit 7-2). Like the Ranchos Los Amigos cognitive function scale, the Glasgow coma scale assigns a numerical value to a patient's responses to stimuli. The sum of the value of these responses is the Glasgow coma score. This scoring system is objective and easy to use. The use of this scale allows healthcare providers to assess and follow the neurological progress of a patient. Most acute care facilities use this objective neurological measurement/assessment system. Assessments with this tool are done frequently. Repetitive scores of 3 over several days indicate a poor prognosis. A score of 3 to 7 indicates a coma, and a score above 8 indicates the patient may benefit from rehabilitation services.

EXHIBIT 7-1 Ranchos Los Amigos Levels of Cognitive Functioning

Level #	Function	Description
I	NO RESPONSE	The patient is totally unresponsive to all stimuli.
II	GENERALIZED RESPONSE	The patient reacts inconsistently and nonpurposefully to environmental stimuli in a nonspecific manner. Responses are generally to deep pain and are likely to be delayed.
III	LOCALIZED RESPONSE	The patient reacts specifically but inconsistently to stimuli. He may respond to discomfort by pulling at tubes or responding to a familiar person by turning his head toward the person.
IV	CONFUSED/AGITATED	The patient is confused and excited. He can't process all that is said or done; his attention span is short. His speech may not make sense, he usually cannot cooperate in his treatment plan, and he tires easily.
V	CONFUSED/INAPPROPRIATE	The patient is alert and able to respond to simple commands. He responds best to familiar people. He requires structure, may wander, and his memory may be impaired.
VI	CONFUSED/APPROPRIATE	The patient demonstrates goal-directed behavior but still requires structure. He has an increased awareness of the environment and his own needs; has the ability to learn but requires frequent repetition.
VII	AUTOMATIC/APPROPRIATE	The patient can follow a daily routine automatically but can't deal with unexpected situations. He has a vague understanding of his condition but no real insight and is likely to be unrealistic about his future.
VIII	PURPOSEFUL/APPROPRIATE	The patient is alert and oriented but may not function as well as before the injury. Once a skill is learned, he requires no supervision. He is able to function in society but may have occasional problems with unexpected or stressful situations.

Source: Courtesy of Ranchos Los Amigos Medical Center, Downey, California.

Neurological Disabilities

Case Managers can plan more effectively when they know what deficits to expect. Patients who have suffered a stroke or brain trauma will have functional disabilities related to where the injury is located (Exhibit 7-3) in the brain.

Patients with spinal cord injuries/lesions require vastly different treatment plans and equipment depending on the level of the injury. Exhibit 7-4 is a brief guide used to gauge functional ability in patients with spinal cord injuries.

Another tool commonly used in the workers' compensation area is a functional capacity evaluation, which is a comprehensive evaluation to assess a patient's ability to perform work-related activity. A well-designed assessment should be administered with concern for the patient's safety and well-being to minimize any potential injury to the

EXHIBIT 7-2 Glasgow Coma Scale

Examiner's Test		Patient's Response	Assigned Score
Eye opening	Spontaneous	Opens eyes on own	4
	Speech	Opens eyes in response to a loud voice	3
	Pain	Opens eyes when pinched	2
	Pain	Does not open eyes	1
Best motor response	Commands	Follows simple commands	6
	Pain	Pulls examiner's hand away when pinched	5
	Pain	Pulls a part of body away when examiner pinches patient	4
	Pain	Flexes body inappropriately to pain (decorticate posturing)	3
	Pain	Body becomes rigid in an extended position when examiner pinches patient (decerebate posturing)	2
	Pain	No motor response to pain	1
Verbal response	Speech	Carries on a conversation correctly, is oriented to time, place, person	5
	Speech	Seems confused and disoriented	4
	Speech	Speech is clear but makes no sense	3
	Speech	Makes sounds the examiner cannot understand	2
	Speech	No speech or noise	1

Source: Reprinted from M. St. Couer. 1996. *Case management practice guidelines*, pp. 2–14, St. Louis: Mosby.

patient. It should be administered by an objective examiner and include activities that are part of the employee's tasks at work. The exam typically includes the following:

- Balance
- Hand coordination
- Hand grip strength
- Maximum walking, stairs, and stepladder capacity
- Prolonged trunk flexion in sitting and standing
- Prolonged trunk rotation in sitting and standing
- Prolonged crawl, knee, and sustained crouch positions
- Repetitive lifting at various levels
- Repetitive push, pull, and carrying capacities
- Repetitive squatting
- Tolerance for elevated work
- Tolerance for prolonged sitting and standing

The results are generally used as an initial assessment, to reassess progress/status before returning to work, or to determine a work conditioning plan for return to work.

EXHIBIT 7-3 Impaired Functional Abilities of Stroke or Brain Trauma Patients

Left Hemisphere	Right Hemisphere
Speech	Spatial orientation
Language	Picture/pattern sense
Complex motor functions	Performancelike functions
Vigilance	Spatial integration
Paired associate learning	Creative associative thinking
Verbal abilities	Calculation
Linguistic description	Simple language comprehension
Verbal ideation	Nonverbal identification
Conceptual similarities	Facial identification
Time analysis	Recognition of environmental sounds
Detail analysis	Nonverbal paired associate learning
Arithmetic	Tactile perception
Writing	
Calculation	
Finger naming	
Right–left orientation	

EXHIBIT 7-4 Guide to Functional Abilities in Patients with Spinal Cord Injuries

Vertebral Level	Functional Ability
C1–C3	Ventilator dependent No neck control; no movement in upper or lower extremities Cardiac pacer
C4	May need ventilator support (C4—phrenic nerve) Shoulder shrug/neck control
C5	Involvement of both hands Weakness of triceps Severe weakness in trunk and lower extremities
C6	Involvement of upper extremities and hands Normal or good triceps Generalized weakness of the trunk and lower extremities, impairing balance and ambulation
C7	Involvement of upper extremities Normal or good finger flexion and extension Grasp and release No intrinsic hand function Generalized weakness of trunk and lower extremities Poor balance
T1–T5	Total abdominal paralysis or poor muscle strength No useful trunk sitting
T6–T10	Upper abdominal and spinal extension musculature sufficient to provide some element of trunk sitting
T11–L2	No quadriceps or very weak
L2–S5	Moderate to good quadriceps; ambulation with some support (S2–S5—loss of bowel and bladder control)

ORTHOSES, PROSTHESES, AND ASSISTIVE DEVICES

Orthoses

An orthosis is a device added to a person's body to achieve one or more of the following ends:

- Support
- Improve anatomical position
- Immobilization
- Correction of deformities
- Assistance for weak muscles
- Restoration of muscle function
- Modification of muscle tone

The term "orthosis" generally encompasses such devices as slings, braces, and splints. Orthoses are used to support or aid in the functioning of the upper and lower extremities, hands, and feet, as well as the trunk and spine. These devices can be relatively simple affairs, made of cotton and plastic, or can be complex electromechanical appliances replete with steel alloys, cantilevered joints, and servomotors.

Prostheses

A prosthesis is a device that restores all or part of a missing body part. The science of prosthetics addresses the mechanical, physiological, and cosmetic functions of restorations. Whereas orthoses are aimed at assisting the body to restore function, prostheses restore or replace those parts of the human body that are absent or no longer function. The need for replacement and cosmesis rather than a simple increase in functionality stems from a person's need for "wholeness" and a "positive body image." With this in mind, the professional prosthetist's goals are to increase both functionality and cosmesis for his or her patient.

Although most laypersons associate the term *prosthesis* with artificial arms and legs, the field is much larger, encompassing many specialties. Prostheses run the gamut from highly functional devices, such as a lens implant after cataract surgery or an artificial hip for a hip fracture, to highly cosmetic devices, such as breast implants after a mastectomy, wigs (a cranial prosthesis) after chemotherapy, and an artificial eye after an enucleation. Choosing a successful prosthetic device for a patient is not like choosing a good suit of clothes "off the rack," as it were. Following the clothing simile, choosing a prosthetic device is more like a formal fitting for a custom-tailored suit. The prosthesis is individualized both for its looks and for its functionality. It takes into account not only such superficialities as size and color but also seeks to meet the individual's needs within the limitations of technology and the individual's ability to compensate. For example, the properties of a prosthetic leg of a 24-year-old athlete will be markedly different from that of the 75-year-old sedentary individual. The athlete will require a leg whose materials can tolerate the impacts of running and jumping, will include biomechanical devices that add "spring" to ankle flexion and extension by conserving energy during weight bearing, and allow for variable swing speeds during the gait. The sedentary individual would benefit from lighter weight materials (which may be less impact resistant) and biomechanical devices in the prosthesis that trade flexibility and energy conservation for increased stability.

Complexities of a Prosthesis "Fitting"

To gain a better understanding of the complexities the patient faces when getting a prosthesis, it is instructive for the Case Manager to review the process for fitting one of the more common types of prosthesis, called transtibial prostheses. The transtibial prosthesis is created for individuals who have suffered a below-the-knee amputation.

Fitting Process

Soon after the wound on the patient's "stump" or "residual limb" has matured, it is casted with plaster bandages. While the plaster is drying, the prosthetist hand-molds the cast by pushing in on those softer prominences composed of skin and muscle tissue while avoiding the bony prominences. When the cast has dried completely, it is removed from the patient and filled with plaster. When the plaster is dry, the cast is removed, and the model of the residual limb is left.

Model

The prosthetist marks all the bony prominences at the distal end of the model and may modify the model by building up plaster over the sensitive bony areas and shaving off plaster over the more tolerant soft tissue prominences. This allows a transfer of weight from those sensitive bony prominences to those tissues that can better tolerate weight bearing. The residual limb does not bear weight on its distal end but rather on those soft tissue areas around the distal end.

Interface

The interface is the part of the prosthesis that touches the residual limb. A good interface is critical to the prosthesis. It should perform the following functions:

- Helps to hold and stabilize the prosthesis to the residual limb
- Comfortably bears the body weight
- Protects the residual limb from damage associated with friction and weight bearing

To begin the process of creating the interface, an "evaluation interface" is made. The evaluation interface is made by vacuum sealing a layer of clear plastic around the plaster mold. The clear plastic interface is then tried on the residual limb. Clear plastic allows the prosthetist to see how the residual limb "seats" within the interface. With the evaluation interface inserted into a temporary prosthetic leg, the patient is asked to sit, stand, and walk; during these exercises the interface is evaluated by the patient and the prosthetist. The plastic interface has the additional properties of being heat malleable. If the interface is not an exact fit, it can be heated in warm water and hand-molded to a more comfortable fit.

Alignment

The alignment of the prosthesis with the interface is also vitally important. With the patient wearing the temporary prosthesis, the prosthetist makes careful measurements and adjustments of the prosthesis in relation to the interface and in relation to its parts (e.g., leg to ankle, foot to toe). Such measurements as height, degree of "toe-in or toe-out," and walking dynamics are inspected. The alignment of the interface and the prosthesis, as well as the various moving parts of the prosthesis to each other, may be adjusted to allow for better walking.

Definitive Prosthesis

After the fitting of the interface and the aligning of the prosthesis are finished, the definitive prosthesis may be made. An average amputee can be fully functional with his prosthesis within a year of his amputation.

Repair and Replacement

Complex prostheses require ongoing adjustment and maintenance. Replacement of the prosthesis is a common and predictable event. Many factors influence replacement frequency; for example, lower extremity prostheses bear weight, sustain high impact, and are exposed to the elements. Damage to the prostheses acquired by these activities demands maintenance, repair, and replacement. Replacement frequency depends on the activity level of the patient and the demands put on the prosthesis, as well as the complexity of the prosthesis and the properties of the materials used. Further, an individual's prosthetic needs may change. For example, a sedentary individual may become more active, requiring a new prosthesis with more features and flexibility. Conversely, an active individual may become more sedentary with advancing age or disease, requiring a replacement prosthesis that is lighter and more stable. Finally, the younger patient will require successively larger prostheses to compensate for growth.

Individuals who fit and produce prosthetics and orthotics are highly trained and certified professionals. Case Managers should ensure the prosthetist they refer patients to has this training and certification.

Assistive Devices

Assistive or adaptive devices are products that substitute for an impaired function and allow the individual to perform an activity more independently. For example, these devices can aid in mobility/ambulation (ambulatory aids), activities of daily living, and self-care as well as improve impaired voice, hearing, vision, and increasing patient safety. Ambulatory aids (e.g., canes, crutches, walkers) are an extension of the upper extremities that transmit body weight and provide support for the patient. Assistive devices for activities of daily living and as for self-care and leisure activities range from simple objects for daily use (e.g., plate guards, spoons with built-up handles, elastic shoelaces, doorknobs with rubber levers) to complex electronic devices, such as voice-activated environmental control systems.

Adaptive devices should be used only if other methods of performing the task are not available or cannot be learned. A reasonable effort should be made to teach the patient a method of performing the task in question with his or her disabilities before an adaptive device is suggested. Mastery of a task (e.g., walking) allows the patient greater independence and flexibility in that he or she does not need a wheelchair to move around and is not limited by lack of ramps. The device may serve as a useful supplement or permit a function to be performed if the adapted method cannot be learned or requires too much effort.

The type of assistive device required is determined by the needs of the individual patient, his or her abilities and functional limitations, and the restrictions of his or her environment. The Case Manager should be aware of all these parameters before authorizing an assistive device. Such common mistakes as a walker being too heavy for a frail elderly woman, a room being too small for a hospital bed, or doorways too narrow for a wheelchair to pass through plague the inexperienced Case Manager.

The device should have proven reliability and safety. A Case Manager should be aware of a product's safety and efficacy record before recommending it to a client. Simple devices such as crutches and walkers have resulted in injuries due to falls; improperly fitted wheelchairs have resulted in decubitus ulcers. The Case Manager should make sure the patient and, when appropriate, family and caregivers receive the appropriate training. This training is often offered by the equipment vendor or by physical or occupational rehabilitation specialists.

The patient and family or caregivers should be involved in the selection of adaptive devices and should be trained in their use. A Case Manager who attends to these issues increases the likelihood that the device is the one desired by the patient, meets the patient's needs, and will be fully used. Exhibit 7-5 lists some examples of assistive devices.

ERGONOMICS

Ergonomics has been an important science in manufacturing for more than 50 years. In the last 20 years it has gained wide acceptance in the fields of rehabilitation, industrial hygiene, worker injury prevention, and workplace design. A Case Manager must be familiar with the basics if he or she is to be successful.

History of Ergonomics

Ergonomics comes from two Greek words, *ergon*, meaning "work," and *nomos*, meaning "laws." The study of ergonomics did not gain much public attention until World War II, when accidents with military equipment were thought to be caused by human error but were then found by investigations to be caused by poorly designed controls. Engineers and designers became aware that making the equipment easier for people to work with could save lives. From this realization the science of ergonomics was born. Ergonomics has also been referred to as human engineering and human factor engineering.

Definition of Ergonomics

Ergonomics is an applied science concerned with designing and arranging things people use, so that the people and things interact most efficiently and safely. Put more simply, it is the application of human sciences to the optimization of people's working environments. This definition emphasizes the important triad of ergonomic elements:

- Health
- Comfort
- Productivity

Ergonomics draws on many disciplines to adapt the design of products and workplaces to people's sizes and shapes and their physical, intellectual, and emotional strengths and limitations. The following disciplines are used by ergonomists:

- Anatomy
- Physiology
- Psychology
- Sociology
- Physics
- Industrial engineering

EXHIBIT 7-5 Examples of Assistive Devices

Visual Aids

- Glasses
- Contact lenses
- Implantable lenses
- Magnifying glasses
- Large-print books
- Audio books
- Braille books
- Seeing-eye dogs
- Text-to-speech synthesizers
- Text-to-Braille translation devices
- Optical character recognition computer software

Hearing

- Hearing aids
- Phone receiver with volume control
- TDD telephone services

Speaking/Communicating

- Picture boards
- Text-to-voice synthesizer
- Computer-augmented speech systems

Orientation to Time, Place, and Person

- Memory books
- Cue cards
- Orientation blackboards
- Calendars
- Clocks/watches/alarms

Memory

Treatment of memory deficits focuses on compensatory aids:
- Memory books
- To-do lists
- Cue cards

Ambulation/Locomotion

- Cane
- Quad cane
- Folding cane chair
- Crutches
- Walker
- Rolling walker
- Wheelchair (nonmotorized)
- Wheelchair (motorized)

(continues)

EXHIBIT 7-5 Examples of Assistive Devices (continued)

Eating Devices

- Built-up handles on eating utensils for weak or incompetent grasp
- Handles on cups and glasses
- Nonskid mats to stabilize plate for eating with one hand
- Rocker knife for one-handed cutting
- Partitions in plates and bowls for eating one-handed

Dressing Devices

- Button hook for buttoning clothes
- Velcro closures on clothes and shoes/boots
- Long-handled shoe horn when reach is limited

Toileting Aids

- Bedside commode, urinal, bedpan
- Built-up toilet and commode seat
- Grab bars next to toilet
- Toilet seat with rails

Shower and Tub Aids

- Long-handled sponge for patients with limited reach
- Washcloth or sponge mitt for patients with weak grasp
- Grab bars in tub
- Tub bench or tub chair
- Handheld shower nozzle

Transfer Devices

- Plastic or wooden transfer board for sliding transfers
- Gait/transfer belt for use by caregiver, if indicated
- Hydraulic lifts for bed, chair, tub, or car transfers
- Hydraulic or electric stair lifts for patients unable to climb stairs
- Chairs modified with higher seats for patients unable to lift out of chair

Recreation

- Large-print playing cards
- Large-print books
- Books on audio tape
- Video games
- Specialized wheelchairs (e.g., racing wheelchairs)
- Swimming flotation devices
- Fishing pole harnesses
- Gardening tools with built-up handles
- Specially designed golf clubs

- Occupational health
- Anthropometry (the science of human measurement)
- Biomechanics (the application of engineering mechanics to biological and medical systems)
- Job task and skill analysis

Goals of Ergonomics

At its most basic, ergonomics seeks to adapt a person's work to a person's physical and psychological capabilities and limitations. By adapting the job to the worker, ergonomics can achieve

- More efficient work
- Higher quality products
- Happier, healthier workforce
- Safer work environments

Ergonomists also work with the U.S. Occupational Safety and Health Administration to develop ergonomic guidelines, standards, and regulations to ensure the safety and comfort of American workers.

Ergonomics and Repetitive Stress Injuries

According to the U.S. Bureau of Labor Statistics, more than 60% of workplace illnesses reported each year are associated with repetitive stress injuries. These injuries result from continuous repetition of the same motion, for instance, repetitive lifting, screwing, or twisting on an assembly line. The injury may be exacerbated by awkward postures, such as bending or reaching. The following are common examples of repetitive stress injuries:

- Carpal tunnel syndrome
- Rotator cuff injuries
- Knee and elbow bursitis
- Low back pain syndrome
- Neck pain

Carpal tunnel syndrome is a common example of a repetitive stress injury. It is a painful and often debilitating swelling of the connective tissue in the wrist. This swelling leads to nerve compression, pain, and disability. Carpal tunnel syndrome results from overuse of the hands and wrists. Common occupations associated with carpal tunnel syndrome are typing on a computer keyboard, cutting meat, or turning knobs and levers. Low back pain is associated with frequent, unassisted heavy lifting. Nurses who move hospital patients in and out of beds are particularly susceptible to this injury.

Not all repetitive stress injuries are the result of lifting, pushing, or flexing. Noise-induced hearing loss resulting from continuous exposure to excessive noise is another type of repetitive stress injury, as are headaches and eyestrain due to improper workplace lighting or poorly positioned computer screens. Workers constantly exposed to vibrations can suffer from sensory neuropathies.

Injury prevention is a top priority for ergonomic engineers when they design workplaces. Offices, assembly lines, tools, and work garments are all designed with injury prevention in mind. These engineers position tools and machinery to be accessible to workers without twisting, reaching, or bending. They design adjustable workbenches, desks, and chairs to comfortably accommodate workers of many different sizes, preventing the need to continuously lean or overextend the arms. The environment of workers is also a concern of the ergonomist. They must establish the correct temperature, lighting, noise, and ventilation to ensure that workers perform under optimal conditions. In the setting of returning an injured worker to his or her job, ergonomists can be employed to redesign a workplace to accommodate a worker's new disabilities or limitations. Alternatively, ergonomists are consulted by vocational specialists to examine injured workers for new jobs, in what is called a job-fit analysis.

Where Do Case Managers and Ergonomics Fit?

It is in the health and safety of workers that Case Managers primarily interact with ergonomics. In working in the field of ergonomics, Case Managers become part of the multidisciplinary team that includes industrial hygienists, safety engineers, and occupational medicine physicians. This team is concerned with identifying health and safety threats to workers and implementing changes in the work environment to eliminate them.

Case Managers have three opportunities for intervention when a safety issue has been identified:

- *Identify and report:* In this role the Case Manager may identify worker injuries and illnesses as being related to unsafe conditions on the job. This information is reported to the ergonomic department, industrial hygienist, and occupational medicine department for further evaluation.
- *Referral agent:* When the Case Manager is notified that a job environment cannot be adequately modified to suit the worker's current limitations, the Case Manager may refer the worker to several areas. Some examples of referrals include rehabilitation for strength and endurance training, work hardening, vocational assessment, and retraining.
- *Patient advocate:* This is a familiar role for the Case Manager. In the industrial setting the Case Manager becomes aware of information that the worker's managers may not have. The Case Manager must make the employers aware of the worker's new limitations as a result of the injury or illness and seek accommodations to the job or additional therapies to make the transition for debilitation to full employment easier. Some examples are
    - Recommending "light duty" or reduced hours for an employee who returns to work and is still in pain from his or her injury
    - Recommending continued therapy to increase a worker's strength and endurance when the worker has a physically demanding job to which he or she is not ready to return
    - Suggesting a job-fit analysis when an injury has left a worker permanently disabled for his or her current job

ASSISTIVE TECHNOLOGY GLOSSARY

Assistive devices are products that increase a patient's functionality and independence by substituting for an impaired function. Assistive technology products are designed to provide additional accessibility to individuals who have physical or cognitive disabilities. The following is a list of common assistive devices:

- *Alternate keyboard:* A computer appliance used to input data. It consists of matrix keys, which are switches that allow easier manipulation than the regular keyboard.
- *Augmentative and alternative communication device:* An electronic device that assists, augments, or supplements a person's ability to communicate. These devices can range from a simple "picture board" with pictures of the desired items or activities that can be pointed to, to computerized systems that can change input from a keyboard, alternate keyboard, head stick, or eye gaze switch into synthesized speech.
- *Chinwand or chinstick:* A pointer or extension device that is mounted to a headpiece and extends from the center of the mandible and angles outward. It is usually coupled with a direct selection input device to aid people with good head mobility but poor upper body strength.
- *Dial scan:* A selection or data input device that resembles a clock with one hand. The single hand on the clock face is used to point to pictures or symbols around the perimeter of the clock face. By pointing the hand to one of the symbols or pictures and actuating a switch, a selection can be made.
- *Direct selection:* A selection made with a single action by directly activating a letter, picture, or other item on an input device. Examples of direct selection are pressing a key on a keyboard, touching a symbol or picture on a touch screen, an eye gaze selection system, or an optical head pointer system.
- *Durable medical equipment:* A product is considered durable medical equipment if it meets the following characteristics:
  - It is reusable (not disposable).
  - It is primarily used for a medical or therapeutic purpose.
  - It has little or no use to a person in the absence of illness.
- *Environmental control systems:* A device (usually electronic) that allows the user to control other devices in his or her environment. Thus, the disabled operator is able to (remotely) control such systems as heating and cooling, lighting, security, opening windows and doors, and turning on televisions without having to be able to perform the tasks physically. The control unit may be mounted on a bed or a wheelchair for ease of access.
- *Ergonomics* (from the Greek words *ergon*, meaning work, and *nomos*, meaning laws): The study of how humans interact with their working environments. It uses the applied science of equipment design for the workplace. The intended object of the study is to maximize productivity by reducing operator fatigue and discomfort. Ergonomics is also called human factors engineering.
- *Headwand or headstick:* A pointer or extension device that is mounted to a headpiece and extends from the center of the forehead and angles downward. It is usually coupled with a direct selection input device to aid people with good head mobility but poor upper body strength.
- *Joystick:* A movable control lever. By tilting the joystick in different directions, the user can control mechanical devices, such as a motorized wheelchair.
- *Keyboard emulating interface:* A piece of either hardware or software that is connected to a computer. It allows the computer to accept the input from a nonstandard input device, as if it were coming from a standard input device (e.g., keyboard).

- *On-screen keyboard:* A virtual keyboard provided on the computer monitor by specific software. The on-screen keyboard can be used with an "alternate input device," such as an alternate keyboard, an optical head pointer, or a sip and puff switch, to input data.
- *Screen reading software:* A computer program capable of reading menus, format commands, and punctuation, as well as text, on the computer monitor.
- *Speech digitizer or speech recognition system:* A device that allows digitally recorded speech to be analyzed and converted into electronic patterns. These patterns can be used as computer commands or to create text.
- *Speech recognition programs:* These programs allow patients to give commands and enter data in computers using only their voices. These programs can be used to create text documents such as letters or e-mail messages, browse the Internet, and navigate among applications and menus by voice.
- *Speech synthesizer:* A computer output device that has the capacity to translate text characters into the spoken word.
- *Telecommunications Device for the Deaf (TDD):* A device that allows the severely hearing impaired to communicate via the phone. It consists of a small computer monitor or display screen, a modem, a connection to a phone line, and some means of input (keyboard). E-mail and cell phone texting are largely supplanting this device in younger patients.
- *Text-to-speech synthesis:* A function of a computer that allows text to be translated into speech sounds.
- *Touch screen:* A special type of computer monitor that acts as an input device. By touching the pictures or symbols on a computer screen monitor, a user is able to make selections.
- *Voice recognition system:* A method for inputting data or making selections on a computerized system. Voice recognition systems translate speech into digital signals. These digital signals can then be used to make selections or to operate a computer or other electronic devices.

REFERENCES

1. Fishback, P. V., & Kantor, S. E. (2000). *A prelude to the welfare state: The origins of workers' compensation.* Chicago: University of Chicago Press.

Appendix 7-A

Rehabilitation Questions

1) When placing a patient who needs assistive devices due to a knowledge deficit in an alternative care setting, the most important thing a Case Manager should consider
   A. Whether the patient can self-feed
   B. Patient safety
   C. Location in relation to family
   D. Whether the facility has activities the patient enjoys

2) Which of the following is (are) true regarding the purposes of an orthosis?
   1. It can be used to support body parts.
   2. It can be used to position body parts.
   3. It can be used to immobilize body parts.
   4. It can be used to modify muscle tone.
      A. 1, 3
      B. 2, 4
      C. 1, 2, 3
      D. All of the above
      E. None of the above

3) Which of the following is (are) true regarding the purposes of an orthosis?
   1. It can be used to replace body parts.
   2. It can be used to position body parts.
   3. It can be used to amputate body parts.
   4. It can be used to modify muscle tone.
      A. 1, 3
      B. 2, 4
      C. 1, 2, 3
      D. All of the above
      E. None of the above

4) Which of the following is (are) not true regarding the purposes of an orthosis?
   1. It can be used to replace body parts.
   2. It can be used to position body parts.
   3. It can be used to amputate body parts.
   4. It can be used to modify muscle tone.
      A. 1, 3
      B. 2, 4
      C. 1, 2, 3
      D. All of the above
      E. None of the above

5) Which of the following is (are) true regarding a prosthesis?
   1. It may restore or replace all or part of a missing body part.
   2. It may improve a person's sense of wholeness or body image.
   3. It has as its goals increased function and cosmesis.
   4. It may result in injury or illness if improperly fitted.
      A. 1, 3
      B. 2, 4
      C. 1, 2, 3
      D. All of the above
      E. None of the above

6) Which of the following is (are) true regarding a prosthesis?
   1. The term *prosthesis* refers only to artificial arms and legs.
   2. It may improve a person's sense of wholeness or body image.
   3. Cosmesis is not an issue when fitting a prosthesis.
   4. It may result in injury or illness if improperly fitted.
      A. 1, 3
      B. 2, 4
      C. 1, 2, 3
      D. All of the above
      E. None of the above

7) Which of the following is (are) not true regarding a prosthesis?
   1. The term *prosthesis* refers only to artificial arms and legs.
   2. It may improve a person's sense of wholeness or body image.
   3. Cosmesis is not an issue when fitting a prosthesis.
   4. It may result in injury or illness if improperly fitted.
      A. 1, 3
      B. 2, 4
      C. 1, 2, 3
      D. All of the above
      E. None of the above

8) Which of the following is (are) true regarding assistive devices?
   1. They are products that substitute for an impaired function.
   2. They are a substitute for rehabilitation services.
   3. They allow an individual to perform an activity more independently.
   4. When prescribing one, little input is needed from the patient or patient's family.
      A. 1, 3
      B. 2, 4
      C. 1, 2, 3
      D. All of the above
      E. None of the above

9) **Which of the following is (are) true regarding the prescribing of an assistive device?**
   1. An evaluation of the patient's interest and abilities is important.
   2. An evaluation of the patient's home and work environment is important.
   3. Training the patient on the device is important.
   4. Training family members on the device is sometimes important.
      A. 1, 3
      B. 2, 4
      C. 1, 2, 3
      D. All of the above
      E. None of the above

10) **Which of the following is (are) not true regarding the prescribing of an assistive device?**
    1. An evaluation of the patient's home and work environment is important.
    2. An evaluation of the patient's interest and abilities is unnecessary.
    3. Training the patient on the device is important.
    4. Training family members on the device is always unnecessary.
       A. 1, 3
       B. 2, 4
       C. 1, 2, 3
       D. All of the above
       E. None of the above

11) **Which of the following statements is (are) true regarding repair and replacement of prosthetic devices?**
    1. Well-made prostheses should not require replacement. A request for replacement is an indication of shoddy workmanship.
    2. Complex prostheses require ongoing adjustment and maintenance.
    3. Good prostheses are strong and durable, and require no repair or maintenance.
    4. Prostheses may need to be replaced frequently.
       A. 1, 3
       B. 2, 4
       C. 1, 2, 3
       D. All of the above
       E. None of the above

12) **Which of the following statements is (are) not true regarding repair and replacement of prosthetic devices?**
    1. Well-made prostheses should not require replacement. A request for replacement is an indication of shoddy workmanship.
    2. Complex prostheses require ongoing adjustment and maintenance.
    3. Good prostheses are strong and durable, and require no repair or maintenance.
    4. Prostheses may need to be replaced frequently.
       A. 1, 3
       B. 2, 4
       C. 1, 2, 3
       D. All of the above
       E. None of the above

376 CHAPTER SEVEN

13) Which of the following factors may influence the rate of prosthesis replacement?
   1. Activity level
   2. Age of user
   3. Type of prosthesis
   4. Impact resistance of materials used
      A. 1, 3
      B. 2, 4
      C. 1, 2, 3
      D. All of the above
      E. None of the above

14) Which of the following factors do not influence the rate of prosthesis replacement?
   1. Activity level
   2. Educational achievements of the user
   3. Type of prosthesis
   4. Patient's social status
      A. 1, 3
      B. 2, 4
      C. 1, 2, 3
      D. All of the above
      E. None of the above

15) Which of the following factors may influence the rate of prosthesis replacement?
   1. Activity level
   2. Educational achievements of the user
   3. Type of prosthesis
   4. Patient's social status
      A. 1, 3
      B. 2, 4
      C. 1, 2, 3
      D. All of the above
      E. None of the above

16) Which of the following statements is (are) true regarding prostheses, orthoses, and assistive devices?
   1. They require individual customization to the patient's needs and likes as well as to his or her dimensions.
   2. Successful and safe use requires patient training.
   3. Their successful implementation depends on a thorough evaluation of the patient's interests, abilities, and goals.
   4. Patient adaptation is short and requires little patient effort.
      A. 1, 3
      B. 2, 4
      C. 1, 2, 3
      D. All of the above
      E. None of the above

17) Which of the following statements is (are) not true regarding prostheses, orthoses, and assistive devices?
   1. They require individual customization to the patient's needs and likes as well as to his or her dimensions.
   2. Even patients who are disinterested in using these devices should be fitted for them.
   3. Their successful implementation depends on a thorough evaluation of the patient's interests, abilities, and goals.
   4. Patient adaptation is short and requires little patient effort.
      A. 1, 3
      B. 2, 4
      C. 1, 2, 3
      D. All of the above
      E. None of the above

18) Which of the following is (are) considered an assistive device?
   1. Text-to-speech synthesizer
   2. Phone receiver volume control
   3. Quad cane
   4. Grab bars in the tub
      A. 1, 3
      B. 2, 4
      C. 1, 2, 3
      D. All of the above
      E. None of the above

19) Which of the following is (are) considered an assistive device?
   1. A "cock-up" splint for the wrist
   2. Phone receiver volume control
   3. A sling to hold a plegic and atrophied arm in place
   4. Grab bars in the tub
      A. 1, 3
      B. 2, 4
      C. 1, 2, 3
      D. All of the above
      E. None of the above

20) Which of the following is (are) not considered an assistive device?
   1. A "cock-up" splint for the wrist
   2. Phone receiver volume control
   3. A sling to hold a plegic and atrophied arm in place
   4. Grab bars in the tub
      A. 1, 3
      B. 2, 4
      C. 1, 2, 3
      D. All of the above
      E. None of the above

21) Which of the following is (are) considered a prosthetic device?
   1. A wig for a person suffering from alopecia totalis
   2. A lens implant after a cataract removal
   3. An artificial hip after a hip fracture
   4. Dentures
       A. 1, 3
       B. 2, 4
       C. 1, 2, 3
       D. All of the above
       E. None of the above

22) Which of the following is (are) considered a prosthetic device?
   1. A built-up shoe to accommodate leg shortening
   2. A lens implant after a cataract removal
   3. Leg braces to assist walking after a spinal injury
   4. Artificial knee joint for severe osteoarthritis
       A. 1, 3
       B. 2, 4
       C. 1, 2, 3
       D. All of the above
       E. None of the above

23) Which of the following is (are) not considered a prosthetic device?
   1. A built-up shoe to accommodate leg shortening
   2. A lens implant after a cataract removal
   3. Leg braces to assist walking after a spinal injury
   4. Artificial knee joint for severe osteoarthritis
       A. 1, 3
       B. 2, 4
       C. 1, 2, 3
       D. All of the above
       E. None of the above

24) Assistive devices include which of the following?
   1. Rolling walker, bedside commode, transfer board
   2. Prosthetic arm, hearing aid
   3. Quad cane, grab bars, long-handled shoehorn, built-up utensil handles
   4. Knee brace
       A. 1, 2
       B. 2, 3
       C. 1, 3
       D. 2, 4

25) A railroad worker who is injured on the job receives compensation under which of the following legislations?
   A. The Mann Act
   B. The Jones Act
   C. Federal Employers' Liability Act (FELA)
   D. Americans with Disabilities Act

26) Which of the following workers are covered under the Federal Employees' Compensation Act (FECA)?
  1. Railroad employees
  2. Postal workers
  3. U.S. seamen and women
  4. Federal employees
     A. 1, 3
     B. 2, 4
     C. 1, 2, 3
     D. All of the above

27) The Case Manager is following a patient with a complaint and diagnosis of back pain. The patient has not been at work for more than 2 weeks, has no documented pathology, and has no specific treatment plan other than "rest." What should the Case Manager recommend at this point?
  1. A functional capacity study
  2. A nerve conduction test
  3. A magnetic resonance image of the area
  4. A second opinion
  5. An independent medical exam
     A. 1, 2
     B. 2, 3
     C. 3, 4
     D. 4, 5
     E. All of the above

28) A Case Manager can expect an amputee with a new prosthesis to experience which of the following?
  A. Balance and gait difficulties
  B. Functional issues
  C. Body image acceptance
  D. All of the above
  E. None of the above

29) The Case Manager receives a referral for a patient with a spinal cord injury at C1-4. When would the Case Manager expect the patient to be ready for discharge home?
  A. When the patient can direct his or her own care
  B. When the patient is independent in self-care
  C. When the patient reaches functional independence at wheelchair level
  D. All of the above
  E. None of the above

30) A patient has an arthrogram scheduled. The Case Manager knows the following is true of this procedure:
  A. An arthrogram aids in the diagnosis of spinal stenosis.
  B. Crepitus is a potential complication of this procedure.
  C. Arthrograms aid in diagnosis of injured bursa or cartilage.
  D. Radiopaque solutions are injected with this procedure.

31) The Case Manager is working on discharging a brain-injured patient to the home setting with family care. When reviewing the patient's readiness for discharge, in relation to the adaptive equipment, which of the following is (are) the most important issue(s)?
   A. The length of time the patient requires the equipment
   B. Whether or not the family has been trained in its use
   C. Whether there are structural barriers to using the equipment in the home
   D. All of the above
   E. None of the above

32) The Case Manager has been following an amputee in an inpatient rehabilitation program. She has been instructed in using her prosthesis and in caring for it and her limb. She is now ready for discharge. What need is most often overlooked when discharging this type of patient?
   A. A follow-up appointment with the prosthetist
   B. A follow-up appointment with the surgeon
   C. The ability to drive a car
   D. The ability to solve problems for herself

33) The Case Manager with a patient who is a paraplegic because of a spinal cord injury recognizes that a major early problem will be
   A. Use of ambulation aids
   B. Patient education
   C. Bladder control
   D. All of the above
   E. None of the above

34) _____ are a variety of implements or equipment used to aid individuals in performing tasks or movements.
   A. Prosthetics
   B. Orthotics
   C. Durable medical equipment
   D. Assistive devices

35) _____ is the paralysis of the lower half of the body and both legs.
   A. Hemiplegia
   B. Paraplegia
   C. Quadriplegia
   D. Hemiparesis

36) _____ is the paralysis of all four limbs.
   A. Hemiplegia
   B. Paraplegia
   C. Quadriplegia
   D. Quadripara

37) _____ is the paralysis of one side of the body.
   A. Hemiplegia
   B. Paraplegia
   C. Quadriplegia
   D. Quadripara

38) The Case Manager can expect which of the following after ACL reconstruction surgery?
   A. Jogging by the 12th postoperative week
   B. Full weight bearing and range of motion by the 4th postoperative week
   C. Bent-knee raises and isometric exercises on the affected leg for the 1st postoperative week while immobilized in a hinged-type brace
   D. All of the above

39) A Case Manager is frustrated by his inability to get the patient to agree to occupational therapy. The patient was involved in a high-speed motor vehicle accident and suffered severe head injuries. When encouraged to attend therapy sessions, the patient refuses, becomes verbally abusive, and hangs up. Likely reason(s) for this patient's reaction is (are)
   A. Head injuries can result in emotional lability.
   B. Head injuries can result in cognitive impairments.
   C. Head injuries can result in prolonged head pain and a depressed mood.
   D. All of the above
   E. None of the above

40) A patient with damage to the spinal cord at C6-7 is referred for case management. Before contacting the patient the Case Manager can expect the patient will experience which of the following symptoms?
   1. Respiratory paralysis
   2. Quadriplegia
   3. Paralysis of the legs, wrists, and hands but retains motion in the elbows and shoulders
   4. Aphasia
      A. 1, 4
      B. 2, 3
      C. 3
      D. All of the above
      E. None of the above

41) After a patient injures her back, it is important for the Case Manager to communicate to the providers of care and those involved in the care plan the physical requirements of the patient's job so that
   1. The treatment team can meet the patient's needs.
   2. Appropriate treatment goals can be identified.
   3. Vocational rehabilitation can begin immediately.
   4. Disability papers can be filed.
      A. 1, 2
      B. 1, 2, 3
      C. 1, 3
      D. All of the above
      E. None of the above

NOTES

Appendix 7-B

Rehabilitation Answers

1) **ANSWER: B**
   Patient safety is the most important issue in this case.

2) **ANSWER: D**
   An orthosis is a device that is added to a person's body to achieve one or more of the following ends: support, position, immobilization, correction of deformities, assistance for weak muscles, restoration of muscle function, and modification of muscle tone.
   The term *orthosis* generally encompasses such devices as slings, braces, and splints. Orthoses are used to support or aid in the functioning of the upper and lower extremities, hands, and feet, as well as the trunk and spine. These devices can be relatively simple affairs, made of cotton belts and plastic splints, or they can be complex electromechanical appliances replete with steel alloys, cantilevered joints, and servomotors.

3) **ANSWER: B**
   An orthosis is a device that is added to a person's body to achieve one or more of the following ends: support, position, immobilization, correction of deformities, assistance for weak muscles, restoration of muscle function, and modification of muscle tone.
   The term *orthosis* generally encompasses such devices as slings, braces, and splints. Orthoses are used to support or aid in the functioning of the upper and lower extremities, hands, and feet, as well as the trunk and spine. These devices can be relatively simple affairs, made of cotton belts and plastic splints, or they can be complex electromechanical appliances replete with steel alloys, cantilevered joints, and servomotors. The replacement of body parts is a function of prostheses.

4) **ANSWER: A**
   An orthosis is a device that is added to a person's body to achieve one or more of the following ends: support, position, immobilization, correction of deformities, assistance for weak muscles, restoration of muscle function, and modification of muscle tone.
   The term *orthosis* generally encompasses such devices as slings, braces, and splints. Orthoses are used to support or aid in the functioning of the upper and lower extremities, hands, and feet, as well as the trunk and spine. These devices can be relatively simple affairs, made of cotton belts and plastic splints, or they can be complex electromechanical appliances replete with steel alloys, cantilevered joints, and servomotors. The replacement of body parts is a function of prostheses.

5) **ANSWER: D**
   A prosthesis is a device that restores or replaces all or part of a missing body part. The science of prosthetics addresses the mechanical, physiological, and cosmetic functions of

restorations. Although orthoses are aimed at assisting the body to restore function, prostheses restore or replace those parts of the human body that are absent or no longer function. The need for replacement and cosmesis rather than a simple increase in functionality stems from a person's need for "wholeness" and a "positive body image." With this in mind, the professional prosthetist has as his or her goals increasing both functionality and cosmesis. Poorly fitted prostheses can cause injury or illness.

6) **ANSWER: B**

A prosthesis is a device that restores or replaces all or part of a missing body part. The science of prosthetics addresses the mechanical, physiological, and cosmetic functions of restorations. Although orthoses are aimed at assisting the body to restore function, prostheses restore or replace those parts of the human body that are absent or no longer function. The need for replacement and cosmesis rather than a simple increase in functionality stems from a person's need for "wholeness" and a "positive body image." With this in mind, the professional prosthetist has as his or her goals increasing both functionality and cosmesis. Poorly fitted prostheses can cause injury or illness. Although most laypersons associate the term *prosthesis* with artificial arms and legs, the field is much larger, encompassing many specialties. Prostheses run the gamut from highly functional devices, such as a lens implant for cataracts or an artificial hip for a hip fracture, to highly cosmetic devices, such as breast implants after a mastectomy, wigs (a cranial prosthesis) after chemotherapy, and an artificial eye after an enucleation.

7) **ANSWER: A**

A prosthesis is a device that restores or replaces all or part of a missing body part. The science of prosthetics addresses the mechanical, physiological, and cosmetic functions of restorations. Although orthoses are aimed at assisting the body to restore function, prostheses restore or replace those parts of the human body that are absent or no longer function. The need for replacement and cosmesis rather than a simple increase in functionality stems from a person's need for "wholeness" and a "positive body image." With this in mind, the professional prosthetist has as his or her goals increasing both functionality and cosmesis. Poorly fitted prostheses can cause injury or illness. Although most laypersons associate the term *prosthesis* with artificial arms and legs, the field is much larger, encompassing many specialties. Prostheses run the gamut from highly functional devices, such as a lens implant for cataracts or an artificial hip for a hip fracture, to highly cosmetic devices, such as breast implants after a mastectomy, wigs (a cranial prosthesis) after chemotherapy, and an artificial eye after an enucleation.

8) **ANSWER: A**

Assistive or adaptive devices are products that substitute for an impaired function and allow the individual to perform an activity more independently. Adaptive devices should be used only if other methods of performing the task are not available or cannot be learned. A reasonable effort should be made to teach the patient a method of performing the task in question before an adaptive device is suggested. Mastery of a task (e.g., walking) allows the patient greater independence and flexibility in that he or she does not need a wheelchair to move around and is not limited by lack of ramps. The device may serve as a useful supplement, however, or permit a function to be performed if the adapted method cannot be learned or requires too much effort. The type of assistive device is determined by the needs of the individual patient, his or her abilities and functional limitations, and the environment.

9) **ANSWER: D**

The type of assistive device is determined by the needs of the individual patient, his or her abilities and functional limitations, and the environment. Such common mistakes as a walker being too heavy for a frail elderly patient, a room being too small for a hospital bed, or doorways too narrow for a wheelchair plague the inexperienced Case Manager. Even simple devices such as crutches and walkers have resulted in injuries due to falls, whereas improperly fitted wheelchairs have resulted in decubitus ulcers. The Case Manager should make sure the patient is properly fitted to the equipment and trained in its use. When appropriate, family and caregivers should also receive the appropriate training. The patient, family, and caregivers should be involved in the selection of the adaptive device and should be trained in its use. A Case Manager who attends to these issues will increase the likelihood that the device is wanted, meets the patient's needs, and will be fully used.

10) **ANSWER: B**
The type of assistive device is determined by the needs of the individual patient, his or her abilities and functional limitations, and his or her environment. Such common mistakes as a walker being too heavy for a frail elderly patient, a room being too small for a hospital bed, or doorways too narrow for a wheelchair plague the inexperienced Case Manager. Even simple devices such as crutches and walkers have resulted in injuries due to falls, whereas improperly fitted wheelchairs have resulted in decubitus ulcers. The Case Manager should make sure the patient is properly fitted to the equipment and trained in its use. When appropriate, family and caregivers should also receive the appropriate training. The patient, family, and caregivers should be involved in the selection of adaptive devices and should be trained in their use. A Case Manager who attends to these issues will increase the likelihood that the device is wanted, meets the patient's needs, and will be fully used.

11) **ANSWER: B**
Complex prostheses require ongoing adjustment and maintenance. Prostheses may even need to be replaced with frequency. Many factors influence replacement frequency. For example, lower extremity prostheses bear weight, sustain high impact, and are exposed to the elements. Damage to the prostheses acquired by these activities demands maintenance, repair, and replacement. Further, an individual's prosthetic needs may change. For example, a sedentary individual may become more active. Conversely, an active individual may become more sedentary with advancing age or disease. Each of these changes may require the individual to acquire a prosthesis with different properties to accommodate these changes. Finally, the younger patient will require successively larger prostheses to compensate for growth.

12) **ANSWER: A**
Complex prostheses require ongoing adjustment and maintenance. Prostheses may even need to be replaced with frequency. Many factors influence replacement frequency. For example, lower extremity prostheses bear weight, sustain high impact, and are exposed to the elements. Damage to the prostheses acquired by these activities demands maintenance, repair, and replacement. Further, an individual's prosthetic needs may change. For example, a sedentary individual may become more active. Conversely, an active individual may become more sedentary with advancing age or disease. Each of these changes may require the individual to acquire a prosthesis with different properties to accommodate these changes. Finally, the younger patient will require successively larger prostheses to compensate for growth.

13) **ANSWER: D**
Many factors influence replacement frequency. For example, lower extremity prostheses bear weight, sustain high impact, and are exposed to the elements. Damage to the prostheses acquired by these activities demands maintenance, repair, and replacement. Replacement frequency depends on the activity level of the patient and the demands he or she puts on the prosthesis, as well as the complexity of the prosthesis and the properties of the materials

used. Further, an individual's prosthetic needs may change. For example, a sedentary individual may become more active, requiring a new prosthesis with more features and flexibility. Conversely, an active individual may become more sedentary with advancing age or disease, requiring a replacement prosthesis that is lighter and more stable. Finally, the younger patient will require successively larger prostheses to compensate for growth.

14) **ANSWER: B**
Many factors influence replacement frequency. For example, lower extremity prostheses bear weight, sustain high impact, and are exposed to the elements. Damage to the prostheses acquired by these activities demands maintenance, repair, and replacement. Replacement frequency depends on the activity level of the patient and the demands he or she puts on the prosthesis, as well as the complexity of the prosthesis and the properties of the materials used. Further, an individual's prosthetic needs may change. For example, a sedentary individual may become more active, requiring a new prosthesis with more features and flexibility. Conversely, an active individual may become more sedentary with advancing age or disease, requiring a replacement prosthesis that is lighter and more stable. Finally, the younger patient will require successively larger prostheses to compensate for growth. There is no association between a patient's educational achievements or social status and prosthesis replacement.

15) **ANSWER: A**
Many factors influence replacement frequency. For example, lower extremity prostheses bear weight, sustain high impact, and are exposed to the elements. Damage to the prostheses acquired by these activities demands maintenance, repair, and replacement. Replacement frequency depends on the activity level of the patient and the demands he or she puts on the prosthesis, as well as the complexity of the prosthesis and the properties of the materials used. Further, an individual's prosthetic needs may change. For example, a sedentary individual may become more active, requiring a new prosthesis with more features and flexibility. Conversely, an active individual may become more sedentary with advancing age or disease, requiring a replacement prosthesis that is lighter and more stable. Finally, the younger patient will require successively larger prostheses to compensate for growth. There is no association between a patient's educational achievements or social status and prosthesis replacement.

16) **ANSWER: C**
Prostheses, orthoses, and assistive devices are aimed at increasing a patient's independence and functionality. These devices require attention to the abilities, interests, and goals of the individual and should be customized to accommodate them. Most devices require training of the patient and sometimes the family members. Adaptation to these devices is difficult, and mastery of them takes time and effort.

17) **ANSWER: B**
Prostheses, orthoses, and assistive devices are aimed at increasing a patient's independence and functionality. These devices require attention to the abilities, interests, and goals of the individual and should be customized to accommodate them. Most devices require training of the patient and sometimes the family members. Adaptation to these devices is difficult, and mastery of them takes time and effort.

18) **ANSWER: D**

19) **ANSWER: B**
Assistive devices substitute for impaired function and promote independence; therefore, a volume control device on a phone receiver and grab bars are assistive devices. Orthoses are devices that are added to the body to support, position, immobilize, and assist weak muscles. A cock-up splint and an arm sling are considered orthoses.

20) **ANSWER: A**
Assistive devices substitute for impaired function and promote independence; therefore, a volume control device on a phone receiver and grab bars are assistive devices. Orthoses are devices that are added to the body to support, position, immobilize, and assist weak muscles. A cock-up splint and an arm sling are considered orthoses.

21) **ANSWER: D**
Prostheses are devices designed to replace absent body parts and restore functioning and cosmesis to the patient.

22) **ANSWER: B**
Prostheses are devices designed to replace absent body parts and restore functioning and cosmesis to the patient. Braces, splints, slings, and special shoes are considered orthotic devices.

23) **ANSWER: A**
Prostheses are devices designed to replace absent body parts and restore functioning and cosmesis to the patient. Braces, splints, slings, and special shoes are considered orthotic devices.

24) **ANSWER: C**
Assistive or adaptive devices are products that substitute for an impaired function and allow the individual to perform an activity more independently. For example, these devices can aid in mobility/ambulation (ambulatory aids), activities of daily living, and self-care as well as improve impaired voice, hearing, vision, and increasing patient safety. Ambulatory aids (e.g., canes, crutches, walkers) are an extension of the upper extremities that transmit body weight and provide support for the patient. Assistive devices for activities of daily living and for self-care and leisure activities range from simple objects for daily use (e.g., plate guards, spoons with built-up handles, elastic shoelaces, doorknobs with rubber levers) to complex electronic devices, such as voice-activated environmental control systems. A prosthetic arm and a hearing aid are prostheses. A knee brace is an orthosis, not an assistive device.

25) **ANSWER: C**
Railroad employees who are injured while working are covered under the statutes of the Federal Employers Liability Act, or FELA. The Jones Act covers seamen injured while working in the maritime industry and the American's with Disabilities Act is an equal employment law that protects workers with disabilities. The Mann Act prohibited White slavery and the interstate transport of females for "immoral purposes."

26) **ANSWER: B**
The Federal Employees' Compensation Act covers federal workers and postal employees for injuries suffered on the job. Railroad workers are covered under the Federal Employers Liability Act, or FELA. U.S. seamen and women are covered under the Merchant Marine Act (a.k.a. the Jones Act).

27) **ANSWER: D**
A second opinion or an independent medical exam is warranted to determine if further diagnostic testing or treatment is medically necessary. The maximum amount of time away from work expected with a nonspecific complaint of back pain, no objective findings, and a patient at rest is 2 weeks.

28) **ANSWER: D**

29) **ANSWER: A**
The patient with an injury at C1-4 is dependent for care and must be instructed in care needs so he or she may direct his or her own care.

30) **ANSWER: C**
Arthrograms are not performed on the spine but are used in injuries to bursa or cartilage.

31) **ANSWER: D**
The family must know how to use the equipment safely, there should be no barriers to its safe use, and the length of time the equipment is needed is a factor in arranging for and selecting the equipment.

32) **ANSWER: D**
Rehabilitation programs often overlook the fact that this patient will have many problems occur because of such things as falls, weight gain or loss, and weather conditions. All these things and others can affect the way the prosthesis fits and her ability to function. The Case Manager should explore the patient's ability to cope with her disability and potential problems. She or he should review typical scenarios and have the physical therapy department have the patient practice getting up off the floor and other difficult situations. The nursing department should review possible scenarios with the fit of the prosthesis, any causes of irritation to the limb, and when to seek out the physician or prosthetist.

33) **ANSWER: C**
The micturition reflex center is located in the sacral region of the spinal cord. As a result, bladder function may be impaired with a lower spinal cord injury.

34) **ANSWER: D**

35) **ANSWER: B**

36) **ANSWER: C**

37) **ANSWER: A**

38) **ANSWER: C**
Postoperatively, the knee is immobilized in a hinged brace in a flexed position.

39) **ANSWER: D**

40) **ANSWER: C**
The other answers require a higher spinal cord injury or brain trauma.

41) **ANSWER: A**
Vocational training may not be necessary, and it certainly does not begin immediately after the back injury. Likewise, disability papers may need to be filed, but that is not the reason for communicating with the providers of care. The primary reason for communicating the physical job requirements to the providers of care is to choose appropriate treatment goals, therein meeting the patient's specific individual needs.

CHAPTER 8

Posttest

1) Of the following, which is (are) not a common cause(s) of malpractice litigation?
   1. Discourteous behavior by the professional
   2. Poor clinical outcomes
   3. Lack of patient understanding
   4. Substandard medical care
      A. 1, 3
      B. 2, 4
      C. 1, 2, 3
      D. All of the above
      E. None of the above

2) Case Managers may decrease the legal liability associated with patient discharges through which of the following activities?
   1. Decreasing the average length of stay of their clients
   2. Confirming the integrity of the patient's support network
   3. Reducing the per-member, per-month medical costs of their clients
   4. Confirming the adequacy of follow-up outpatient care
      A. 1, 3
      B. 2, 4
      C. 1, 2, 3
      D. All of the above
      E. None of the above

3) Case Managers are committed to informed consent, providing options for the patient to choose from, and educating the patient to make independent decisions. This principle is known as
   A. Veracity
   B. Beneficence
   C. Autonomy
   D. Nonmaleficence

4) In a malpractice suit the plaintiff must prove two points:
   1. His or her compliance with the prescribed treatment plan
   2. Negligence on the part of the Case Manager
   3. Injury from the Case Manager's negligence
   4. Intent on the part of the Case Manager
      A. 1, 4
      B. 2, 3
      C. None of the above
      D. All of the above

5) Communication failures, lack of information given to the family, lack of patient understanding, and discourteous behavior are all causes of
   A. Lack of patient compliance
   B. Patient injuries
   C. Patient complaints
   D. Malpractice litigation

6) Of the following statements, which is (are) not true regarding ethics, as they relate to case management?
   1. They are rules of conduct that govern a person or members of a profession.
   2. They are thoughts that govern a person's conduct.
   3. They are a society's ideal for a person's conduct.
   4. They are the minimal acceptable standards for a person's conduct.
      A. 1, 3
      B. 2, 4
      C. 1, 2, 3
      D. All of the above
      E. None of the above

7) Which of the following should be disclosed to the patient when a provider is obtaining consent for a medical, surgical, or psychological intervention?
   1. The projected or desired outcomes of the proposed treatment and the likelihood of success
   2. Reasonably foreseeable risks or hazards inherent in the proposed treatment or care (which must be done in a manner that the patient can understand)
   3. Alternatives to the proposed care or treatment plan
   4. Consequences of forgoing the treatment
      A. 1, 3
      B. 2, 4
      C. 1, 2, 3
      D. All of the above
      E. None of the above

8) Which of the following is (are) a requirement for obtaining informed consent?
   1. The patient may consent voluntarily or may be coerced if uncooperative.
   2. The patient must have the capacity to give consent.
   3. The patient must be an adult; however, emancipated minors must have parents' consent.
   4. In the event that the patient is a minor or adult without capacity to give consent, parents, attorneys, or legal guardians may give consent.
      A. 1, 3
      B. 2, 4
      C. 1, 2, 3
      D. All of the above
      E. None of the above

9) As a result of the case of *Wickline v. the State of California*, the following are true:
   1. Providers can be held accountable for negative outcomes when they discharge patients solely at the request of the insurer or payer.
   2. Case Managers can be held liable for negative outcomes as a consequence of their denials.
   3. Insurers or utilization review firms can be held liable for negative outcomes as a consequence of their denials.
   4. If a provider appeals an adverse determination and a negative outcome occurs, the liability may be passed to the insurer.
      A. 1, 2, 3
      B. 2, 3, 4
      C. All of the above
      D. None of the above

10) Which of the following statements is (are) true regarding the legal term *tort*?
    1. It comes from a Latin word that means "twist."
    2. It implies that testimony has been given falsely.
    3. It refers to damage or injury that is done willfully or negligently.
    4. It refers only to medical malpractice cases.
       A. 1, 3
       B. 2, 4
       C. 1, 2, 3
       D. All of the above
       E. None of the above

11) A Case Manager is frustrated by her inability to get her patient to agree to occupational therapy. The patient was involved in a high-speed motor vehicle accident and suffered severe head injuries. When encouraged to attend therapy sessions, the patient refuses, becomes verbally abusive, and hangs up. Which of the following is (are) a likely reason(s) for this patient's reaction?
    A. Head injuries can result in emotional lability.
    B. Head injuries can result in cognitive impairments.
    C. Head injuries can result in prolonged head pain and mood depression.
    D. All of the above
    E. None of the above

12) Of the following diagnoses, which should trigger an inquiry for potential case management services?
    1. Blepharitis
    2. Verruca vulgaris
    3. Coryza
    4. Pedis planus
       A. 1, 3
       B. 2, 4
       C. 1, 2, 3
       D. All of the above
       E. None of the above

13) Of the following, which utilization figure for an individual's medical claims would make an appropriate financial threshold for case management evaluations?
    A. Claims exceeding $500 per year
    B. Claims exceeding $1,000 per year
    C. Claims exceeding $10,000 per year
    D. Claims exceeding $100,000 per year
    E. Claims exceeding $1,000,000 per year

14) A Case Manager is told by a paraplegic, "I feel like half a person." The Case Manager's response should be to
   A. Distract the patient from self-pity.
   B. Help the patient explore personal feelings.
   C. Ignore the comment.
   D. Actively discourage negative comments.

15) The Case Manager has a patient who continues to focus on her functional loss. Which of the following is (are) the best response(s) by the Case Manager?
   1. "You should be making faster progress than this in PT."
   2. "Your last physical therapy report states you have increased your strength and flexibility."
   3. "Other patients with this injury returned to work 2 weeks ago."
      A. 1, 2
      B. 2, 3
      C. 2
      D. All of the above
      E. None of the above

16) A patient has just had a full diagnostic workup of his condition. The need for surgery has been ruled out, and the condition has been diagnosed as chronic. Which of the following is (are) true of the patient's follow-up needs?
   A. The patient should be followed every 2 months by the surgeon, in case his condition changes and he requires surgery.
   B. Several other opinions should be sought to confirm the first diagnosis.
   C. Follow-up with the patient's primary care physician is indicated to obtain any needed treatment, monitoring, or medications required for the chronic condition.
   D. All of the above
   E. None of the above

17) The Case Manager has a patient with a recent amputation. The patient expresses concern that his wife will no longer find him attractive. The Case Manager should realize that
   A. The patient is in a grieving stage.
   B. The patient is experiencing self-pity, which will pass.
   C. After a severe illness, injury, or major surgery patients can have a distorted body image.
   D. All of the above
   E. None of the above

18) Case Managers know that motivating a patient with a knowledge deficit can be problematic. As the Case Manager evaluating the duration and progress of occupational services, what questions would you ask if informed a patient was making little progress and was noncompliant with his or her instructions?
   1. Has anyone explored the reasons for his or her resistance?
   2. Has anyone discussed his or her lack of progress and cooperation with the family?
   3. What time of day is he or she receiving teaching?
   4. Is there a time of day when he or she is more cooperative and compliant?
      A. 1, 2, 3
      B. 2, 3, 4
      C. All of the above
      D. None of the above

19) Which of the following statements is (are) true regarding the psychological aspects of chronic disease and disability?
   1. Only catastrophic illnesses, such as cancer and spinal cord injuries, have psychological ramifications.
   2. Even injuries that are usually considered minor can have severe social and psychological ramifications.
   3. Psychological reactions, such as euphoria and mania, are common in catastrophic illnesses.
   4. Psychological reactions, such as depression and dependency, are common in catastrophic illnesses.
      A. 1, 3
      B. 2, 4
      C. 1, 2, 3
      D. All of the above
      E. None of the above

20) Which of the following organizations must comply with the mandates of the Americans with Disabilities Act?
   1. Small businesses with fewer than 100 employees
   2. The federal government
   3. Multinational corporations with headquarters in the United States
   4. Native American tribes
      A. 1, 3
      B. 2, 4
      C. 1, 2, 3
      D. All of the above
      E. None of the above

21) Which of the following would help to define the "essential functions of the job" under the mandates of the Americans with Disabilities Act?
   1. The job function takes up the majority of the employee's time.
   2. The job function is described in the collective bargaining agreement.
   3. The job function is recorded in the written job description.
   4. The job function in question is considered "essential" to the jobs of others in the same or similar job.
      A. 1, 3
      B. 2, 4
      C. 1, 2, 3
      D. All of the above
      E. None of the above

22) Which of the following statements is (are) true regarding the Women's Health and Cancer Rights Act?
   1. It ensures rehabilitative therapies, such as physical therapy, to postmastectomy patients.
   2. It ensures coverage for surgery of the contralateral breast to provide a symmetrical appearance after mastectomy.
   3. It ensures coverage for postsurgical care, such as lymphedema treatment.
   4. It ensures coverage for breast prostheses after mastectomy.
      A. 1, 3
      B. 2, 4
      C. 1, 2, 3
      D. All of the above
      E. None of the above

394 CHAPTER EIGHT

23) Which of the following statements is (are) true regarding unemployment insurance?
   1. Financing of unemployment benefits varies from state to state.
   2. Unemployment compensation benefits guarantee a replacement of 50% of salary.
   3. Benefits may be extended past the usual maximum length of benefit, during periods of heavy unemployment.
   4. All states pay a minimum of 46 weeks of unemployment benefits.
      A. 1, 3
      B. 2, 4
      C. 1, 2, 3
      D. All of the above
      E. None of the above

24) Which of the following statements about the workers' compensation insurance program is (are) true?
   1. The cost of workers' compensation insurance is borne by the employer only.
   2. The employee is expected to contribute 3% of his or her earned income toward workers' compensation premiums.
   3. The workers' compensation program was intended to provide an impetus for an increase in employer safety programs.
   4. Employer safety programs have dramatically decreased the industrial accident rate.
      A. 1, 3
      B. 2, 4
      C. 1, 2, 3
      D. All of the above
      E. None of the above

25) Which of the following statements is (are) true regarding third-party administrators (TPAs)?
   1. The TPA usually operates in the environment of the self-insured employer.
   2. The TPA is an agent of the insurer.
   3. The TPA is not party to the insurance contract and is not liable for losses incurred by employees.
   4. The TPA's sole function is to provide "insurance-type" administrative services to the employer.
      A. 1, 3
      B. 2, 4
      C. 1, 2, 3
      D. All of the above
      E. None of the above

26) Which of the following characteristics is (are) common to victims of automobile accidents?
   1. Senescence
   2. Seriousness of injuries
   3. Low incidence of head injuries
   4. High incidence of spinal injuries
      A. 1, 3
      B. 2, 4
      C. 1, 2, 3
      D. All of the above
      E. None of the above

27) Which of the following is (are) true regarding peer review organizations (PROs)?
1. They were established under the Tax Equity and Fiscal Responsibility Act.
2. They are entities selected by CMS to reduce medical costs.
3. They are entities selected by CMS to ensure quality of care and appropriateness of admissions, readmissions, and discharges.
4. PROs concern themselves with the care of Medicare and Medicaid patients.
    A. 1, 3
    B. 2, 4
    C. 1, 2, 3
    D. All of the above
    E. None of the above

28) Which of the following individuals is (are) not protected under the Pregnancy Discrimination Act?
1. A pregnant but unwed employee
2. A part-time employee
3. An independent contractor
4. An employee of a successor corporation
    A. 1, 2
    B. 3, 4
    C. 1, 2, 3
    D. All of the above
    E. None of the above

29) Which of the following mental health benefit limitations are allowable under the tenets of the Mental Health Parity Act?
1. Annual dollar limit for mental health care
2. Limited number of annual outpatient visits
3. Lifetime dollar limit on mental health care
4. Limited number of inpatient days annually
    A. 1, 3
    B. 2, 4
    C. 1, 2, 3
    D. All of the above
    E. None of the above

30) Arranging for continuity of care upon discharge from the hospital is also known as
    A. Discharge status
    B. Effective utilization review
    C. Discharge planning
    D. Timeliness

31) Case management documentation should
1. Be done upon closure of the case
2. Be done as close to the time of all contacts as possible
3. Be thorough
4. Reflect the patient's level of involvement in care planning
    A. 1, 2, 3
    B. 1, 3, 4
    C. 2, 3, 4
    D. 1, 2, 3, 4

32) Assessment, planning, implementation, coordination, monitoring, and evaluation are referred to as
   A. The nursing process
   B. The scientific method
   C. The six essential activities of case management
   D. None of the above

33) Accurate, thorough case management documentation
   A. Limits or reduces liability
   B. Is a legal medical record subject to state record retention laws
   C. Is confidential
   D. None of the above
   E. All of the above

34) The role of the Case Manager is that of
   A. Educator, facilitator, and insurance advocate
   B. Assessor, planner, educator, facilitator, and patient advocate
   C. Claims adjuster, planner, educator, and facilitator
   D. Assessor, medical planner, and facilitator

35) Which of the following is not true about case management?
   A. It is a new profession.
   B. It is an area of practice within an individual's profession.
   C. It is performed by a variety of healthcare providers.
   D. It is performed in a variety of settings.

36) Case Managers work in a variety of settings. Which of the following is (are) part of the provider sector?
   1. Insurance company
   2. Infusion company
   3. Rehabilitation center
   4. Hospital
      A. 1, 2, 3
      B. 2, 3, 4
      C. None of the above
      D. All of the above

37) Although Case Managers work in a variety of settings, they all have a common denominator of patient advocacy, educating patients, and facilitating patients' optimal outcomes. But the focal point of their work is
   A. Empowering physicians to be gatekeepers
   B. Empowering patients to be active decision makers in their health care
   C. Mandating care plans to patients and their families
   D. Mandating services to be provided by their physicians

38) Case Managers deal with vocational activity most often in a(n)
   A. Subacute setting
   B. Acute care facility
   C. Rehabilitation center
   D. None of the above

39) Which of the following is (are) true regarding the practice of case management?
1. It is a relatively new profession.
2. Certification ensures appropriate care plans.
3. All Case Managers are nurses.
4. Case management is based on the premise that when an individual reaches his or her optimal level of wellness and functional capability, everyone benefits.
    A. 1
    B. 2
    C. 1, 3
    D. 2, 4
    E. All of the above

40) Which of the following is (are) true regarding the purposes of an orthosis?
1. It can be used to replace body parts.
2. It can be used to position body parts.
3. It can be used to amputate body parts.
4. It can be used to modify muscle tone.
    A. 1, 3
    B. 2, 4
    C. 1, 2, 3
    D. All of the above
    E. None of the above

41) Which of the following is (are) true regarding a prosthesis?
1. The term *prosthesis* refers only to artificial arms and legs.
2. It may improve a person's sense of wholeness or body image.
3. Cosmesis is not an issue when fitting a prosthesis.
4. It may result in injury or illness if improperly fitted.
    A. 1, 3
    B. 2, 4
    C. 1, 2, 3
    D. All of the above
    E. None of the above

42) Which of the following is (are) true regarding the prescribing of an assistive device?
1. An evaluation of the patient's interests and abilities is important.
2. An evaluation of the patient's home and work environment is important.
3. Training the patient on the device is important.
4. Training family members on the device is sometimes important.
    A. 1, 3
    B. 2, 4
    C. 1, 2, 3
    D. All of the above
    E. None of the above

43) Which of the following factors do not influence the rate of prosthesis replacement?
1. Activity level
2. Educational achievements of the user
3. Type of prosthesis
4. Patient's social status
    A. 1, 3
    B. 2, 4
    C. 1, 2, 3
    D. All of the above
    E. None of the above

44) Which of the following is (are) considered assistive devices?
1. A "cock-up" splint for the wrist
2. Phone receiver volume control
3. A sling to hold a plegic and atrophied arm in place
4. Grab bars in the tub
    A. 1, 3
    B. 2, 4
    C. 1, 2, 3
    D. All of the above
    E. None of the above

45) Introductions, empowerment, trust, active listening, questioning, and testing discrepancies are all part of
    A. Determining functional status
    B. Interviewing
    C. The communication process
    D. None of the above

46) The Case Manager will find which of the following services difficult to arrange at home?
1. Tocolytic therapy
2. Respiratory therapy
3. Infusion therapy
4. Blood transfusions
5. Dialysis
    A. 1, 2, 3
    B. 2, 3, 4
    C. 1, 4
    D. 4, 5
    E. None of the above

47) When the Case Manager is arranging for transfer from the acute care setting to a traumatic brain injury or rehabilitation facility, she or he needs to verify that the facility
    A. Can provide the therapies required by the patient
    B. Has a medical director who is board-certified
    C. Is accredited by JCAHO and CARF
    D. A, C
    E. All of the above

48) _____ are facilities that provide lower cost alternatives for complex cases that do not require the services of an acute care facility or specialized care center but require more care than can be provided at home.
   A. Subacute care centers
   B. Long-term care facilities
   C. Rehabilitation hospitals
   D. Convalescent hospitals

49) A thorough interview and assessment enables the Case Manager to assist the patient and family to
   A. Make informed healthcare decisions
   B. Make informed financial decisions
   C. Cope with the complex healthcare system
   D. All of the above

50) Under the terms of the Tax Equity and Fiscal Responsibility Act (TEFRA), which of the following medical specialties was exempted from the diagnosis-related groups (DRGs) program?
   A. Cardiology
   B. Endocrinology
   C. Rehabilitation medicine
   D. Radiation oncology
   E. Family medicine

NOTES

Appendix 8-A

Answers to Posttest

1) **ANSWER: B**
   For some, it is surprising that poor clinical outcomes and negligent medical care are not common causes of malpractice litigation. In fact, studies have demonstrated that patients rarely identify most substandard medical care.

2) **ANSWER: B**
   The Case Manager has an obligation of "reasonable care" to the patient. Failing to ensure the discharge is "safe" is negligent on the part of the Case Manager.

3) **ANSWER: C**

4) **ANSWER: B**

5) **ANSWER: D**
   The items on this list are the common causes for malpractice litigation.

6) **ANSWER: B**
   Ethics are the rules or standards that govern the conduct of a person or members of a profession. Ethical rules describe a society's ideal of how a person or a professional should conduct him- or herself. Thoughts that govern a person's conduct are not necessarily ethical or virtuous.

7) **ANSWER: D**

8) **ANSWER: B**
   Emancipated minors are considered adults under most states' law. Consent must be given freely, without coercion.

9) **ANSWER: C**
   Therefore, Case Managers should aggressively seek all data necessary to make an informed decision that is in the best interests of their patients.

10) **ANSWER: A**
    The word *tort* comes from the Latin *torquêre*, to twist, and implies injury. In law, a tort is a damage, an injury, or a wrongful act done willfully, negligently, or in circumstances involving strict liability—a legal wrong committed upon the person or property independent of contract. It may be a direct invasion of some legal right of the individual, an infraction of some public duty by which special damage accrues to the individual, or the violation of some private obligation by which like damage accrues to the individual. Torts are not specific to medical malpractice cases.

11) **ANSWER: D**

12) **ANSWER: E**

Coryza is a common cold, and blepharitis is a minor infection of the eyelid. Pedis planus are flat feet, and verruca vulgaris are common warts. None of these conditions requires the services of a Case Manager.

13) **ANSWER: C**

Screening all patients with claims over $500 and $1,000 per year would yield too many claims and too few catastrophic illnesses. Those patients with claims of $100,000 and over would no doubt be well known to the insurers and Case Managers long before the patients hit those thresholds. Thresholds of $5,000 to $10,000 are most commonly seen in the industry.

14) **ANSWER: B**

The Case Manager should permit and encourage the patient to explore his or her feelings without judgment, punishment, or rejection.

15) **ANSWER: C**

The Case Manager should be motivating the patient by focusing on his or her progress, not lack of progress.

16) **ANSWER: C**

Chronic conditions not requiring surgery can be handled by the primary care physician, who can then make referrals when the patient's condition changes or he or she deems referrals are medically necessary.

17) **ANSWER: C**

Many patients who survive illness, injury, or major surgery perceive their change in body image to be greater and more embarrassing than it would be to an objective observer. These patients become profoundly ashamed of their bodies, which can lead to social isolation.

18) **ANSWER: C**

All the previous questions can help shed light on the reason for the patient's resistance and assist the team in formulating a more effective care plan.

19) **ANSWER: B**

The illness need not be as "catastrophic" as a closed head injury, a cervical spinal injury, or cancer to cause serious changes in a person's life. A carpenter who loses the use of a hand, a dancer who suffers from vertigo, and a professional athlete who injures a knee are examples of patients whose injuries, although not considered catastrophic by most, have serious effects beyond the physical realm and into the social and psychological spheres. These patients have not just suffered a serious and painful injury but have also lost careers, hopes, dreams, social status, and income. As a result of the life changes precipitated by major illness and injury, patients commonly experience loss, anger, fear and anxiety, depression, and dependency.

20) **ANSWER: A**

The exceptions to the ADA are as follows:

- Religious organizations or private membership clubs, except when these organizations sponsor a public event
- The federal government, or corporations owned by the federal government
- Native American tribes
- When compliance with this Act can prove a hardship for small employers. Therefore, if an employer has fewer than 15 employees, he or she is exempt. (Note: Because an accommodation is expensive for an employer does not automatically make it a "hardship.")

21) **ANSWER: D**
The following are rules of thumb to help determine whether a job function is an "essential function" of the job:

- Essential job functions recorded in the written job descriptions, prepared before advertising for the job or interviewing candidates, are considered evidential when determining the essential functions of the job.
- The job function in question takes up the majority of the job's time.
- The job function in question is considered "essential" to the jobs of others in the same or similar job.
- The job function is described in a collective bargaining agreement.

22) **ANSWER: D**
The Women's Health and Cancer Rights Act is a law that was enacted as part of an Omnibus Appropriations Bill and is effective for plan years beginning on or after October 21, 1998. This Act amended ERISA to require group health plans, including self-insured plans, which provide coverage for mastectomies, to provide certain reconstructive and related services following mastectomies. The services mandated by the Act include the following:

- Reconstruction of the breast upon which the mastectomy has been performed
- Surgery and reconstruction of the other breast to produce a symmetrical appearance
- Prosthesis and treatment for physical complications attendant to the mastectomy, for example, lymphedema

23) **ANSWER: A**
State financing and benefit laws vary widely. In general, unemployment compensation benefits under state laws are intended to replace about 50% of an average worker's previous wages. Maximum weekly benefits provisions, however, result in benefits of less than 50% for most higher-earning workers. All states pay benefits to some unemployed persons for 26 weeks. In some states the duration of benefits depends on the amount earned and the number of weeks worked in a previous year. In others, all recipients are entitled to benefits for the same length of time. During periods of heavy unemployment, federal law authorizes extended benefits, in some cases up to 39 weeks; in 1975 extended benefits were payable for up to 65 weeks. Extended benefits are financed in part by federal employer taxes.

24) **ANSWER: A**
The cost of workers' compensation insurance premiums is borne by the employer, with no contribution by the employee. The authors of the Workers' Compensation Act intended that the significant cost of this compulsory insurance would provide an incentive to employers to increase workers' safety programs and result in decreased work-related injuries. Stringent safety programs instituted by major corporations have, nevertheless, failed to stop the rise in industrial accident rates. It is estimated that industrial accidents have cost U.S. manufacturers more than $11 billion per year.

25) **ANSWER: D**
Third-party administrators (or TPAs) usually operate in the environment of the self-insured employer. Although they may act as an agent of the "insurer," the TPA is not party to the insurance contract between the employer and the employee. The TPA does not incur any risk for employer or employee losses. A TPA's sole function is to perform "insurance-type" administrative services for self-insured employers. These services include, but are not limited to, performing claims adjudication and payment, maintaining all records, providing utilization and quality management, case management, and managing the provider network.

26) **ANSWER: B**
Automobile accident victims are characterized by their youth and the seriousness of their injuries, which include closed head trauma, spinal trauma, and permanent disability.

27) **ANSWER: D**
Under TEFRA, peer review organizations (PROs) were established. A PRO is an entity that is selected by CMS to reduce costs associated with the hospital stays of Medicare and Medicaid patients. Further, they are charged with conducting reviews of hospital-based care on these patients to ensure quality of care and appropriateness of admissions, readmissions, and discharges. Through this review procedure, PROs can maintain and/or lower admission rates and reduce lengths of stay, while ensuring against inadequate treatment.

28) **ANSWER: E**

29) **ANSWER: B**
Although annual or lifetime dollar limits cannot be set under the provisions of the Mental Health Parity Act, other limits are allowed. Examples of other allowable limits are as follows:

- Limited number of annual outpatient visits
- Limited number of inpatient days annually
- A per-visit fee limit
- Higher deductibles and copayments for mental health benefits under MHPA, without parity in medical and surgical benefits

If an employer does not offer medical benefits, he or she does not have to offer mental health benefits; said differently, if an employer chooses not to offer mental health benefits, he or she must also choose not to offer medical benefits.

30) **ANSWER: C**

31) **ANSWER: D**
Proper documentation will minimize a Case Manager's liability risk.

32) **ANSWER: C**

33) **ANSWER: E**

34) **ANSWER: B**
Case Managers are patient advocates, not insurance advocates. They neither adjust claims nor are they medical planners; that is the physician's role.

35) **ANSWER: A**
Case management by itself is not a profession but an area of practice within an individual's profession.

36) **ANSWER: B**
HMOs, insurance companies, and third-party administrators are examples of the payer sector.

37) **ANSWER: B**

38) **ANSWER: C**

39) **ANSWER: D**

40) **ANSWER: B**
An orthosis is a device added to a person's body to achieve one or more of the following ends: support, position, immobilization, correction of deformities, assistance with weak muscles,

restoration of muscle function, and modification of muscle tone. Prostheses are aimed more at replacement of body parts. The term *orthosis* generally encompasses such devices as slings, braces, and splints. Orthoses are used to support or aid in the functioning of the upper and lower extremities, hands, and feet, as well as the trunk and spine.

41) **ANSWER: B**
A prosthesis is a device that restores or replaces all or part of a missing body part. The science of prosthetics addresses the mechanical, physiological, and cosmetic functions of restorations. Although orthoses are aimed at assisting the body to restore function, prostheses restore or replace those parts of the human body that are absent or no longer function. The need for replacement and cosmesis, rather than a simple increase in functionality, stems from a person's need for "wholeness" and a "positive body image." With this in mind the professional prosthetist's goal is to increase both functionality and cosmesis. Poorly fitted prostheses can cause injury or illness. Although most laypersons associate the term *prosthesis* with artificial arms and legs, the field is much larger, encompassing many specialties. Prostheses run the gamut from highly functional devices, such as a lens implant for cataracts and an artificial hip for a hip fracture, to highly cosmetic devices, such as breast implants after a mastectomy, wigs (a cranial prosthesis) after chemotherapy, and an artificial eye after an enucleation.

42) **ANSWER: D**
The type of assistive device is determined by the needs of the individual patient, her or his abilities and functional limitations, and her or his environment. Such common mistakes as a walker being too heavy for a frail elderly patient, a room being too small for a hospital bed, or doorways being too narrow for a wheelchair plague the inexperienced Case Manager. Even simple devices such as crutches and walkers have resulted in injuries due to falls, and improperly fitted wheelchairs have resulted in decubitus ulcers. The Case Manager should make sure the patient is properly fitted to the equipment and trained in its use. When appropriate, family and caregivers should also receive the appropriate training. The patient and family or caregivers should be involved in the selection of adaptive devices and should be trained in their use. A Case Manager who attends to these issues will increase the likelihood that the device is wanted, meets the patient's needs, and will be fully used.

43) **ANSWER: B**
Many factors influence replacement frequency. For example, lower extremity prostheses bear weight, sustain high impact, and are exposed to the elements. Damage to the prostheses acquired by these activities demands maintenance, repair, and replacement. Replacement frequency depends on the activity level of the patient and the demands he or she puts on the prosthesis, as well as the complexity of the prosthesis and the properties of the materials used. Further, an individual's prosthetic needs may change. For example, a sedentary individual may become more active, requiring a new prosthesis with more features and flexibility. Conversely, an active individual, with advancing age or disease, may become more sedentary, requiring a replacement prosthesis that is lighter and more stable. Finally, the younger patient will require successively larger prostheses to compensate for growth. There is no association between a patient's educational achievements or social status and prosthesis replacement.

44) **ANSWER: B**
Assistive devices substitute for impaired function and promote independence; therefore, a volume control device on a phone receiver and grab bars are assistive devices. Orthoses are devices that are added to the body to support, position, immobilize, and assist weak muscles. A cock-up splint and an arm sling are considered orthoses.

45) **ANSWER: B**

46) **ANSWER: D**
Blood transfusions are not usually done at home due to the risk of transfusion reaction. Dialysis may be done at home, but due to the associated risks it is generally not done at home unless the patient is truly homebound.

47) **ANSWER: E**

48) **ANSWER: A**

49) **ANSWER: D**
A thorough interview and assessment allow for the collection of data required to assist the patient in formulating his or her case management plan.

50) **ANSWER: C**
Under TEFRA, medical rehabilitation was exempted from the DRGs. Rehabilitation would continue to be a cost-based reimbursement system, subject to certain limits.

APPENDIX A

Consent Agreement Form

Re: Patient: _____

   Plan: _____

   Insured: _____

   Social Security #: _____

Case Management Agreement

To ensure appropriate medical case management services, I, *patient name*, authorize my physician, hospital, or any other healthcare professional involved with my care or treatment to disclose all medical, hospital, vocational, or related information to *Name of Case Management Company*. I further authorize that this information be shared (as necessary) only with professionals, agencies, or insurance companies who will be involved in the coordination, provision, or payment of services. I understand that this is a benefit provided to all *Insured Group's Name* employees and their dependents by *Insured Group's Name*.

_____   _____

Patient Signature   Date

_____   _____

Witness   Date

Source: Adapted from "Legal and Ethical Responsibilities of the Case Management Profession," by C. M. Mullahy, 1998, *The Case Manager's Handbook*, 2nd ed., p. 68, Jones and Bartlett.

APPENDIX B

Patient Case Report

Employer Group Name
Case Management Status Report
September 1–September 30, 1998

Employee:	Employee #1 (Patient is not identified to maintain confidentiality.)
Relationship:	Employee/Spouse/Dependent
Insurance Data:	Name of Insurer
Social:	25-year-old male who lived alone prior to accident. Lives with mother in rural area after accident.
Past Medical History:	Unremarkable
Current Status:	Paraplegia. Lives at home with home care services.

INTERVENTION

The Case Manager monitored the patient's clinical status while the patient was hospitalized and arranged for him to transfer from the acute care unit to a skilled nursing unit for rehabilitation. On 7/17/98, the patient was transferred to the skilled nursing facility for physical therapy, occupational therapy, and wound care. The patient was not able to participate in an acute rehabilitation program at this time due to poor endurance and his extensive wounds. Progress at the subacute level was slow, but steady. While the patient was in the skilled nursing facility, the Case Manager worked with the family members, physician, discharge planner, social worker, and other providers to facilitate a discharge to the patient's mother's home. The Case Manager also was contacted by the employer because the employer wanted the Case Manager to be aware of the fact that this employee's job was waiting for the patient and that the plant he worked in was totally handicapped accessible.

On 8/14/98, the patient was discharged to his mother's home. He refused to be admitted for acute rehabilitation, preferring to receive home care services. The Case Manager arranged for:

- Daily skilled nursing visits for wound care
- Physical therapy three times a week to:
  - strengthen upper extremity and trunk
  - teach transfers
  - teach dressing and sitting skills
- Social work counseling to:
  - encourage him to engage in community activities
  - motivate the patient to utilize community resources
  - assist the patient in coping with this traumatic injury
  - assist in the transition, eventually, for returning to work

COST SAVINGS ANALYSIS

By transferring the patient to a skilled nursing facility after he was stabilized, the Case Manager was able to shorten the length of stay at the acute care facility. Additionally, she was able to provide the appropriate level of care at a subacute facility at negotiated fees. Discharging the patient to his mother's home, she was able to provide quality, therapeutic care while shortening his skilled nursing facility stay and negotiating for the services provided at home. Because he was at his mother's home, he also did not require as extensive hours of care (shifts) as he would have had he gone home alone.

The difference in cost between this case being case managed and not is as follows:

Projected Expenses Without Case Management

Hospital stay	approximately $1,450/day × 24 days	$34,800
Skilled nursing facility	approximately $700/day × 7 days	$ 4,900
Total:		$39,700

Actual Expenditures

Hospital stay:	approximately $1450/day × 6 days	$ 8,700
Skilled nursing facility:	approximately $500/day × 18 days	$ 9,000
Home care:		
Skilled Nursing	$125/visit negotiated to $80/visit × 6	$ 480
Physical Therapy	$175/visit negotiated to $80/visit × 2	$ 160
Social Worker	$145/visit negotiated to $100/visit × 2	$ 200
Durable medical equipment		
ROHO Mattress Rental	$667/month rental negotiated to $400/month	$ 400
Hospital Bed	$1,500 purchase price negotiated to $1,000	$ 1,000
Total:		$19,940
Total Savings:		$19,760

CONCLUSION

The patient will continue to be followed by the Case Manager. Skilled nursing visits, physical therapy, and social work counseling will continue at home to prevent him from being readmitted, to heal his wounds, to prepare him to live with his paraplegia, and to return the patient to work as soon as feasible.

Respectfully Submitted,

Denise Fattorusso RN, CCM, BS

APPENDIX C

Vendor Progress Report

VENDOR NAME

Employee Name:
Identification number: 111-22-3333
Employer Group Name:
Report Period: March 2012

This patient has been receiving occupational therapy, cognitive therapy, and speech/language therapy since January 2012.

GOALS FOR THE LAST REPORTING PERIOD

1. Improve sensory awareness of right upper extremity.
2. Normalize tone throughout right upper extremity.
3. Improve shoulder stability and AROM of right upper extremity.
4. Improve motor planning skills.
5. Improve gross and fine motor coordination of right upper extremity.
6. Increase ADL independence:
   - To be able to shave with right hand.
   - To be able to write more fluently with his right hand.
7. To improve task tolerance with minimal encouragement.
8. To improve delayed sequential recall with 75% accuracy.
9. To increase selective attention and attention to detail for lengthy/complex material.
10. Complete word-finding tasks with 85% accuracy provided with minimal cues.
11. Retell a short paragraph presented verbally in three to five sentences.
12. Improve oral reading skills at the short paragraph level.
13. Follow two-step, two-item written directives to 85% accuracy independently.
14. Utilize a strategy per session to compensate for communication deficits.
15. Improve lingual strength, coordination, and proprioception by executing oral motor activities with clinician and at home.
16. Complete reading comprehension skills three to four sentences in length.
17. Complete simple deductive reasoning tasks with 80% accuracy.

Occupational Therapy/Physical Status:

Static sitting balance	Good
Dynamic sitting balance	Good
Static standing balance	Good
Dynamic standing balance	Good

Status of Right Upper Extremity:

Range of motion of RUE has significantly improved. Mr. X does not appear to present with any physical limitations. He continues to have difficulty with shoulder elevation, supination, and opposition to 5th digit.

This is probably due to motor planning difficulties. He continues to use his right upper extremity more spontaneously during all functional activities. He continues to exhibit difficulty with shaving using his right hand. This is most likely due to motor planning difficulties. His handwriting continues to improve; however, he is hesitant to practice writing on a continual basis.

Fine motor coordination was assessed with the Purdue Pegboard Test. He was able to place 4 pegs in the board in 30 seconds with his right hand (severe impairment) and 16 pegs with his left nondominant hand (intact). This is an improvement—when he first began therapy, he was unable to manipulate the pegs. There has been no change with fine motor coordination on timed tests.

GOALS FOR THE NEXT REPORTING PERIOD (1 MONTH)

1. Improve sensory awareness of RUE.
2. Normalize tone throughout RUE.
3. Improve motor planning skills to be able to use right hand for shaving.
4. Improve gross and fine motor coordination of RUE as demonstrated by placing 6 pegs in the board (Purdue Pegboard Test) with his right hand.
5. Increase ADL independence:
   - To be able to shave with his right hand.
   - To be able to write more fluently with his right hand.
   - To use his right hand during simple meal preparation.

Cognitive Status

A. Stamina/Endurance	NA 1 2 3 4 5
B. Concentration/Attention	NA 1 2 3 4 5
C. Orientation to Person, Place, and Time	NA 1 2 3 4 5
D. Memory	
1. Long term/remote	NA 1 2 3 4 5
2. Immediate	NA 1 2 3 4 5
a. Visual	NA 1 2 3 4 5
b. Verbal	NA 1 2 3 4 5
3. Delayed	NA 1 2 3 4 5
a. Visual	NA 1 2 3 4 5
b. Verbal	NA 1 2 3 4 5
4. Use of compensatory strategies	NA 1 2 3 4 5
Comments: Continues to require moderate cues in order to utilize recommended strategies.	
5. Ability to complete functional memory assignments	NA 1 2 3 4 5
E. Visual Processing	
1. Scanning	NA 1 2 3 4 5
2. Compensating for visual neglect	NA 1 2 3 4 5
3. Visual-spatial skills	NA 1 2 3 4 5

F. Academic Tasks
  1. Reading
     a. Estimated pre-injury level   NA 1 2 3 4 5
     b. Current   NA 1 2 3 4 5
     Comments: Aphasia. Continues to demonstrate reduced attention to details, moderate cues required. Note: Mr. X perseverates on word read in a previous sentence. Paraphasias noted during oral reading.
  2. Math
     a. Estimated pre-injury level   NA 1 2 3 4 5
     b. Current   NA 1 2 3 4 5
     Comments: Mr. X requires minimal cues to complete simple banking task.
  3. Writing   NA 1 2 3 4 5
     Comments: Severe difficulty secondary to right dominant involvement.
G. Problem Solving
  1. Verbal problem solving   NA 1 2 3 4 5
     Comments: Aphasia. Mr. X's word-finding difficulties have improved but continue to affect his verbal problem-solving ability as he displays difficulty expressing himself in complete sentences.
  2. Visual problem solving   NA 1 2 3 4 5
H. Executive functions
  1. Initiation   NA 1 2 3 4 5
  2. Planning   NA 1 2 3 4 5
  3. Organization   NA 1 2 3 4 5
  4. Flexibility   NA 1 2 3 4 5
  5. Follow-through   NA 1 2 3 4 5

GOALS FOR THE NEXT REPORTING PERIOD (1 MONTH)

1. Improve reading comprehension of moderate length/complexity by increasing attention to details, given minimal cues.
2. Improve task tolerance with minimal encouragement.
3. Improve delayed sequential recall of auditory and visual information with 75% accuracy.
4. Utilize strategies once per session, given moderate cues.

Speech/Language Status

A. Receptive Language
  1. Follows directions
     a. Oral   NA 1 2 3 4 5
     b. Written   NA 1 2 3 4 5
     Comments: Reduced attention to details continues when directives are more complex. Continues to demonstrate difficulty with reading on a written directional task.
  2. Auditory comprehension—words/sentences/paragraphs   NA 1 2 3 4 5
B. Expressive Language
  1. Word
     a. Naming   NA 1 2 3 4 5
     Comments: Mr. X presents with aphasia/apraxia. However, confrontational naming tasks continue to improve.

b. Finding　　　　　　　　　　　　　　　　　　　NA 1 2 3 4 5
　　　Comments: Mr. X presents with aphasia with increased frustration. Continues to require moderate prompts to utilize strategies. Word finding is moderately to severely reduced during conversational discourse.
　　　c. Fluency　　　　　　　　　　　　　　　　　　　NA 1 2 3 4 5
　　　Comments: Mr. X presents with apraxia/aphasia. He continues to demonstrate decreased oral fluency. Improvement has been noted.
　　2. Syntax　　　　　　　　　　　　　　　　　　　　　NA 1 2 3 4 5
　　3. Verbal organization and sequencing　　　　　　　　NA 1 2 3 4 5
　　　Comments: Reduced thought organization, word-finding difficulties, and mild apraxia compromise verbal organization and sequencing during storytelling. In addition, Mr. X has difficulty repairing breakdowns due to reduced verbal organization. Mr. X is able to sequence accurately three to four sentences given moderate cues.
　　4. Deductive/abstract reasoning　　　　　　　　　　　NA 1 2 3 4 5
C. Motor Speech
　　1. Strength/function of oral musculature
　　　Comments: Lingual of oral musculature　　　　　　NA 1 2 3 4 5
　　2. Dysphasia　　　　　　　　　　　　　　　　　　　NA 1 2 3 4 5
　　3. Dysarthria　　　　　　　　　　　　　　　　　　　NA 1 2 3 4 5
　　4. Apraxia (verbal, oral)　　　　　　　　　　　　　　NA 1 2 3 4 5
　　5. Speech intelligibility　　　　　　　　　　　　　　　NA 1 2 3 4 5
D. Pragmatic Language
　　1. Body posture/facial expression　　　　　　　　　　NA 1 2 3 4 5
　　2. Verbal initiation　　　　　　　　　　　　　　　　　NA 1 2 3 4 5
　　　Comments: Verbal initiation has improved.
　　3. Lexicon selection　　　　　　　　　　　　　　　　NA 1 2 3 4 5
　　　Comments: Apraxia/aphasia. Reduced word-finding skills confound lexical selection.
　　4. Topic (introduce, maintain, change)　　　　　　　　NA 1 2 3 4 5
　　　Comments: Mr. X introduces topics and maintains those introduced by self and others.

GOALS FOR THE NEXT REPORTING PERIOD (1 MONTH)

1. Increase selective attention and attention to detail for lengthy/complex material.
2. Retell a short paragraph presented verbally in three to five sentences.
3. Complete word-finding tasks with 90% accuracy, provided with minimal cues.
4. Improve oral reading skills at the short paragraph level.
5. Follow two-step, two-item written directives to 85% accuracy independently.
6. Utilize one strategy per session to compensate for communication deficits.
7. Improve lingual strength, coordination, and proprioception by executing oral motor activities with clinician and at home.
8. Increase reading comprehension skills four sentences in length.
9. Complete moderately difficult deductive reasoning tasks with 90% accuracy.
10. Repair a communication breakdown by revising intended message one time per session.

APPENDIX D

Alternate Benefit Plan Form

Benefit Agreement

Plan Contact: _____

Plan: _____

Fax Number: _____

Re: Patient: _____

Insured: _____

Social Security #: _____

Plan Number: _____

Dear <u>Plan Contact</u>:

This is to confirm our conversation today regarding the above-mentioned patient. <u>Patient's Name</u> requires the following:

_____
_____
_____

I would appreciate it if you would sign below, acknowledging your approval of benefit reimbursement for <u>Specific Services.</u>

My fax number is ___-___-___.

If you have any questions, do not hesitate to contact me at ___-___-___. Thank you for your cooperation.

Sincerely,

_____, RN, CCM

Case Manager

I have reviewed and am in agreement with the above case management plan.

_____   _____
(Plan's HR Representative)   (Date)

415

APPENDIX E

CMSA 1996 Statement Regarding Ethical Case Management Practice

INTRODUCTION

This statement is intended to provide guidance to the individual case manager in the development and maintenance of an environment in which case management practice is conducted ethically. Such an environment is one in which morality prevails and there is support for right (good) decisions and actions.

The statement sets forth ethical principles for case management practice. When applied in practice, these principles underlie right decisions and actions. Thus, they can be utilized by individuals or peers to judge the morality of particular decisions and/or actions.

Ethics is inherently intertwined with morality. In the practice of the healthcare professions, ethics traditionally has dealt with the interpersonal level between provider (e.g., Case Manager) and client, rather than the policy level, which emphasized the good of society. Ethics deals with ferreting out what is appropriate in situations that are labeled "dilemmas" because there are no really good alternatives and/or where none of the alternatives is particularly desirable. Thus, ethics addresses the judgment of right and wrong or good and bad.

ETHICAL PRINCIPLES IN CASE MANAGEMENT PRACTICE

As professionals emanating from a variety of healthcare disciplines, Case Managers adhere to the code of ethics for their profession of origin. In all healthcare practices certain principles of ethics apply. Case management is guided by the principles of autonomy, beneficence, nonmaleficence, justice, and veracity.

Autonomy is defined as "a form of personal liberty of action when the individual determines his or her own course in accordance with a plan chosen by himself or herself." This is the fundamental ethical principle of case management practice. The role of Case Manager as client advocate arises from a commitment to the concept of client autonomy. The needs of the client, as perceived by the client, are preeminent. The Case Manager collaborates with the autonomous client with the goal of fostering and encouraging the client's independence and self-determination. This leads the Case Manager to educate and empower the client/family to promote growth and development of the individual and family so that self-advocacy and self-direction are achieved. This implies informing and supporting clients in their options and decisions related to their health care.

From application of the principle of autonomy, the practice of case management is concerned with preservation of the dignity of the client and family. The Case Manager is knowledgeable about and respects the rights of the individual and family, which arises from human dignity and worth, including consent and privacy. The case management plan is individualized and constantly changing based on the needs of the specific client and family. The Case Manager does not discriminate based on social or economic status, personal attributes, or the nature of the health problems of the client.

Beneficence is "the obligation or duty to promote good, to further a person's legitimate interests, and to actively prevent or remove from harm." In ethical case management practice the application of beneficence is balanced with the interests of autonomy in order to prevent paternalism and promote self-determination. The definition of the principle of nonmaleficence is related to beneficence. Nonmaleficence means refraining from doing harm to others. The realization of this principle in case management practice involves emphasis on quality outcomes.

Although uniformity of thought about the practical application of the principle within our society does not exist, Frankens defines justice as maintenance of what is right and fair. The concept of distributive justice deals with the moral basis for dissemination of goods and evils, burdens and benefits. The concept of justice raises such public healthcare policy questions as: Who should receive services? Based on what criteria? Who should pay for services for the poor? What services should benefit from government funding?, etc. Case management practice brings the issue of comparative treatment of individuals into sharp focus because on a daily basis it deals with allocation of healthcare resources on an individual level. Case Managers know first hand the dilemmas related to relative access to care based on such factors as geography and ability to pay.

Decisions regarding such goods and benefits as access to healthcare services within a society with limited resources are initially analyzed based on individual need. Where a fundamental need exists, that is, in situations in which an individual will be harmed if a product or a service is not provided, the Case Manager advocates for the individual to receive it. The Case Manager applies concepts of fairness so as to maximize the individual's ability to carry out reasonable life plans.

Veracity means truth telling. This is an essential operational principle for the Case Manager in order to develop trust. Trust is an essential forerunner of collaborative relationships between Case Manager and clients/families and among Case Manager, providers, and payers. Truth telling also is basic to the exercise of self-determination by the autonomous client/family.

CONCLUSION

The professional Case Manager strives for a moral environment and practice in which ethical principles can be actualized. Ethical dilemmas are identified and reasonable solutions sought through appropriate consultation and moral action. The ethical Case Manager is accountable to the client as well as peers, the employer/payor and to him/herself and to society for the results of his/her decisions and actions.

CMSA Standards of Practice Committee
February 1996

DEFINITIONS

Client: The individual who is ill, injured, or disabled who collaborates with the Case Manager to receive services.
Payor: The individual or entity that purchases case management services.
Family: Family members and/or those significant to the client.

APPENDIX F

Global Assessment of Functioning (GAF) Scale

Consider psychological, social, and occupational functioning on a hypothetical continuum of mental health illness. Do not include impairment in functioning due to physical (or environmental) limitations.

Code	(Note: Use intermediate codes when appropriate, e.g., 45, 68, 72.)
91–100	Superior functioning in a wide range of activities. Life's problems never seem to get out of hand; is sought out by others because of his or her many positive qualities. No symptoms.
81–90	Absent or minimal symptoms (e.g., mild anxiety before an exam), good functioning in all areas, interested and involved in a wide range of activities, socially effective, generally satisfied with life, no more than everyday problems or concerns (e.g., an occasional argument with family members).
71–80	If symptoms are present, they are transient and expectable reactions to psychosocial stressors (e.g., difficulty concentrating after family argument); no more than slight impairment in social, occupational, or school functioning (e.g., temporarily falling behind in school work).
61–70	Some mild symptoms (e.g., depressed mood and mild insomnia) OR some difficulty in social, occupational, or school functioning (e.g., occasional truancy or theft within the household), but generally functioning pretty well; has some meaningful interpersonal relationships.
51–60	Moderate symptoms (e.g., flat affect and circumstantial speech, occasional panic attacks) OR moderate difficulty in social, occupational, or school functioning (e.g., few friends, conflicts with peers or coworkers).
41–50	Serious symptoms (e.g., suicidal ideation, severe obsessional rituals, frequent shoplifting) OR any serious impairment in social, occupational, or school functioning (e.g., no friends, unable to keep a job).
31–40	Some impairment in reality testing or communication (e.g., speech is at all times illogical, obscure, or irrelevant) OR major impairment in several areas, such as work or school, family relations, judgment, thinking, or mood (e.g., depressed man avoids friends, neglects family, and is unable to work; child frequently beats up younger children, is defiant at home, and is failing at school).
21–30	Behavior is considerably influenced by delusions or hallucinations OR serious impairment in communication or judgment (e.g., sometimes incoherent, acts grossly inappropriately, suicidal preoccupation) OR inability to function in almost all areas (e.g., stays in bed all day; no job, home, or friends).
11–20	Some danger of hurting self or others (e.g., suicide attempts without clear expectation of death, frequently violent, manic excitement) OR occasionally fails to maintain minimal personal hygiene (e.g., smears faeces) OR gross impairment in communication (e.g., largely incoherent or mute).
1–10	Persistent danger of severely hurting self or others (e.g., recurrent violence) OR persistent inability to maintain minimal personal hygiene OR serious suicidal act with clear expectation of death.
0	Inadequate information.

Source: Table adapted from *DSM-IV-TR*, American Psychiatric Association, Washington, DC, 2000.

APPENDIX G
DSM-IV Multiaxial Classification

Axis I: Clinical Disorders, Other Disorders That May Be a Focus of Clinical Attention

Disorders Usually First Diagnosed in Infancy, Childhood, or Adolescence (*excluding Mental Retardation, which is diagnosed on Axis II*)
Delirium, Dementia, and Amnestic and Other Cognitive Disorders
Mental Disorders Due to a General Medical Condition
Substance-Related Disorders
Schizophrenia and Other Psychotic Disorders
Mood Disorders
Anxiety Disorders
Somatoform Disorders
Factitious Disorders
Dissociative Disorders
Sexual and Gender Identity Disorders
Eating Disorders
Sleep Disorders
Impulse-Control Disorders Not Elsewhere Classified
Adjustment Disorders
Other Conditions That May Be a Focus of Clinical Attention

Axis II: Personality Disorders, Mental Retardation

Paranoid Personality Disorder
Narcissistic Personality Disorder
Schizoid Personality Disorder
Avoidant Personality Disorder
Antisocial Personality Disorder
Obsessive-Compulsive Personality Disorder
Borderline Personality Disorder
Personality Disorder Not Otherwise Specified
Histrionic Personality Disorder
Mental Retardation

Axis III: General Medical Conditions (with ICD-9-CM codes)

Infectious and Parasitic Diseases (001–139)
Neoplasms (140–239)
Endocrine, Nutritional, and Metabolic Diseases and Immunity Disorders (240–279)
Diseases of the Blood and Blood-Forming Organs (280–289)
Diseases of the Nervous System and Sense Organs (320–389)
Diseases of the Circulatory System (390–459)

Diseases of the Respiratory System (460–519)
Diseases of the Digestive System (520–579)
Diseases of the Genitourinary System (580–629)
Complications of Pregnancy, Childbirth, and the Puerperium (630–676)
Diseases of the Skin and Subcutaneous Tissue (680–709)
Diseases of the Musculoskeletal System and Connective Tissue (710–739)
Certain Conditions Originating in the Perinatal Period (760–779)
Symptoms, Signs, and Ill-Defined Conditions (780–779)
Injury and Poisoning (800–999)

Axis IV: Psychological and Environmental Problems

Problems with primary support group
Problems related to the social environment
Educational problems
Occupational problems
Housing problems
Economic problems
Problems with access to healthcare services
Problems related to interaction with the legal system/crime
Other psychosocial and environmental problems

Axis V: Global Assessment of Functioning

Please refer to Appendix F: Global Assessment of Functioning (GAF) Scale

Source: American Psychiatric Association. 2000. *Diagnostic and Statistical Manual of Mental Disorders,* 4th ed. Washington, DC: American Psychiatric Association.